ADVANCES IN

Surgery

Editor-in-Chief
John L. Cameron, MD

ELSEVIER

PHILADELPHIA LONDON TORONTO MONTREAL SYDNEY TOKYO

ADVANCES IN
Surgery

VOLUMES 1 THROUGH 44 (OUT OF PRINT)

VOLUME 48

1. Inguinal Hernia: Follow or Repair? *by Bala Ramanan, Brittney J. Maloley, and Robert J. Fitzgibbons Jr*
2. Is It Safe to Follow Side Branch IPMNs? *by Giovanni Marchegiani and Carlos Fernàndez-del Castillo*
3. Endoscopic Myotomy for Achalasia *by Christy M. Dunst, Ashwin A. Kurian, and Lee L. Swanstrom*
4. Can Interventionalists do Endovascular Aortic Aneurysm Repair As Well As Vascular Surgeons? *by Tazo Inui and Dennis F. Bandyk*
5. Does Walking Speed Predict Postoperative Morbidity? *by Nicole T. Townsend and Thomas N. Robinson*
6. Does Close Temperature Regulation Affect Surgical Site Infection Rates? *by Ira L. Leeds, Elizabeth C. Wick, and Genevieve B. Melton*
7. The Utility of the Robot in Pancreatic Resections *by Amer H. Zureikat, Melissa E. Hogg, and Herbert J. Zeh III*
8. Current Treatment for Small (<5 cm) Hepatocellular Carcinoma: Evolving Roles for Ablation and Resection *by Amudhan Pugalenthi, C. Suzanne Cutter, and Yuman Fong*
9. Screening for Pancreatic Cancer *by Katherine E. Poruk, Matthew A. Firpo, and Sean J. Mulvihill*
10. Tissue Engineering *by Ravi S. Katari, Andrea Peloso, and Giuseppe Orlando*
11. Acute Cholecystitis: Early Versus Delayed Surgery *by Werner Hartwig and Markus W. Büchler*
12. Gastrointestinal Stromal Tumors: Who Should Get Imatinib and for How Long? *by Vinod P. Balachandran and Ronald P. DeMatteo*

13. Readmission After Surgery *by Donald J. Lucas and Timothy M. Pawlik*

14. What Is Wrong with the Training of General Surgery? *by Daniel T. McKenna and Samer G. Mattar*

15. Aspirin, Clopidogrel, and the Surgeon *by Prakash A. Patel and Lee A. Fleisher*

16. Islet Autotransplantation and Total Pancreatectomy *by Piotr Witkowski, Omid Savari, and Jeffrey B. Matthews*

17. Liver Transplantation for Metastatic Neuroendocrine Tumors *by Haniee Chung and William C. Chapman*

18. Irreversible Electroporation: A Novel Therapy for Stage III Pancreatic Cancer*by Matthew J. Weiss and Christopher L. Wolfgang*

VOLUME 47

1. Repair of Giant Ventral Hernias *by Jai Bikhchandani and Robert Joseph Fitzgibbons Jr*

2. Laparoscopic Colon Resection: Is It Being Utilized? *by Sean Joseph Langenfeld, Jon S. Thompson, and Dmitry Oleynikov*

3. Safety of Surgical Resident Training *by Usama Ahmed Ali and Jon D. Vogel*

4. Current Management of the Zollinger-Ellison Syndrome *by Geoffrey W. Krampitz and Jeffrey A. Norton*

5. What Laboratory Tests Are Required for Ambulatory Surgery? *by Jaime Benarroch-Gampel and Taylor S. Riall*

6. Factors Affecting Readmission After Pancreaticoduodenectomy *by Callisia N. Clarke, Jeffrey J. Sussman, Daniel E. Abbott, and Syed A. Ahmad*

7. Should Peritoneal Lavage Be Used with Suction During Laparoscopic Appendectomy for Perforated Appendicitis? *by Shawn D. St. Peter and George W. Holcomb III*

8. Appendicitis: Changing Perspectives *by Pedro G.R. Teixeira and Demetrios Demetriades*

9. Readmission After Abdominal Aortic Aneurysm Repair: What Does it Mean? *by David Yu Greenblatt, Sara Fernandes-Taylor, and K. Craig Kent*

10. Duodenal Switch for Morbid Obesity: Is it Safe? *by Rodney J. Mason*

11. Is Propranolol of Benefit in Pediatric Burn Patients? *by Celeste C. Finnerty and David N. Herndon*

12. What Is the Optimal Means of Staging Colon Cancer? *by Elizabeth A. Arena and Anton J. Bilchik*

13. The Effect of Do-Not-Resuscitate Status on Postoperative Mortality in the Elderly Following Emergency Surgery *by John E. Scarborough and Theodore N. Pappas*

14. Incidental Gall Bladder Cancer *by Anu Behari and Vinay K. Kapoor*

15. General Surgery Residency Training Issues *by Mary E. Klingensmith and Frank R. Lewis*

16. Is the Abdominal Aortic Aneurysm Rupture Rate Decreasing? *by Andy M. Lee and Elliot L. Chaikof*

17. Stress-induced Hyperglycemia: Is It Harmful Following Trauma? *by Patrick L. Bosarge and Jeffrey D. Kerby*

18. Improvement in the Diagnosis of Appendicitis *by Frederick Thurston Drake and David Reed Flum*

VOLUME 46

1. Who Should Have or Not Have an Axillary Node Dissection with Breast Cancer? *by Richelle T. Williams, David P. Winchester, Katharine Yao, and David J. Winchester*

2. Intestinal Stomas: Indications, Management, and Complications *by Sean T. Martin and Jon D. Vogel*

3. Zero Surgical Site Infections: Is It Possible? *by C. Daniel Smith*

4. Does Simulation Training Improve Outcomes in Laparoscopic Procedures? *by Benjamin Zendejas, Roberto Hernandez-Irizarry, and David R. Farley*

5. Hypertonic Resuscitation After Severe Injury: Is it of Benefit? *by Eileen M. Bulger and David B. Hoyt*

6. What is the Prognosis After Retransplantation of the Liver? *by Ali Zarrinpar and Johnny C. Hong*

7. Screening for Abdominal Aortic Aneurysms *by Joseph L. Bobadilla and K. Craig Kent*

8. Novel Management Strategies in the Treatment of Severe *Clostridium difficile* Infection *by Ibrahim Nassour, Evie H. Carchman, Richard L. Simmons, and Brian S. Zuckerbraun*

9. The Genetic Counselor: An Important Surgical Ally in the Optimal Care of the Cancer Patient *by Erin Salo-Mullen and Jose Guillem*

10. Readmission Rates after Abdominal Surgery: Can They Be Decreased to a Minimum? *by Thomas J. Lee and Robert C.G. Martin II*

11. Superiority of Minimally Invasive Parathyroidectomy *by John W. Kunstman and Robert Udelsman*

12. Current Treatment of Papillary Thyroid Microcarcinoma *by Xiao-Min Yu, Ricardo Lloyd, and Herbert Chen*

13. Use of Computed Tomography in the Emergency Room to Evaluate Blunt Cerebrovascular Injury *by Nancy A. Parks and Martin A. Croce*

14. How Important is Glycemic Control During Coronary Artery Bypass? *by Harold L. Lazar*

15. Capillary Leak Syndrome in Trauma: What is it and What are the Consequences? *by Deborah M. Stein and Thomas M. Scalea*

16. Morbidity and Effectiveness of Laparoscopic Sleeve Gastrectomy, Adjustable Gastric Band, and Gastric Bypass for Morbid Obesity *by Timothy D. Jackson and Matthew M. Hutter*

17. Are Cancer Trials Valid and Useful for the General Surgeon and Surgical Oncologist? *by Waddah B. Al-Refaie and Selwyn M. Vickers*

18. The Current Management of Pancreatic Neuroendocrine Tumors *by Trevor A. Ellison and Barish H. Edil*

VOLUME 45

1. Current Management of Small Bowel Obstruction *by Martin Donald Zielinski and Michael Patrick Bannon*

2. Screening for Colorectal Cancer *by Jin He and Jonathan E. Efron*

3. Varicose Vein: Current Management *by Beejay A. Feliciano and Michael C. Dalsing*

Editor: John Vassallo
Developmental Editor: Meredith Clinton

Editorial Office:
Elsevier
1600 John F. Kennedy Blvd,
Suite 1800
Philadelphia, PA 19103-2899

International Standard Serial Number: 0065-3411
International Standard Book Number: 978-0-323-35543-8

ADVANCES IN
Surgery

CONTRIBUTORS

KAREEM ABU-ELMAGD, MD, PhD, Professor of Surgery, Cleveland Clinic Lerner College of Medicine; Director, Center for Gut Rehabilitation and Transplantation, Transplant Center, Cleveland Clinic, Cleveland, Ohio

KARL Y. BILIMORIA, MD, MS, Assistant Professor, Department of Surgery; Vice Chair of Quality; Director, Surgical Outcomes and Quality Improvement Center, Center for Healthcare Studies, Northwestern Memorial Hospital, Feinberg School of Medicine, Northwestern University, Chicago, Illinois

JUAN J. BLONDET, MD, Minimally Invasive and Bariatric Surgery Fellow, University of California Irvine Medical Center, Orange, California

RICHARD J. BOLD, MD, Division of Surgical Oncology, UC Davis Cancer Center, Sacramento, California

MURRAY F. BRENNAN, MFB, MD, FACS, Vice President of International Affairs; Benno C. Schmidt Chair in Clinical Oncology, Sarcoma Disease Management Team, Department of Surgery, Memorial Sloan Kettering Cancer Center, New York, New York

ERIN G. BROWN, MD, Department of General Surgery, UC Davis Medical Center, Sacramento, California

TIMOTHY I. CARTER, MD, Department of Surgery, SUNY Downstate Medical Center, New York, New York

GUILHERME COSTA, MD, Staff, Thomas E. Starzl Transplantation Institute, University of Pittsburgh Medical Center, Pittsburgh, Pennsylvania

AIMEE M. CRAGO, MD, PhD, FACS, Assistant Attending Surgeon, Sarcoma Disease Management Team, Department of Surgery, Memorial Sloan Kettering Cancer Center, New York, New York

LOUISE DE LA MOTTE, MD, PhD, Department of Vascular Surgery, Rigshospitalet, University of Copenhagen, Copenhagen, Denmark

GERARD DOHERTY, MD, FACS, Utley Professor and Chair of Surgery, Department of Surgery, Boston Medical Center, Boston University School of Medicine, Boston, Massachusetts

TIMOTHY C. FABIAN, MD, Department of Surgery, University of Tennessee Health Science Center, Memphis, Tennessee

MICHAEL B. FARNELL, MD, Section of Hepato-Pancreatic-Biliary Surgery, Division of Subspecialty General Surgery, Department of Surgery, Mayo Clinic, Rochester, Minnesota

DOUGLAS L. FRAKER, MD, FACS, Division of Endocrine and Oncologic Surgery, Hospital of the University of Pennsylvania, Philadelphia, Pennsylvania

MASATO FUJIKI, MD, PhD, Staff, Center for Gut Rehabilitation and Transplantation, Transplant Center, Cleveland Clinic, Cleveland, Ohio

KOJI HASHIMOTO, MD, PhD, Staff, Center for Gut Rehabilitation and Transplantation, Transplant Center, Cleveland Clinic, Cleveland, Ohio

CHRISTA L. JILLARD, MD, Fellow, Section of Endocrine Surgery, Department of Surgery, Duke University School of Medicine, Durham, North Carolina

GEORGE KASOTAKIS, MD, MPH, Assistant Professor, Section of Trauma, Acute Care Surgery and Surgical Critical Care, Department of Surgery, Boston Medical Center, Boston University School of Medicine, Boston, Massachusetts

HENRIK KEHLET, MD, PhD, FACS (Hon), Section for Surgical Pathophysiology, Rigshospitalet, University of Copenhagen, Copenhagen, Denmark

RACHEL R. KELZ, MD, MSCE, FACS, Division of Endocrine and Oncologic Surgery, Hospital of the University of Pennsylvania, Philadelphia, Pennsylvania

MICHAEL L. KENDRICK, MD, Section of Hepato-Pancreatic-Biliary Surgery, Division of Subspecialty General Surgery, Department of Surgery, Mayo Clinic, Rochester, Minnesota

GREGORY D. KENNEDY, MD, PhD, Associate Professor, Department of Surgery, University of Wisconsin School of Medicine and Public Health, Madison, Wisconsin

K. CRAIG KENT, MD, A.R. Curreri Professor of Surgery; Chairman, Department of Surgery, University of Wisconsin School of Medicine and Public Health, Madison, Wisconsin

AJAI KHANNA, MD, PhD, Staff, Center for Gut Rehabilitation and Transplantation, Transplant Center, Cleveland Clinic, Cleveland, Ohio

CHERYL LAU, MD, FRCS(Edin), Jurong Health Services, Singapore, Singapore

HARISH LAVU, MD, Associate Professor; Section Chief HPB Surgery, The Jefferson Pancreas Biliary and Related Cancer Center, Thomas Jefferson University, Philadelphia, Pennsylvania

DANIEL E. LEVIN, MD, Administrative Chief Resident, Department of General Surgery, University of Rochester Medical Center, Rochester, New York

ANTHONY A. MEYER, MD, PhD, Chair, Department of Surgery, UNC School of Medicine, University of North Carolina at Chapel Hill, Chapel Hill, North Carolina

CHRISTINA A. MINAMI, MD, Post-Doctoral Research Fellow and Housestaff, Department of Surgery, Surgical Outcomes and Quality Improvement Center, Center for Healthcare Studies, Northwestern Memorial Hospital, Feinberg School of Medicine, Northwestern University, Chicago, Illinois

JOHN M. MORTON, MD, MPH, FACS, FASMBS, Chief, Bariatric and Minimally Invasive Surgery, Stanford School of Medicine, Stanford, California

BAO-NGOC NGUYEN, MD, Assistant Professor, Department of Surgery, George Washington University, Washington, DC

NINH T. NGUYEN, MD, Professor of Surgery, University of California Irvine Medical Center, Orange, California

MANISH PARIKH, MD, Associate Professor, Department of Surgery, NYU Medical Center; Director of Bariatric Surgery, Bellevue Hospital Center, New York, New York

WALTER PEGOLI Jr, MD, Surgeon-in-Chief, Department of General Surgery, Golisano Children's Hospital; Joseph M. Lobozzo II Professor in Pediatric Surgery, University of Rochester Medical Center, Rochester, New York

EDWARD PHILLIPS, MD, FACS, Director, Division of General Surgery; Professor and Vice Chair, Department of Surgery; Chair Holder, Storz Chair in MIS, Cedars-Sinai Medical Center, Los Angeles, California

CRISTIANO QUINTINI, MD, Staff, Center for Gut Rehabilitation and Transplantation, Transplant Center, Cleveland Clinic, Cleveland, Ohio

TIMOTHY S. SADIQ, MD, Assistant Professor, Division of GI Surgery, UNC School of Medicine, University of North Carolina at Chapel Hill, Chapel Hill, North Carolina

RANDALL P. SCHERI, MD, Assistant Professor of Surgery, Section of Endocrine Surgery, Duke University School of Medicine, Durham, North Carolina

TORBEN V. SCHROEDER, MD, DMSc, Center for Clinical Education, Rigshospitalet, University of Copenhagen, Copenhagen, Denmark

MONICA SETHI, MD, Research Fellow, Department of Surgery, NYU Medical Center; Bellevue Hospital, New York, New York

ANTON N. SIDAWY, MD, MPH, Professor and Lewis B. Saltz Chair, Department of Surgery, George Washington University, Washington, DC

JULIE ANN SOSA, MD, MA, Professor of Surgery and Medicine (Oncology); Chief, Section of Endocrine Surgery; Leader, Endocrine Neoplasia Diseases Group, Department of Surgery, Duke University School of Medicine, Durham, North Carolina

MAY C. TEE, MD, MPH, Section of Hepato-Pancreatic-Biliary Surgery, Division of Subspecialty General Surgery, Department of Surgery, Mayo Clinic, Rochester, Minnesota

SARAH E. TEVIS, MD, Surgical Resident, Department of Surgery, University of Wisconsin School of Medicine and Public Health, Madison, Wisconsin

JORDAN A. WEINBERG, MD, Department of Surgery, University of Tennessee Health Science Center, Memphis, Tennessee

CHARLES J. YEO, MD, Samuel D. Gross Professor and Chair, Department of Surgery, The Jefferson Pancreas Biliary and Related Cancer Center, Thomas Jefferson University, Philadelphia, Pennsylvania

ADVANCES IN
Surgery

CONTENTS

VOLUME 49 • 2015

Advances in Surgery 49 (2015) 1–13

ADVANCES IN SURGERY

What Are the Indications for Resection After an Episode of Sigmoid Diverticulitis?

Anthony A. Meyer, MD, PhD[a], Timothy S. Sadiq, MD[b,*]

[a]Department of Surgery, UNC School of Medicine, University of North Carolina at Chapel Hill, 4001 Burnett-Womack Building, Chapel Hill, NC 27599-7050, USA; [b]Division of GI Surgery, UNC School of Medicine, University of North Carolina at Chapel Hill, 4035 Burnett-Womack, CB 7081, Chapel Hill, NC 27599-7081, USA

Keywords

• Diverticulitis • Recurrent diverticulitis • Laparoscopic peritoneal lavage
• Complicated diverticulitis • Hartmann procedure

Key points

- Diverticulitis is a common and costly health care problem that has received renewed attention over the past decade, particularly with regard to surgical management.
- The historical indication for sigmoid resection after a recurrent episode of uncomplicated diverticulitis has been replaced by an individualized approach.
- The role of the Hartmann procedure in the management of acute diverticulitis complicated by perforation is diminishing in favor of antibiotics with or without percutaneous drainage followed by elective single stage resection in Hinchey I/IIA disease and in favor of resection with primary anastomosis/protecting loop ileostomy in Hinchey III/IV cases.
- Although much has been learned over the past 10 years, it has largely been through retrospective analysis.

Sigmoid diverticulitis is a common problem, requiring patients to interface with both medical and surgical disciplines across various primary and secondary care settings. The diagnosis and treatment of sigmoid diverticulitis utilizes significant health care resources. According to data from the 2010 National Hospital Discharge Survey, colonic diverticulitis accounts for more than 200,000 annual admissions and more than 1 million days of inpatient care per

Disclosure: The authors have nothing to disclose.

*Corresponding author. *E-mail address*: tim_sadiq@med.unc.edu

0065-3411/15/$ – see front matter
http://dx.doi.org/10.1016/j.yasu.2015.03.005

year [1] with an estimated annual direct cost to payers of $1.8 billion [2]. Despite its commonness and financial impact on the US health care system, sigmoid diverticulitis management remains abstruse, largely because of the dearth of high-quality data to guide clinicians. This lack of knowledge has significant widespread implications, particularly with regard to modern surgical management. This article discusses the available data to clarify the role of surgical resection in this population.

THE EVOLUTION OF SURGERY FOR DIVERTICULITIS IN THE TWENTIETH CENTURY

By the early twentieth century the cause, manifestations, and complications of diverticular disease were well characterized [3]. Treatment was medical, consisting largely of bed rest and saline enemas with the addition of antibiotics once they became widely available in the 1930s. During this time, surgery was used almost exclusively to treat complications of diverticulitis such as perforation, abscess, fistula, or obstruction. Typical therapy was nonresectional, consisting of abscess drainage and creation of a proximal transverse diverting colostomy, often followed by colostomy closure without resection once symptoms had resolved. However, the results were poor [4].

In his provocative 1942 article, Smithwick [4] reported the experience of The Massachusetts General Hospital showing that the "outlook for patients with severe forms of diverticulitis is not very bright" when nonresectional procedures were performed. In contrast, his cohort that was operated on with sigmoid resection had better long-term outcomes, suggesting that resectional therapy "appears to offer the patient suffering from a severe form of diverticulitis the greatest hope for relief...." That article and others popularized the 3-stage resection for diverticulitis.

Subsequent articles called for a more aggressive surgical mentality, arguing that surgery should not be reserved only for cases with complications but rather should be used to intervene before complications ensued [5]. Over the decades that followed, surgical progress was steady: 3-stage surgery for complicated disease was replaced by 1-stage and 2-stage resections [6,7], and elective resection for recurrent uncomplicated diverticulitis was routinely performed because of the belief that recurrence was common and increasingly likely to result in complicated disease if allowed to continue unchecked.

PARADIGM SHIFT IN THE TWENTY-FIRST CENTURY

However, over the past decade, every aspect of colonic diverticulitis has been examined, challenging long-held beliefs. Disordered colonic motility resulting in oversegmentation and diverticula that perforate when obstructed by fecaliths has long been the accepted etiopathogenesis of diverticulitis but it is being challenged by new theories that altered gut microbiota may be responsible for the inflammation that manifests clinically as acute colonic diverticulitis [8]. The mainstay of medical therapy for uncomplicated diverticulitis has always been antibiotics but this too is being questioned by randomized clinical trial data showing that no advantage is conferred to patients treated with antibiotics compared with those treated without antibiotics [9]. Surgical treatment, however, has had the greatest paradigm shift, particularly in terms of who should be operated.

INDICATIONS FOR SIGMOID RESECTION

Historically, the indications for surgical resection in the setting of sigmoid diverticulitis have been clear: emergently in the case of free perforation/peritonitis, after a single episode of acute complicated diverticulitis, and after 2 episodes of acute uncomplicated diverticulitis [10,11]. The problem is that these entrenched rules were not data driven; some may have existed despite contradictory data [12]. Over the last decade or more, data have emerged contesting these widely held maxims, making the question of indications for resection as relevant in 2014 as it was in the early twentieth century.

RECURRENT UNCOMPLICATED DIVERTICULITIS

For years it has been recommended that elective sigmoid resection be performed following 2 episodes of uncomplicated diverticulitis [10,11]. The data that led to this recommendation are difficult to pinpoint, although they are usually attributed to Parks [13]. In 1969, he reported on 455 patients admitted with diverticulitis, of whom 138 required surgery on that admission and 317 were treated medically and discharged. Of the medically treated patients, 78 (24.6%) were readmitted for a second attack, 12 (3.8%) with a third episode, and 5 (1.6%) with a fourth attack. Of these 78 readmissions, 6 (7.7%) died as a result of recurrent disease and another 20 patients required surgery. Parks [13] wrote that, "Medical treatment of recurrent disease was less rewarding than treatment of the presenting attack, and more than half of the patients continued to have symptoms after discharge from the hospital." The interpretation of these data and remarks was one of medical futility and likely led to or became the justification for the enthusiasm for prophylactic surgical resection after 2 uncomplicated episodes that has followed. However, it is unlikely that Parks himself intended such a simplistic rule. In a 1970 article reporting that more than 20% of surgically treated patients continued to have pain despite surgery, he espoused a more nuanced view, "Since this follow up of surgical patients reveals that symptoms are not uncommon after resection, prophylactic resection could be advised only after very careful selection" [14].

Parks' data were not the only or even the major driver of this 2-episode policy. The collective mentality was likely also propelled by assumptions that have served as the justification for interval prophylactic sigmoid resection for decades but recently have come under intense scrutiny.

Assumption 1: recurrence is common after successful medical treatment of uncomplicated diverticulitis

Quantifying the risk of recurrence after an episode of diverticulitis is difficult because available studies suffer from incomplete follow-up, a reliance on discharge data, poor capture of outpatient events, and the dependence on retrospective analysis of treatment decisions rather than prospective randomized datasets. Despite this, modern data have benefitted from the wide availability of computed tomography (CT), which objectifies recurrence in a way that was not possible when the primary means of diagnosis was clinical evaluation and barium enema. As a result, abdominal pain in a patient with a history of diverticulitis is not automatically attributed to recurrence but can be assessed by CT, likely leading to fewer diagnoses of recurrent diverticulitis after successful medical therapy. Recent studies report recurrence after an initial episode of uncomplicated diverticulitis to be 13% to 36% (Table 1) [15–20], and the few studies that provide data on rerecurrence [16,17] reveal it to be uncommon and not particularly virulent. Therefore, the natural history of diverticulitis does not seem as progressive and inevitably recurrent as was historically believed, and has dampened enthusiasm for resection after 2 episodes of diverticulitis.

Assumption 2: recurrent attacks are more severe and lead to more complicated disease and need for emergency surgery

It therefore follows that interval colectomy after recurrent diverticulitis would prevent morbidity by intervening before the development of complications, particularly emergency surgery requiring a stoma. However, modern data have shown that complicated recurrence is uncommon, occurring in up to 5% of recurrent cases, and rarely requires emergency surgery or a stoma (Table 2) [15,16,19,21,22]. In fact, an easier argument can be made for the virulence of the first episode than for recurrent episodes. Humes and West [23] reported UK population data showing that 72.3% of patients admitted with complicated diverticulitis did not have a previous history of diverticulitis. Ritz and colleagues [24] reported outcomes of 934 patients admitted with acute diverticulitis and found that those presenting with a first episode were more likely to have free perforation and require emergency surgery than those with a history of prior disease (25.3% vs 7.9%; $P<.001$). Even among patients with recurrence, risk of free perforation decreased with number of previous episodes of diverticulitis. Similarly, Pittet and colleagues [25] retrospectively compared 202 patients presenting with a first episode of diverticulitis with 69 patients presenting with recurrent

Table 1
Recurrence after successful medical therapy for uncomplicated diverticulitis

Study	Patients at risk for recurrence (n)	Recurrence rate (%)	Rerecurrence rate (%)
Parks [13]	317	24.6	5.4
Buchs et al [15]	280	16.4	—
Eglinton et al [16]	320	23.4	4.7
Broderick-Villa et al [17]	2366	13.3	3.9
Binda et al [18]	329	17.2	—
Hall et al [19]	672	36	—
Anaya & Flum [20]	20,136	19	—

Table 2
Complicated recurrence after successful medical treatment of uncomplicated diverticulitis

Study	Patients at risk for recurrence (n)	Complicated recurrence (%)	Need for emergency surgery/stoma (%)
Buchs et al [15]	280	2.1	1.4
Eglinton et al [16]	320	5	0.9
Li et al [21]	14,124	—	1.9
Shaikh & Krukowski [22]	—	—	4.7
Hall et al [19]	672	3.9	—

disease and found that those presenting with an initial episode required emergency surgery more often than those presenting with recurrent disease (15.8% vs 5.8%; $P = .04$). Furthermore, failure of medical therapy, length of hospital stay, frequency of readmission, and 30-day mortality were similar between the two groups, suggesting that recurrent episodes of diverticulitis do not pose increased risk or morbidity. Taken together, these data show that prophylactic surgery for recurrent diverticulitis for the purpose of preventing complicated disease and worse outcomes is misguided and should not be used as justification for resection.

Assumption 3: surgical resection is curative

The unintended consequences of sigmoid resection must be factored into the decision making in surgery for recurrent uncomplicated diverticulitis. Although mortality associated with sigmoid resection is low, overall morbidity is 16%to 19.6% even in the laparoscopic era [26,27], postoperative recurrent diverticulitis ranges from 5.8% to 8.7% [28,29], and ongoing symptoms despite successful surgery are disappointingly common [29,30]. Egger and colleagues [29] reported on 73 patients operated on for uncomplicated disease and found that 15 patients (20.5%) had persistent symptoms on follow-up. Of those with persistent symptoms, review of surgical specimen histopathology revealed acute or chronic inflammation, suggesting that these patients were not mistakenly operated on for irritable bowel syndrome (IBS) but likely had IBS coexisting with diverticular disease or their persistent symptoms were partly the consequence of their postoperative state. Similar findings have been reported in other series [30] as well. Taken together, it is reasonable and necessary to carefully balance the potential curative aspects of surgery against its limitations and against the risks of ongoing observation and medical treatment of recurrent episodes.

The decision to perform elective sigmoid resection should be individualized for each patient.

If rerecurrent diverticulitis is not as likely as was once thought, and those that do multiply recur are not at particular risk for complicated disease and poor outcomes, and surgical outcomes are imperfect, what (if any) are the indications for resection? The most recently updated practice parameters from the American Society of Colon and Rectal Surgeons recommend that the decision to perform elective sigmoid resection following recovery from uncomplicated acute diverticulitis be individualized [31]. The trouble is that again there are few data. As presented in this article, most recent research has focused on debunking historical indications for resection rather than defining those patients prone to recur who would benefit from surgical resection after recovery from recurrent uncomplicated diverticulitis. Family history of diverticulitis and segment of disease longer than 5 cm [19], increased fecal calprotectin following recovery [32], and detection of endoscopic/histologic inflammation on follow-up [33] have been associated with recurrent disease but none have proved to be predictive enough to warrant resection. Research efforts to identify populations prone to complicated recurrence that would benefit from elective surgical resection rather than continued medical therapy have targeted those with young age at disease onset, those with collagen vascular diseases, and those who are chronically immunosuppressed. Although young age at presentation has historically been considered uniquely virulent and subject to lower thresholds to operate [12], the preponderance of recent data suggests otherwise: young patients have a similar presentation, recurrence, and need for emergency surgery as older patients [24,34–36]. As a result, age at disease presentation does not factor into whether surgery should be recommended for recurrent diverticulitis. Immunosuppressed patients have also been singled out as being at higher risk of developing complicated recurrence or need for emergency surgery and targeted for early prophylactic resection. Data supporting this policy are mixed, with some studies reporting a greater risk of perforation in recurrent disease in those with collagen vascular diseases, those using immunosuppression, or those having chronic renal failure [37], whereas other studies have suggested that the high risk attributable to acute diverticulitis in immunosuppressed patients largely manifests during the first episode with higher rates of perforation, need for emergency surgery, and mortality compared with the nonimmunosuppressed but not with subsequent episodes, thus negating any benefit to prophylactic resection in this population [38]. However, the investigators did observe that immunosuppressed patients managed successfully medically for a severe episode have a higher risk to present with severe disease in case of recurrence, potentially representing a scenario in which elective resection after a single episode may be preferred to observation.

Counseling patients with recurrent uncomplicated diverticulitis centers on, firstly, ensuring that the patient understands that the rationale for surgery is not to prevent complex recurrence or need for emergency surgery/stoma but to prevent/minimize future recurrence and its morbidity. Second, a well-informed patient needs to know that the modern literature is not clear on who benefits from elective resection. Third, patients need to understand the risks/benefits/limitations associated with sigmoid resection. Most patients will be satisfied to learn that surgery is not mandatory and will not be interested in pursuing resection, except those who have had severe episodes in the past, have had multiple recurrence episodes in a short period of time, and those who travel for work/pleasure and fear developing recurrent episodes while away. In these patients, patient-specific risk factors should then be factored in to determine whether surgery is best for the patient.

COMPLICATED ACUTE DIVERTICULITIS

Acute diverticulitis associated with free perforation, abscess, obstruction, or fistula (complicated acute diverticulitis) and has always been the domain of the surgeon. In 2015, this remains true for obstruction and fistula because definitive and durable nonoperative or nonresectional therapies have not emerged for these conditions. However, management of acute diverticulitis complicated by perforation has been evolving. The Hinchey classification system for perforated diverticulitis as modified by Sher and colleagues [39] is useful in this context (Box 1).

Patients presenting with peritonitis or sepsis in the setting of acute perforated diverticulitis require emergent surgery for source control, classically in the form of sigmoid resection and proximal end colostomy with distal defunctionalized stump (Hartmann procedure [HP]). There will always be a role for this procedure in life-threatening situations. However, the high morbidity and mortality after an urgent HP [40] and the reality that many patients never achieve colostomy closure [41] has provided the motive to rethink whether the HP is overused, particularly for the treatment of less severe presentations, and can be replaced by less morbid and more effective therapies.

Hinchey III and IV diverticulitis: Hartmann procedure versus primary anastomosis

A case-matched control study [42] of mostly Hinchey III and IV patients comparing HP with primary anastomosis with protecting ileostomy (PAS) showed that the stoma reversal rate was higher with PAS than with HP (96% vs 60%; $P = .001$), with significantly fewer complications (23% vs 66%; $P = .02$). Furthermore, case-matched analysis of Hinchey III patients comparing primary anastomosis with protective ileostomy with those without protective ileostomy showed similar morbidity. The investigators concluded that primary anastomosis with protective ileostomy is superior to HP in acutely perforated left-sided diverticulitis and that an ileostomy many not be necessary for Hinchey III patients.

A subsequent multicenter randomized control trial [43] by the same group 5 years later comparing PAS with HP for Hinchey III and IV diverticulitis

Box 1: Modified Hinchey classification

Modified Hinchey classification for perforated acute diverticulitis

- I: Pericolic abscess
- IIA: Pelvic/distant abscess amenable to percutaneous drainage
- IIB: Complex abscess associated with fistula
- III: Generalized purulent peritonitis
- IV: Generalized fecal peritonitis

From Hinchey E, Schaal PG, Richards GK. Treatment of perforated diverticular disease of the colon. Adv Surg 1978;12:85–109.

showed similar results. Overall complication rates were similar between the two groups, stoma reversal rate was higher with PAS than with HP (90% vs 57%; $P = .005$), and serious complications were reduced with PAS compared with HP (0% vs 20%; $P = .046$). Although this study is limited by its small size, large number of patients not assessed for eligibility, and early termination of the trial based partly on low accrual rates, it does provide data to narrow the indications for HP in favor of primary anastomosis, if only to increase the likelihood of ultimately restoring continuity.

Hinchey III diverticulitis: laparoscopic peritoneal lavage

In 1996, O'Sullivan and colleagues [44] presented 8 patients with generalized peritonitis evaluated with urgent laparoscopy and found to have nonfeculent, purulent diverticulitis (Hinchey III), that was treated with saline irrigation, postoperative antibiotics, and careful observation. All patients recovered without acute diverticulitis-related complications and were not subjected to interval resection. Many small nonrandomized studies followed and a recent systematic review [45] showed that laparoscopic lavage for nonfeculent perforated diverticulitis is efficacious with low mortality, morbidity, and colostomy rates, especially compared with historical management with an urgent HP. Prospective data [46] from 92 patients (Hinchey II, 25 patients; Hinchey III, 67 patients) managed with laparoscopic peritoneal lavage showed 3% mortality and 4% morbidity. Following the procedure, 2 patients required further intervention for pelvic abscess, 1 successfully treated with percutaneous drainage and the other requiring an HP. Following successful treatment, only 2 patients represented with acute diverticulitis, both uncomplicated and successfully treated with antibiotics, at median follow-up of 26 months.

Despite these promising data, there remains considerable criticism and reluctance to adopt laparoscopic lavage [47]. A common concern is that many of these studies are inclusive of patients who could be managed without surgery and that randomized prospective data are needed to justify a treatment that is such a departure from the traditional approach, especially in light of the known failure rate of laparoscopic lavage, which ranges from 2% to 18% in recent studies [48–50]. Accumulated experience suggests that intraoperative assessment to identify and exclude patients with overt (presence of fecal peritonitis or gross defect visible at laparoscopy) or unsuspected (positive hydropneumatic test) perforation from laparoscopic lavage is key to achieving reliably safe outcomes. Even using these strict inclusion criteria, Rossi and colleagues [50] reported that 5 of 44 washouts for Hinchey III diverticulitis (11%) failed to adequately control abdominal sepsis and all required resection, 2 with an HP. Even proponents acknowledge that laparoscopic peritoneal lavage is not a panacea but is a good alternative to traditional resectional approaches in properly selected patients [51]. Multiple prospective randomized trials are underway and the results will help clarify the role of laparoscopic lavage in this difficult patient population [52–54].

Hinchey I and IIA diverticulitis

Improved antibiotics, better disease characterization with CT imaging, and image-guided percutaneous abscess drainage have played a large role in curtailing the use of urgent HP for Hinchey I and IIA diverticulitis. Patients who respond to antibiotics with or without percutaneous abscess drainage are then typically subjected to an elective interval single-stage sigmoid resection [55–58] in accordance with the current recommendations from the American Society of Colon and Rectal Surgeons [31]. This recommendation is attributable to reports of high recurrence rates without surgery [57] and, in part, to surgery having always been the primary treatment of complicated disease. Smithwick's [4] recognition that surgical resection improved outcomes of patients with complicated diverticulitis compared with those managed with medical therapy or lesser surgical procedures strengthened the role of surgery for complicated disease and provides a historical contextual explanation for why this mentality has persisted to the modern day.

However, there is debate about whether interval sigmoid colectomy is necessary in all patients who have successfully recovered from a single episode of complicated diverticulitis. Such questioning is conceptually defensible based on the recurrent uncomplicated diverticulitis literature showing that rerecurrence is low and, when it occurs, is not virulent. In addition, general experience with abscesses following any colorectal resection treated with antibiotics with or without percutaneous abscess drainage commonly results in resolution and reoperation is not often required. Published evidence that are used to answer this question relies largely on small retrospective cohorts of patients with complicated diverticulitis who were managed with antibiotics with or without percutaneous image-guided drainage rather than sigmoid resection because they were too sick to have elective surgery; refused surgery; were not provided adequate surgical follow-up; or, rarely, were recommended not to have surgery because of their excellent response to medical therapy [59–61]. In these highly selected cohorts, studies have shown diverticulitis recurrence rates ranging from 0% to 46.7% [55,59–61] with rare need for subsequent emergency surgery in the case of recurrence [56,59,60,62]. This wide range of recurrence rates reflects the heterogeneous populations (nonstandardized patient selection) within these small series with variable length of follow-up, making it difficult to determine whether nonoperative management is effective. However, Elagili and colleagues' [61] recurrence rate of 47% carries significant weight because it has the longest mean follow-up (60 months), providing sufficient argument that current data are not strong enough to overturn the traditional approach that surgery should follow after a patient has recovered from an episode of complicated diverticulitis [31]. However, it does provide the equipoise necessary to consider expectant nonoperative management in well-selected, informed patients who have responded well to percutaneous abscess drainage and/or antibiotics. Expanding nonoperative treatment to include patients at better risk (those who historically have had interval sigmoid resection) might result in even better results, but this is speculative and prospective studies are needed to more clearly answer this question. In this respect, abscess size greater than 5 cm [56], presence of pelvic abscess as opposed to mesocolic abscess [62], and immunosuppression/renal insufficiency [55] are all associated with poorer outcomes and may be useful in selecting patients who are appropriate for nonoperative treatment.

SUMMARY

Diverticulitis is a common and costly health care problem that has received renewed attention over the past decade, particularly with regard to surgical management. The historical indication for sigmoid resection after a recurrent episode of uncomplicated diverticulitis has been replaced by an individualized approach. The role of HP in the management of acute diverticulitis complicated by perforation is diminishing in favor of antibiotics with or without percutaneous drainage in Hinchey I/IIA disease and in favor of resection with primary anastomosis/protecting loop ileostomy in Hinchey III/IV cases. In addition, laparoscopic peritoneal lavage has been championed as a less morbid but effective therapy for the treatment of Hinchey III diverticulitis. Although much has been learned over the past 10 years, it has largely been through retrospective analysis. Further refinements in surgical therapy for diverticulitis will depend on high-quality prospective study.

References

[1] National Center for Health Statistics. Centers for Disease Control and Prevention Web site. Available at: http://www.cdc.gov/nchs/nhds/nhds_tables.htm#detailed. Accessed October 2, 2014.

[2] Yen L, Davis KL, Hodgkins P, et al. Direct costs of diverticulitis in a US managed care population. Am J Pharm Benefits 2012;4(5):e118–29.

[3] Schoetz DJ. Diverticular disease of the colon. A century old problem. Dis Colon Rectum 1999;42:703–9.

[4] Smithwick RH. Experiences with the surgical management of diverticulitis of the sigmoid. Ann Surg 1942;115:969–85.

[5] Bartlett MK, McDermott WV. Surgical treatment of diverticulitis of the colon. N Engl J Med 1953;248(12):497–9.

[6] Colcock BP. Surgical treatment of diverticulitis. Twenty years' experience. Am J Surg 1968;115:264–70.

[7] Rodkey GV, Welch CE. Changing patterns in the surgical treatment of diverticular disease. Ann Surg 1984;200:466–78.

[8] Daniels L, Philipszoon LE, Boermeester MA. A hypothesis: important role for gut microbiota in the etiopathogenesis of diverticular disease. Dis Colon Rectum 2014;57(4):539–43.

[9] Chabok A, Pahlman L, Hjern F, et al. Randomized clinical trial of antibiotics in acute uncomplicated diverticulitis. Br J Surg 2012;99(4):532–9.

[10] Roberts P, Abel M, Rosen L, et al. Practice parameters for sigmoid diverticulitis. Supporting documentation. Dis Colon Rectum 1995;38(2):126–32.

[11] Wong WD, Wexner SD, Lowry A, et al. Practice parameters for the treatment of sigmoid diverticulitis. Supporting documentation. Dis Colon Rectum 2000;43(3):290–7.

[12] Janes S, Meagher A, Frizelle FA. Elective surgery after acute diverticulitis. Br J Surg 2005;92:133–42.

[13] Parks TG. Natural history of diverticular disease of the colon. A review of 521 cases. BMJ 1969;4:639–45.

[14] Parks TG, Connell AM. The outcome in 455 patients admitted for treatment of diverticular disease of the colon. Br J Surg 1970;57(10):775–8.
[15] Buchs NC, Konrad-Mugnier B, Jannot AS, et al. Assessment of recurrence and complications following uncomplicated diverticulitis. Br J Surg 2013;100:976–9.
[16] Eglinton T, Nguyen T, Raniga S, et al. Patterns of recurrence in patients with acute diverticulitis. Br J Surg 2010;97:952–7.
[17] Broderick-Villa G, Burchette RJ, Collins JC, et al. Hospitalization for acute diverticulitis does not mandate routine elective colectomy. Arch Surg 2005;140:576–83.
[18] Binda GA, Arezzo A, Serventi A, et al. Multicentre observational study of the natural history of left-sided acute diverticulitis. Br J Surg 2012;99:276–85.
[19] Hall JF, Roberts PL, Ricciardi R, et al. Long-term follow-up after an initial episode of diverticulitis: what are the predictors of recurrence? Dis Colon Rectum 2011;54:283–8.
[20] Anaya DA, Flum DR. Risk of emergency colectomy and colostomy in patients with diverticular disease. Arch Surg 2005;140:681–5.
[21] Li D, de Mestral C, Baxter NN, et al. Risk of readmission and emergency surgery following nonoperative management of colonic diverticulitis. Ann Surg 2014;260(3):423–31.
[22] Shaikh S, Krukowski ZH. Outcome of a conservative policy for managing acute sigmoid diverticulitis. Br J Surg 2007;94:876–9.
[23] Humes DJ, West J. Role of acute diverticulitis in the development of complicated colonic diverticular disease and 1-year mortality after diagnosis in the UK: population-based cohort study. Gut 2012;61:95–100.
[24] Ritz JP, Lehmann KS, Frericks B, et al. Outcome of patients with acute sigmoid diverticulitis: multivariate analysis of risk factors for free perforation. Surgery 2011;149(5): 606–13.
[25] Pittet O, Kotzampassakis N, Schmidt S, et al. Recurrent left colonic diverticulitis episodes: more severe than the initial diverticulitis? World J Surg 2009;33:547–52.
[26] Pendlimari R, Touzios JG, Azodo IA, et al. Short-term outcomes after elective minimally invasive colectomy for diverticulitis. Br J Surg 2011;98:431–5.
[27] De Magistris L, Azagra JS, Goergen M, et al. Laparoscopic sigmoidectomy in moderate and severe diverticulitis: analysis of short-term outcomes in a continuous series of 121 patients. Surg Endosc 2013;27:1766–71.
[28] Thaler K, Baig MK, Berho M, et al. Determinants of recurrence after sigmoid resection for uncomplicated diverticulitis. Dis Colon Rectum 2003;46:385–8.
[29] Egger B, Peter MK, Candinas D. Persistent symptoms after elective sigmoid resection for diverticulitis. Dis Colon Rectum 2008;51:1044–8.
[30] Andeweg C, Peters J, Bleichrodt R, et al. Incidence and risk factors of recurrence after surgery for pathology-proven diverticular disease. World J Surg 2008;32:1501–6.
[31] Feingold D, Steele SR, Lee S, et al. Practice parameters for the treatment of sigmoid diverticulitis. Dis Colon Rectum 2014;57:284–94.
[32] Tursi A, Elisei W, Picchio M, et al. Increased faecal calprotectin predicts recurrence in colonic diverticulitis. Int J Colorectal Dis 2014;29:931–5.
[33] Tursi A, Elisei W, Giorgetti GM, et al. Detection of endoscopic and histological inflammation after an attack of colonic diverticulitis is associated with higher diverticulitis recurrence. J Gastrointestin Liver Dis 2013;22(1):13–9.
[34] Hjern F, Josephson T, Altman D, et al. Outcome of younger patients with acute diverticulitis. Br J Surg 2008;95(6):758–64.
[35] Kotzampassakis N, Pittet O, Schmidt S, et al. Presentation and treatment outcome of diverticulitis in younger adults: a different disease than in older patients? Dis Colon Rectum 2010;53(3):333–8.
[36] Nelson RS, Velasco A, Mukesh BN. Management of diverticulitis in younger patients. Dis Colon Rectum 2006;49(9):1341–5.
[37] Klarenbeek BR, Samuels M, van der Wal MA, et al. Indications for elective sigmoid resection in diverticular disease. Ann Surg 2010;251(4):670–4.

[38] Biondo S, Borao JL, Kreisler E, et al. Recurrence and virulence of colonic diverticulitis in immunocompromised patients. Am J Surg 2012;204(2):172–9.
[39] Sher ME, Agachan F, Bortul M, et al. Laparoscopic surgery for diverticulitis. Surg Endosc 1997;11:264–7.
[40] Ince M, Stocchi L, Khomvilai S, et al. Morbidity and mortality of the Hartmann procedure for diverticular disease over 18 years in a single institution. Colorectal Dis 2012;14:e492–8.
[41] Vermeulen J, Coene PP, Van Hout NM, et al. Restoration of bowel continuity after surgery for acute perforated diverticulitis: should Hartmann's procedure be considered a one-stage procedure? Colorectal Dis 2009;11:619–24.
[42] Breitenstein S, Kraus A, Hahnloser D, et al. Emergency left colon resection for acute perforation. Primary anastomosis or Hartmann's procedure? A case-matched control study. World J Surg 2007;31:2117–24.
[43] Oberkofler CE, Rickenbacher A, Raptis DA, et al. A multicenter randomized clinical trial of primary anastomosis or Hartmann's procedure for perforated left colonic diverticulitis with purulent or fecal peritonitis. Ann Surg 2012;256:819–27.
[44] O'Sullivan GC, Murphy D, O'Brien MG, et al. Laparoscopic management of generalized peritonitis due to perforated colonic diverticula. Am J Surg 1996;171:432–4.
[45] Toorenvliet BR, Swank H, Schoones JW, et al. Laparoscopic peritoneal lavage for perforated colonic diverticulitis: a systematic review. Colorectal Dis 2010;12:862–7.
[46] Myers E, Hurley M, O'Sullivan GC, et al. Laparoscopic peritoneal lavage for generalized peritonitis due to perforated diverticulitis. Br J Surg 2008;95:97–101.
[47] De Korte N, Klarenbeek BR, Kuyvenhoven JP, et al. Management of diverticulitis: results of a survey among gastroenterologists and surgeons. Colorectal Dis 2011;13:e411–7.
[48] Rade F, Bretagnol F, Auguste M, et al. Determinants of outcome following laparoscopic lavage for perforated diverticulitis. Br J Surg 2014;101:1602–6.
[49] Swank HA, Mulder IM, Hoofwijk AG, et al. Early experience with laparoscopic lavage for perforated diverticulitis. Br J Surg 2013;100:704–10.
[50] Rossi GL, Mentz R, Bertone S, et al. Laparoscopic peritoneal lavage for Hinchey III diverticulitis: is it as effective as it is applicable? Dis Colon Rectum 2014;57(12):1384–90.
[51] O'Leary DP, Myers E. Laparoscopic lavage for perforated diverticulitis: a panacea? Dis Colon Rectum 2013;56(3):385–7.
[52] Swank HA, Vermeulen J, Lange JF, et al. The Ladies Trial: laparoscopic peritoneal lavage or resection for purulent peritonitis and Hartmann's procedure or resection with primary anastomosis for purulent or faecal peritonitis in perforated diverticulitis. BMC Surg 2010;10:29.
[53] Thornell A, Angenete E, Gonzales E, et al. Treatment of acute diverticulitis laparoscopic lavage vs resection (DILALA): Study protocol for a randomized controlled trial. Trials 2011;12:186.
[54] Hogan A, Winder DC. The LapLAND trial: Laparoscopic lavage for acute non-faeculent diverticulitis. Available at: http://www.clinicaltrials.gov/show/NCT01019239. Accessed November 29, 2014.
[55] Felder SI, Barmparas G, Lynn J, et al. Can the need for colectomy after computed tomography-guided percutaneous drainage for diverticular abscess be predicted? Am Surg 2013;79:1013–6.
[56] Gaertner WB, Willis DJ, Madoff RD, et al. Percutaneous drainage of colonic diverticular abscess: is colon resection necessary? Dis Colon Rectum 2013;56:622–6.
[57] Kaiser AM, Jiang JK, Lake JP, et al. The management of complicated diverticulitis and the role of computed tomography. Am J Gastroenterol 2005;100:910–7.
[58] Brandt D, Gervaz P, Durmishi Y, et al. Percutaneous CT scan-guided drainage vs. antibiotherapy alone for Hinchey II diverticulitis: a case-control study. Dis Colon Rectum 2006;49:1533–8.
[59] Nelson RS, Ewing BM, Wengert TJ, et al. Clinical outcomes of complicated diverticulitis managed nonoperatively. Am J Surg 2008;196(6):969–74.

[60] Bridoux V, Antor M, Schwarz L, et al. Elective operation after acute complicated diverticulitis: is it still mandatory? World J Gastroenterol 2014;20(25):8166–72.
[61] Elagili F, Stocchi L, Ozuner G, et al. Outcomes of percutaneous drainage without surgery for patients with diverticular abscess. Dis Colon Rectum 2014;57:331–6.
[62] Ambrosetti P, Chautems R, Soravia C, et al. Long-term outcome of mesocolic and pelvic diverticular abscesses of the left colon: a prospective study of 73 cases. Dis Colon Rectum 2005;48:787–91.

Advances in Surgery 49 (2015) 15–29

ADVANCES IN SURGERY

ELSEVIER
MOSBY

Hospital Readmissions

Are They Preventable?

Erin G. Brown, MD[a], Richard J. Bold, MD[b,*]

[a]Department of General Surgery, UC Davis Medical Center, 2315 Stockton Boulevard, Sacramento, CA 95817, USA; [b]Division of Surgical Oncology, UC Davis Cancer Center, 4501 X Street, Sacramento, CA 95817, USA

Keywords

• Readmission • Health care reform • Surgery

Key points

- Thirty-day hospital readmission is common after general surgical procedures.
- Complex surgical procedures, preoperative patient comorbidities, and occurrence of postoperative complications are strongly associated with an increased risk of unplanned readmission.
- There is a need for further research to identify successful interventions to decrease readmission rates among surgical patients.

INTRODUCTION

Admission to a health care facility is intended to address an acute change in a person's health (either planned or unplanned), with discharge based on the presumption that the patient has returned to a health status no longer requiring the resources of inpatient level of care. Unfortunately, readmission is a common event with significant impact for both the patient and the health care system. The landmark study by Jencks and colleagues [1] highlights the prevalence of readmissions nationwide. One-fifth of Medicare patients hospitalized for treatment were readmitted within 30 days of discharge. Furthermore, a staggering 67.1% of patients discharged after medical treatment and 51.5% of patients discharged after surgery had either been rehospitalized or died within 1 year of discharge from the index hospitalization. The same study estimated

The authors have nothing to disclose.

*Corresponding author. Division of Surgical Oncology, UC Davis Cancer Center, Suite 3010, 4501 X Street, Sacramento, CA 95817. *E-mail address*: richard.bold@ucdmc.ucdavis.edu

0065-3411/15/$ – see front matter
http://dx.doi.org/10.1016/j.yasu.2015.03.013

the annual financial burden of unplanned readmissions among Medicare patients to be more than $17 billion.

In the face of these sobering numbers, the Affordable Care Act set to reduce unnecessary readmissions by enacting the Hospital Readmissions Reduction Program [2]. Implemented in October of 2012, the program began by reducing reimbursement payments to hospitals with higher than expected 30-day readmission rates for patients with congestive heart failure, myocardial infarction, and pneumonia. For the fiscal year 2015, penalties were set to begin for chronic obstructive pulmonary disease and hip and knee arthroplasty, the first surgical procedures to be included under the measure. Reimbursement cuts for readmission after coronary artery bypass grafts are slated to begin in 2017. These financial penalties are based on a supposition that higher than expected rates of readmission are due to the provision of lower than average quality of care, and can be changed to reduce or avoid the penalties.

This supposition has ignited a flurry of research to characterize, identify causes of, and potentially reduce the prevalence of readmission. However, some have begun to question whether readmission rates are truly a marker of quality medical care. Although it is undeniable that hospital readmissions have a significant impact on our patients and the health care system, it is not entirely clear whether efforts to reduce readmission rates are the best way to improve the quality of care clinicians provide. This article analyzes the current literature on surgical readmissions to characterize the issue and provide insight into whether the rate of hospital readmission can be lowered through the identification of events that truly are preventable.

SURGICAL READMISSIONS

Numerous studies across the United States have investigated hospital readmissions among medical and surgical patients. Readmission rates among medical patients remain consistently higher than those for surgical patients [1,3]. Medical conditions most susceptible to readmission, such as congestive heart failure and chronic obstructive pulmonary disease, are chronic problems characterized by acute exacerbations to be managed, whereas surgery is more often a single intervention aimed at disease elimination. In fact, many rehospitalizations after surgery are attributed to medical conditions unrelated to the index surgical procedure. The interplay between physiologic events attributable to surgery and exacerbation of underlying comorbidities is sufficiently difficult that causal relationships cannot be concretely determined; however, readmission after surgery remains a significant burden to our patients regardless of the cause.

Several studies that have examined readmission rates for general surgery patients have found that the rate of 30-day readmission is anywhere from 7% to 16% (Table 1) [1,4–7]. Tsai and colleagues [7] examined 30-day readmissions among Medicare patients undergoing coronary artery bypass grafting, pulmonary lobectomy, endovascular repair of abdominal aortic aneurysm (AAA), colectomy, and hip replacement, and found that nearly 1 in 7 patients were readmitted within 30 days of discharge. Although readmission rates

Table 1
Readmission rates after general surgical procedures

	Jencks et al [1], 2009	Glance et al [4], 2014	Kassin et al [5], 2012	Kohlnhofer et al [6], 2014	Tsai et al [7], 2013
30-Day readmission rate (%)	15.6	6.8	11.3	9	13.1
Surgical procedures included	Any surgical procedure	General, vascular, and orthopedic surgical procedures	Inpatient general surgery procedures	Inpatient general surgery procedures	Coronary artery bypass graft, pulmonary lobectomy, endovascular AAA repair, colectomy, hip replacement

Abbreviation: AAA, abdominal aortic aneurysm.

among surgical patients may be lower than those for medical patients, the impact of surgical readmissions is clearly widespread.

TRACKING READMISSIONS

Despite the expansive literature surrounding surgical readmissions, there remains significant variation in data-collection methods and even basic definitions. For example, the National Surgical Quality Improvement Project (NSQIP; administered by the American College of Surgeons) reports readmissions within 30 days of the index surgical procedure, whereas the University Healthcare Consortium (UHC) and Medicare report readmissions within 30 days of discharge. For some procedures with significant postoperative inpatient care, these 2 definitions may have different rates, with UHC and Medicare likely reporting higher rates than NSQIP. Other studies extend readmission data beyond a year, and claim that these numbers better reflect the actual impact of readmission on our patients and the health care system.

Not only do definitions vary widely, but data-collection sources also seem to dramatically affect reported rates of readmission. Sacks and colleagues [8] compared readmission diagnoses based on administrative and clinical data to determine how well administrative databases could determine a planned versus an unplanned readmission. The investigators found discordance among 31% of readmissions; furthermore, administrative data misclassified almost 10% of admissions as unplanned when physician review determined them to be planned. Another study comparing readmission data from NSQIP and UHC showed dramatic differences between the 2 systems [9]. Whereas NSQIP better captured readmissions to other facilities, which is estimated to be as high as 50% [10], UHC captured significantly more admissions because of the differences in the readmission time frame. This study also showed that administrative databases were not reliable in determining whether the readmission was related to the index hospitalization based on independent physician review.

With huge financial penalties at stake based on the readmission data collected, it is clear that standardized definitions and data algorithms are needed to fairly and appropriately establish readmission benchmarks. Without uniform, nationwide data reporting, hospitals may be incentivized to underreport data or attribute the readmission to a prior hospitalization. Furthermore, hospitals that reliably and accurately capture data may be unfairly penalized. While administrative databases serve as a starting point for quality improvement, they may not be appropriate tools for implementing penalties at the current time. Adoption of a national registry is one solution to improve quality care across the country.

VARIABLES ASSOCIATED WITH READMISSION

Among the literature focusing on general surgery patients as a whole, the most consistent finding among research on surgical readmissions is their association with postoperative complications. Kassin and colleagues [5] studied readmissions after any inpatient general surgery procedure, and found that nearly half of all readmissions were secondary to complications related to gastrointestinal problems (nausea, vomiting, obstruction) and infection. Patients experiencing a postoperative complication were 4 times more likely to require readmission after discharge. Furthermore, patients experiencing multiple complications were at even higher risk for rehospitalization.

The interaction between postoperative complications, hospital length of stay (LOS), and readmission is complex, but undeniably intertwined. Morris and colleagues [11] examined this relationship by examining almost 60,000 Veterans Affairs patients who underwent major surgery. As expected for this group of patients and procedures, the complication rate was 23%, with 12% of patients being readmitted within 30 days. Although the occurrence of a postoperative complication predicted a higher risk of readmission, it was observed that approximately one-third of complications were diagnosed after discharge from the index hospitalization. In addition, postoperative infection, one of the most common reasons for readmission after surgery, was diagnosed after discharge in most cases.

Does the drive to decrease the LOS with the use of enhanced recovery pathways lead to increased readmissions by sending patients home too soon? Or should we be keeping patients longer after surgery to avoid readmissions? Existing literature is mixed regarding the relationship between LOS and readmission. Some have suggested that a decreased LOS is associated with increased rehospitalization rates [6,12,13]; however, several others have reported the opposite [14–17]. When analyzing readmission rates among patients with cancer undergoing surgery nationwide, the authors found that a shorter LOS actually predicted lower readmission rates [18]. Although the literature on LOS and readmission is conflicting, this likely reflects the complexity of the interaction between LOS, complications, and the timing of the occurrence of postoperative complications with the subsequent readmission.

Socioeconomic and racial factors also play a complicated, but important, role in readmissions. Racial disparities exist in both access to care and surgical outcomes. Girotti and colleagues [19] reported that black patients were more likely than white patients to require rehospitalization after surgery, even after adjusting for other patient and hospital factors. Furthermore, readmissions may be largely affected by social factors such as a lack of social support in the home, lack of access to postdischarge care resources, lower education, and poverty-associated consequences (eg, lack of transportation, health care insurance, or access to a primary care physician) [20]. These findings highlight that the scope of factors affecting readmissions extends beyond patient-related and hospital-related factors to the support systems and communities of patients.

These studies examining global readmission rates and trends for all general surgery patients have provided important characterization of the impact and scope of the issue. However, they also revealed that readmission rates and the causes for readmission are highly variable among different surgical procedures [5,21]. Therefore, these findings have led to increased focus on procedure-specific outcomes.

HEPATOBILIARY READMISSIONS

Pancreaticoduodenectomy (PD) is a complex operation with high rates of morbidity and poor long-term survival, making it an ideal focus for quality improvement research. Similarly, readmission rates after PD are some of the highest among general surgery procedures, with rates ranging between 19% and 59% (Table 2) [22]. With an average estimated cost of $16,000 per readmission, this is a significant financial burden on the health care system [5,23]. Similarly to research for all general surgery patients, multiple studies have demonstrated an increased risk of readmission with the presence of postoperative complications. More specifically, the most common reasons for readmission were gastrointestinal complications, dehydration, pancreatic leak, and infection [14,24,25].

Although most of these studies were single-institution reviews, a large, multi-institutional study reviewing readmission rates within the Central Pancreas Consortium showed that 1 in 5 patients were readmitted within 90 days after pancreaticoduodenectomy [26]. By limiting the data to relatively early postoperative readmission, the investigators likely excluded readmissions secondary to disease progression or planned readmission for chemotherapy, unlike some of the aforementioned studies. However, the findings within this larger group of high-volume hepatobiliary specialists echoed those seen in the smaller studies. On multivariate analysis, they again reported an increased risk of readmission with wound infections and the presence of pancreatic fistulas.

Other studies have identified a relationship between patient comorbidities and increased risk of readmission [10,14,27–30]. In fact, Hyder and colleagues [27] demonstrated that patient factors accounted for 95% of variations in readmission rates among almost 300 hospitals, whereas hospital and physician factors have relatively little impact on readmission rates. Therefore, efforts to reduce readmissions need to focus on identifying patients at increased risk for readmission, and both reducing and more effectively managing postoperative complications.

COLORECTAL READMISSIONS

Colon cancer is one of the most common cancer diagnoses in the United States, with almost 150,000 new cases diagnosed annually [12]. Postoperative readmission after colectomy is common, and the estimated cost of readmission is nearly $13,000 (see Table 2) [31]. Several large studies have examined readmission rates after colectomy. In 2010, Greenblatt and colleagues [12] reviewed the SEER (Surveillance, Epidemiology, and End Results) Medicare database for all patients treated with colectomy for colon adenocarcinoma over a 10-year period and found a 30-day readmission rate of 11%, with the most common time to readmission being a mere 2 days after discharge. Of importance, they showed a mortality rate of 7% during the readmission hospitalization, and a significantly higher risk of death within 1 year for those patients who required rehospitalization. To better understand the differences between those patients readmitted and those not, the 2 groups were compared. Readmitted

Table 2
Readmissions after a variety of surgical procedures

	Pancreaticoduodenectomy	Colectomy	AAA
30-Day readmission rate (%)	19–59 [21]	11–13.5 [12,31]	5–13 [33]
Estimated cost of readmission	$16,000 per readmission [5,22]	$13,000 per readmission [30]	$10,091 per readmission [32]
Reasons for readmission	Gastrointestinal complications, dehydration, pancreatic leak, infection [14,23,24]	Gastrointestinal complications, infection, renal failure, pulmonary embolism [12,31]	Infection, renal failure, gastrointestinal complications (open), graft failure (endovascular) [33]

patients were from lower income households, were less educated, and had more medical comorbidities. Again, they saw a link between postoperative complications and readmission, and the reasons for readmission were similar to those of patients undergoing pancreatic resection, with gastrointestinal complications and infection being the 2 most common reasons for readmission.

Another large study of rehospitalizations after colectomy analyzed data from the NSQIP and Medicare databases, and found a similar 30-day readmission rate of 13.5% [32]. Although readmitted patients had more comorbidities, the most important predictor of readmission was the occurrence of a postoperative complications, and the risk of readmission further increased with an increasing number of complications. This finding suggests an interaction between comorbid disease and the severity of complications; namely, patients with underlying health problems are more likely to require inpatient care for the management of a postoperative complication. Infection was again a common reason for readmission, although renal failure and pulmonary embolism also contributed significantly to the cause for hospital readmission.

VASCULAR READMISSIONS

Patients undergoing vascular surgery procedures are another group known to be at significantly increased risk for readmission. The Medicare Payment Advisory Commission selected 7 groups of index hospitalizations that accounted for approximately one-third of preventable readmissions, one of which was vascular surgical procedures [33]. The same report identified vascular readmissions as the most expensive on a per-patient basis. This result prompted research to characterize and target reducing readmissions after vascular surgery, and the focus has largely focused on AAA repair. Existing studies show varying rates of 30-day readmission between 5% and 13% for both open and endovascular repair (see Table 2) [34]. Again, the most common reason for readmission after AAA repair, either open or endovascular, was for care related to procedure-related complications. The most common indication for readmission was infection, regardless of operative approach. In fact, more than one-third of patients with a wound infection required readmission. Postoperative renal failure was another important predictor of rehospitalization. Again, procedure-specific differences in the cause for readmission were noted, even though the intervention was for the same underlying process: gastrointestinal complications were prevalent among the open group and graft complications were common in the endovascular group. Unlike the readmissions for other surgical procedures, medical comorbidities were not associated with an increased risk of readmission.

Finally, Greenblatt and colleagues [34] found that patients discharged to a skilled nursing facility were 2.5 times more likely to be readmitted than those discharged home with home health resources. In addition, light was shed on the sobering fact that readmitted patients were significantly more likely to die within 1 year (unadjusted 1-year mortality of 23.4% for those readmitted vs 4.5% for those who were not). Even after adjusting for age, gender, comorbidities, and procedure on multivariate analysis, the odds ratio of readmission for 1-year mortality was 5.8, truly highlighting the serious impact of readmission on patients.

PREDICTING PATIENTS AT RISK FOR READMISSION

The first step toward reducing unplanned readmissions is to identify patients at increased risk for rehospitalization after surgery. From the aforementioned literature, we know that the primary drivers of increased risk for readmission come from the complexity of the procedure, the occurrence of a postoperative complication, and the extent of medical comorbidities [35]. Several groups have used these variables to create prediction models in an attempt to better identify those patients at risk for readmission. Bradley and colleagues [36] attempted to predict which patients were at increased risk for readmission by using the Rothman Index (RI), a composite score tallied in the electronic medical record based on patient vitals, laboratory results, and nursing assessments. The investigators discovered that patients with higher RI scores were at greater risk for readmission, and postulated that this may be a way to help physicians allocate outpatient resources to reduce readmissions. Fry and colleagues [37] developed a risk-adjusted, postoperative LOS model to determine outliers within this category. Patients identified as LOS outliers were significantly more likely to experience both postoperative readmission and death. Unfortunately these models may be difficult to implement, as they may identify patients at increased risk for readmission but do not necessarily implicate the cause, and thus allow any guidance for specific interventions to prevent the readmission.

DEFINING PREVENTABLE

There is no consensus as to what, exactly, is a preventable readmission. Are all unplanned readmissions in some way preventable? Or should it be just those whereby identifiable change in medical management may have prevented the readmission?

The literature already cited demonstrates the huge impact of readmissions on our patients and the health care system. There is also an important trend of decreased long-term survival among those patients who are readmitted, further underscoring the dramatic impact rehospitalization can have on patients. One sees a common association between complications and increased readmissions, with infection, dehydration, and gastrointestinal complications being frequent reasons for readmission among many groups. However, despite these common themes, there is wide variability in the definition of a preventable readmission. Dawes and colleagues [38] defined a readmission as preventable if a "reasonable improvement in the health care process could have potentially avoided the need for rehospitalization," and divided these preventable readmissions into 3 categories based on premature hospital discharge, inadequate follow-up, and potential ability to manage the patient on an outpatient basis. Between 2 physician reviewers there was disagreement 10% to 15% of the time, and the investigators found that readmissions were only preventable 21% of the time. Of those that were deemed preventable, dehydration was the most common readmission diagnosis. One study defined preventable as a superficial site infection or dehydration [31] while another deemed those patients readmitted within 7 days of discharge as a target for improvement [26].

The authors performed a retrospective nationwide review of patients with cancer readmitted after surgery, focusing on patients readmitted within 7 days of discharge for nausea, vomiting, dehydration, and postoperative pain (Fig. 1A) [18]. Similarly to others, the authors saw a need for improved patient care coordination as a means to provide care to these patients through closer discharge follow-up, establishment of observational units for administration of fluids, and enhanced palliative care programs. However, looking further into readmissions among this subset of patients treated at their own institution, the authors evaluated how many of the patients had contact with the clinic (either by telephone or clinic visit) between discharge and readmission. Most patients (78% of those readmitted for nausea, vomiting, or dehydration, and 60% of those readmitted for pain) were found to have made contact before readmission, leading the authors to believe that closer follow-up may not be the ideal target for improving transitions of care at their institution (see Fig. 1B). Efforts to enhance coordinated care will be critical at both institutional and national levels to provide quality care in the absence of readmission, but the optimal means to achieve this has yet to be elucidated.

PREVENTING READMISSIONS

Interventions have been successfully implemented to reduce readmissions, but most of these strategies focus on medical patients. For example, palliative care has been shown to both reduce readmission and improve quality of life, but is obviously only appropriate for a specific subset of patients [39]. Others have suggested that closer discharge follow-up may prevent readmissions. However, Weinberger and colleagues [40] found that increased access to primary care among Veterans Affairs patients with diabetes, congestive heart failure, and chronic obstructive pulmonary disease actually increased readmissions; interestingly, although these patients had higher readmission rates, they were also more satisfied with their care. Other studies have investigated medication reconciliation, improved in-hospital discharge education, and postdischarge phone calls and visits. A recent systematic review evaluated these interventions and found that no single act, when implemented alone, was consistently associated with decreased readmission rates [41]. The investigators did find that postdischarge phone calls were a common component among successful bundled interventions, but when tested in isolation such phone calls were not enough to reduce rehospitalization rates.

The benefit of postdischarge phone calls has also been suggested in the surgical literature. Keller and colleagues [42] examined readmissions among patients undergoing ileostomy closure and found a high incidence of readmission for small bowel obstruction and dehydration, but also that readmission

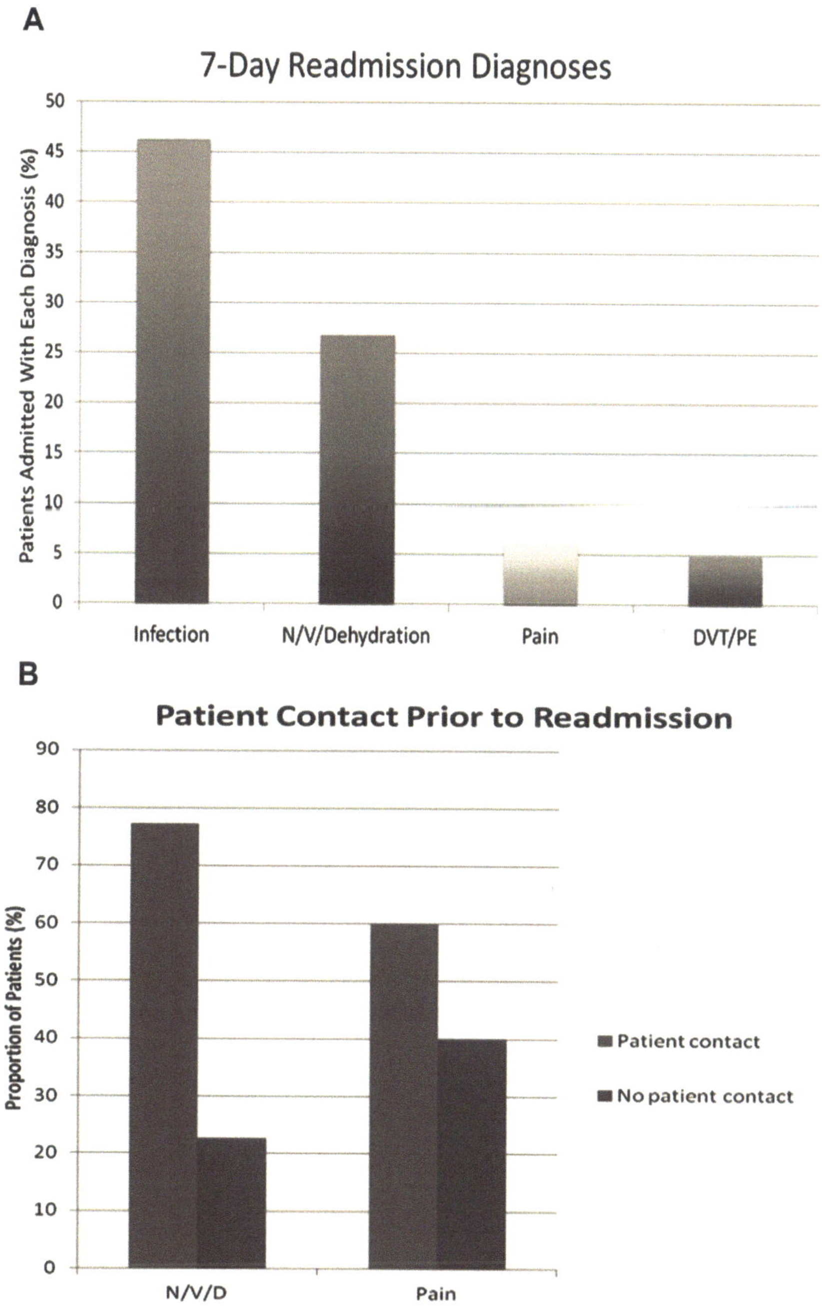

Fig. 1. (*A*) Reasons for readmission within 7 days of discharge among patients with cancer after surgery. (*B*) Most of these patients had contact, by either clinic visit or phone follow-up, before being readmitted. DVT, deep venous thrombosis; N/V/D, nausea/vomiting/dehydration; PE, pulmonary embolism.

most often occurred before the first scheduled follow-up. These investigators have since tailored their enhanced recovery pathway to include telephone follow-up within 7 days of discharge. However, data evaluating the success of the intervention are pending. In another study, a panel of quality and outcomes experts reviewed a total of 34 measures to reduce surgical readmissions, and found that most focused on detailed review of the expected postoperative course, discharge instructions, and improved communication with the patient's primary care physician [43]. Of importance, they also included measures that addressed preoperative and perioperative care. Enhanced recovery pathways encompassing these practices were a common feature of endorsed measures. Although identifying practices that will be agreeable to most physicians is critical to successful implementation, to date no studies have demonstrated the effectiveness of such measures in reducing readmissions for surgical patients.

Bundled interventions and enhanced recovery pathways may help prevent a subset of readmissions and improve patient care coordination for surgical patients. Unfortunately, they often fail to address financial resources, social support, and access to care, which are all critical factors affecting the risk for readmission [44]. Kangovi and Grande [45] proposed a framework to reduce readmissions among high-risk patients by acknowledging the socioeconomic factors associated with rehospitalization; they urge hospitals to screen patients for these issues before discharge and target specific resources for them, in essence providing better transitions in care. Greenblatt and colleagues [34] added to this conceptual model by suggesting inclusion of complications, both in identifying complications and appropriately managing the care of such complications. Such additions are critical when targeting reductions in surgical readmissions. These conceptual models address several important facets of readmission: patient and socioeconomic variables, hospital-based factors, procedure-related aspects, and outpatient resources. Within each area, several issues can be identified as potential targets for interventions to improve readmission rates and patient care coordination.

SUMMARY: READMISSIONS—PENALTIES, PROGRESS, PREVENTION

Rehospitalization places an enormous financial burden on the health care system and patients' quality of life. However, with the threat of financial penalties for surgical readmissions imminently looming, the concept of a surgical readmission as a rescue is extremely important. Readmissions are not always bad, but often represent good judgment and appropriate patient care. Furthermore, financial penalties for medical readmissions have been shown to disproportionately affect larger hospitals, teaching hospitals, and safety-net hospitals, which typically provide care to economically vulnerable patients [46]. As we move forward in attempts to reduce surgical readmissions, conscious efforts will need to be made to avoid unfairly penalizing hospitals that provide care to the underserved. As suggested by Girotti and colleagues [47], penalties should adjust for socioeconomic status but also allow for an acceptable level of readmission rates to prevent hospitals from failing to readmit when it is, in fact, the appropriate course of action.

Readmissions are largely related to more complex surgical procedures and patients with more medical comorbidities, and are strongly associated with postoperative complications. Although some of these represent nonmodifiable factors, there is still a definite need for improved transitions of care within the health care system, and a need for more research to identify successful interventions to decrease readmission rates among surgical patients. Although the entire spectrum of interventions may not universally apply to all hospitals, surgical procedures, or patients, efforts to reduce unnecessary readmissions is critical. Hospital readmission following a surgical procedure may be a necessary component of optimal care, although active engagement at the patient, hospital, and policy levels will be crucial to achieving an appropriate and fair system for administering readmission penalties.

References

[1] Jencks S, Williams MV, Coleman EA. Rehospitalizations among patients in the Medicare fee-for-service program. N Engl J Med 2009;360:1418–28.
[2] Fact sheets: CMS to improve quality of care during hospital inpatient stays August 4, 2014. Available at: http://www.cms.gov/Newsroom/MediaReleaseDatabase/Fact-sheets/2014-Fact-sheets-items/2014-08-04-2.html. Accessed August 13, 2014.
[3] Rosen A, Chen Q, Shin M, et al. Medical and surgical readmissions in the Veterans Health Administration. Med Care 2014;52:243–9.
[4] Glance LG, Kellermann AL, Osler TM, et al. Hospital readmission after noncardiac surgery: the role of major complications. JAMA Surg 2014;149(5):439–45.
[5] Kassin M, Owen R, Perez S, et al. Risk factors for 30-day hospital readmission among general surgery patients. J Am Coll Surg 2012;215(3):322–30.
[6] Kohlnhofer BM, Tevis SE, Weber SM, et al. Multiple complications and short length of stay are associated with postoperative readmissions. Am J Surg 2014;207(4):449–56.
[7] Tsai TC, Joynt KE, Orav EJ, et al. Variation in surgical-readmission rates and quality of hospital care. N Engl J Med 2013;369(12):1134–42.
[8] Sacks GD, Dawes AJ, Russell MM, et al. Evaluation of hospital readmissions in surgical patients: do administrative data tell the real story? JAMA Surg 2014;149(8):759–64.
[9] Hechenbleikner EM, Makary MA, Samarov DV, et al. Hospital readmission by method of data collection. J Am Coll Surg 2013;216(6):1150–8.
[10] Yermilov I, Bentrem D, Sekeris E, et al. Readmissions following pancreaticoduodenectomy for pancreas cancer: a population-based appraisal. Ann Surg Oncol 2009;16(3):554–61.
[11] Morris MS, Deierhoi RJ, Richman JS, et al. The relationship between timing of surgical complications and hospital readmission. JAMA Surg 2014;149(4):348–54.
[12] Greenblatt DY, Weber SM, O'Connor ES, et al. Readmission after colectomy for cancer predicts one-year mortality. Ann Surg 2010;251(4):659–69.
[13] McAleese P, Odling-Smee W. The effect of complications on length of stay. Ann Surg 1994;220(6):740–4.
[14] Emick DM, Riall TS, Cameron JL, et al. Hospital readmission after pancreaticoduodenectomy. J Gastrointest Surg 2006;10(9):1243–52 [discussion: 1252–3].
[15] Gawlas I, Sethi M, Winner M, et al. Readmission after pancreatic resection is not an appropriate measure of quality. Ann Surg Oncol 2013;20(6):1781–7.
[16] Martin RC, Brown R, Puffer L, et al. Readmission rates after abdominal surgery. Ann Surg 2011;254(4):591–7.

[17] Reddy DM, Townsend CM Jr, Kuo YF, et al. Readmission after pancreatectomy for pancreatic cancer in Medicare patients. J Gastrointest Surg 2009;13(11):1963–74 [discussion: 1974–5].
[18] Brown EG, Burgess D, Li CS, et al. Hospital readmissions: necessary evil or preventable target for quality improvement. Ann Surg 2014;260(4):583–91.
[19] Girotti ME, Shih T, Revels S, et al. Racial disparities in readmissions and site of care for major surgery. J Am Coll Surg 2014;218(3):423–30.
[20] Arbaje AI, Wolff JL, Yu Q, et al. Postdischarge environmental and socioeconomic factors and the likelihood of early hospital readmission among community-dwelling Medicare beneficiaries. Gerontologist 2008;48:495–504.
[21] Lee TJ, Martin RC. Readmission rates after abdominal surgery. Adv Surg 2012;46(1): 155–70.
[22] Clarke CN, Sussman JJ, Abbott DE, et al. Factors affecting readmission after pancreaticoduodenectomy. Adv Surg 2013;47(1):99–110.
[23] Kent T, Sachs TE, Callery MP, et al. Readmission after major pancreatic resection: a necessary evil? J Am Coll Surg 2011;213:515–23.
[24] Kastenberg ZJ, Morton JM, Visser BC, et al. Hospital readmission after a pancreaticoduodenectomy: an emerging quality metric? HPB (Oxford) 2013;15(2):142–8.
[25] Brown EG, Yang A, Canter RJ, et al. Outcomes of pancreaticoduodenectomy: where should we focus our efforts to improve outcomes? JAMA Surg 2014;149:694–9.
[26] Ahmad SA, Edwards MJ, Sutton JM, et al. Factors influencing readmission after pancreaticoduodenectomy: a multi-institutional study of 1302 patients. Ann Surg 2012;256(3): 529–37.
[27] Hyder O, Dodson RM, Nathan H, et al. Influence of patient, physician, and hospital factors on 30-day readmission following pancreatoduodenectomy in the United States. JAMA Surg 2013;148(12):1095–102.
[28] Rosemurgy A, Bloomston M, Serafini F, et al. Frequency with which surgeons undertake pancreaticoduodenectomy determines length of stay, hospital charges, and in-hospital mortality. J Gastrointest Surg 1995;5(1):21–6.
[29] Schneider EB, Hyder O, Brooke BS, et al. Patient readmission and mortality after colorectal surgery for colon cancer: impact of length of stay relative to other clinical factors. J Am Coll Surg 2012;214(4):390–8 [discussion: 398–9].
[30] Grewal SS, McClaine RJ, Schmulewitz N, et al. Factors associated with recidivism following pancreaticoduodenectomy. HPB (Oxford) 2011;13(12):869–75.
[31] Keller DS, Swendseid B, Khorgami Z, et al. Predicting the unpredictable: comparing readmitted versus non-readmitted colorectal surgery patients. Am J Surg 2014;207(3): 346–51.
[32] Lawson EH, Hall BL, Louie R, et al. Identification of modifiable factors for reducing readmission after colectomy: a national analysis. Surgery 2014;155(5):754–66.
[33] Medicare Payment Advisory Commission. Report to the Congress: promoting greater efficiency in Medicare. Washington, DC: Medicare Payment Advisory Commission; 2007.
[34] Greenblatt DY, Fernandes-Taylor S, Kent KC. Readmission after abdominal aortic aneurysm repair. Adv Surg 2013;47(1):141–52.
[35] Wiseman JT, Guzman AM, Fernandes-Taylor S, et al. General and vascular surgery readmissions: a systematic review. J Am Coll Surg 2014;219(3):552–69.e2.
[36] Bradley EH, Yakusheva O, Horwitz LI, et al. Identifying patients at increased risk for unplanned readmission. Med Care 2013;51(9):761–6.
[37] Fry DE, Pine M, Pine G. Medicare post-discharge deaths and readmissions following elective surgery. Am J Surg 2014;207(3):326–30 [discussion: 330].
[38] Dawes AJ, Sacks GD, Russell MM, et al. Preventable readmissions to surgical services: lessons learned and targets for improvement. J Am Coll Surg 2014;219(3):382–9.
[39] Slamowicz RE, Erbas B, Sundararajan V, et al. Predictors of readmission after elective coronary artery bypass graft surgery. Ausr Health Rev 2008;32:677–83.

[40] Weinberger M, Oddone EZ, Henderson WG. Does increased access to primary care reduce hospital readmissions? N Engl J Med 1996;334:1441–7.
[41] Hansen LO, Young RS, Hinami K, et al. Interventions to reduce 30-day rehospitalization: a systemic review. Ann Intern Med 2011;155:520–8.
[42] Keller DS, Swendseid B, Khan S, et al. Readmissions after ileostomy closure: cause to revisit a standardized enhanced recovery pathway? Am J Surg 2014;208(4):650–5.
[43] Halverson AL, Sellers MM, Bilimoria KY, et al. Identification of process measures to reduce postoperative readmission. J Gastrointest Surg 2014;18(8):1407–15.
[44] Weissman JS, Stern RS, Epstein AM. The impact of patient socioeconomic status and other factors on readmission: a prospective study in four Massachusetts hospitals. Inquiry 1994;31:163–72.
[45] Kangovi S, Grande D. Hospital readmissions—not just a measure of quality. JAMA 2011;306:1796–7.
[46] Joynt KE, Jha AK. Characteristics of hospitals receiving penalties under the hospital readmissions reduction program. JAMA 2013;309:341–2.
[47] Girotti ME, Shih T, Dimick JB. Rethinking hospital readmission as a surgical quality measure. JAMA Surg 2014;149:757–8.

Advances in Surgery 49 (2015) 31–63

ADVANCES IN SURGERY

Recent Advances in Intestinal and Multivisceral Transplantation

Koji Hashimoto, MD, PhD[a], Guilherme Costa, MD[b], Ajai Khanna, MD, PhD[a], Masato Fujiki, MD, PhD[a], Cristiano Quintini, MD[a], Kareem Abu-Elmagd, MD, PhD[a,*]

[a]Center for Gut Rehabilitation and Transplantation, Transplant Center, Cleveland Clinic, 9500 Euclid Avenue, Cleveland, OH 44195, USA; [b]Thomas E. Starzl Transplantation Institute, University of Pittsburgh Medical Center, 200 Lothrop Street, Pittsburgh, PA 15261, USA

Keywords

• Intestinal and multivisceral transplantation • Long-term outcome • Quality of life • Chronic rejection • Intestinal rehabilitation • Nutritional failure

Key points

- Early seeking for multidisciplinary comprehensive medical and surgical rehabilitative measures, including transplantation, should always be considered for all patients dependent on home parenteral nutrition.
- Gut rehabilitation with early restoration of nutritional autonomy has been shown to be associated with better survival and quality-of-life outcomes.
- With transplantation, and despite the observed improvement in overall survival, further enhancement in long-term outcomes is still needed particularly of the liver-free allografts.
- Until full clinical achievement of allograft tolerance, further innovations in immunosuppression and immunomodality studies are required including better HLA match, effective DSA management, and other innovative tactics.

INTRODUCTION

The successful development of clinical intestinal and multivisceral transplantation is one of the most important milestones in the recent history of organ

The authors have nothing to disclose.

*Corresponding author. *E-mail address:* abuelmk@ccf.org

0065-3411/15/$ – see front matter
http://dx.doi.org/10.1016/j.yasu.2015.04.003

transplantation. Despite early disappointments, the 3 main types of visceral transplantation (Fig. 1) have evolved to be the standard of care for patients with nutritional failure and complex abdominal pathology. As with other organs, evolution of this procedure is expected to be the result of continual interplay between new advances in surgical techniques, novel immunosuppressive strategies, and better postoperative management [1,2]. With new insights into mechanisms of drug-free allograft acceptance and other important predictors of long-term functional survival, further progress is expected with achievement of less challenging postoperative management and better long-term therapeutic efficacy particularly of the liver-free visceral allograft [3,4].

With the 1989 University of Pittsburgh Medical Center clinical introduction of tacrolimus and the initial encouraging results with intestinal and multivisceral transplantation, a wave of clinical interest in the field was witnessed across North America and Europe [5–9]. With continual efforts to improve outcome, the clinical practicality of the procedure has gradually increased with promising outlook [10–14]. Such an achievement was fortified by the 2000 approval of the Health Care Financing Administration, currently known as the Centers for Medicare and Medicaid Services (CMS) considering the intestinal, liver-intestinal, and multivisceral transplantation procedures as the standard of care for patients with irreversible intestinal failure who no longer can be maintained on home parenteral nutrition (HPN) [15].

Since our 2002 coming-of-age *Advances in Surgery* publication, the field of visceral transplantation has witnessed major achievements and faced new challenges [1,15]. This report provides an-in-depth and up-to-date review of the recent developments in clinical practice, surgical techniques, immunosuppression, and postoperative care. The multifaceted challenges are addressed in the milieu of the current long-term outcomes beyond the 5-year milestone, including survival, quality of life (QOL), and value of health care. In addition, new insights are highlighted to further advance the field, particularly with the current wave of health reform [4].

CURRENT CLINICAL PRACTICE

Nomenclature

With increased practicality, visceral transplantation has been successfully used for patients with different varieties of end-stage gastrointestinal disorders. Accordingly, different combinations of en bloc abdominal visceral organ replacement have been more frequently used [1,16,17]. As a result, various innovative techniques have been introduced to both donor and recipient operation to reduce morbidity and mortality [1,13,18–21]. Subsequently, controversies concerning the original nomenclature have emerged [22]. The issue was then addressed and laid to rest by evidence-based classification preserving the 3 main "icons" of the transplant procedure: intestinal, liver-intestine, and multivisceral with the adoption of a new subclassification according to the type of added organs, as shown in Table 1 [23]. Accordingly, the heritage of such an orphan field including more than 2 decades of clinical experience is

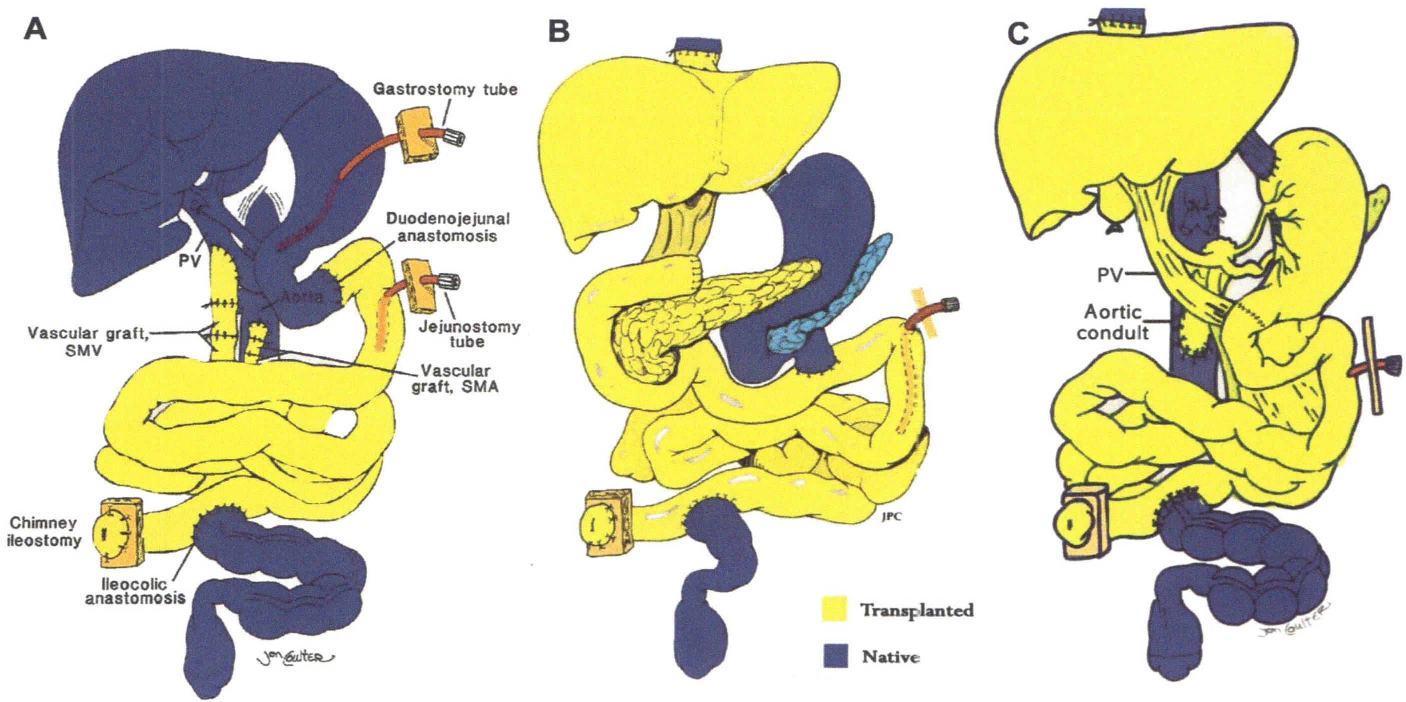

Fig. 1. Prototypes of visceral transplantation. (*A*) Isolated intestine, (*B*) liver-intestine, and (*C*) multivisceral. The liver-intestine cllograft includes the pancreas and duodenum. Transplanted allografts are yellow.

Table 1
The nomenclature of the different types of the small bowel–contained allografts

Classification	I-intestine	II-liver-intestine	III-multivisceral: Full	III-multivisceral: Modified
Main types	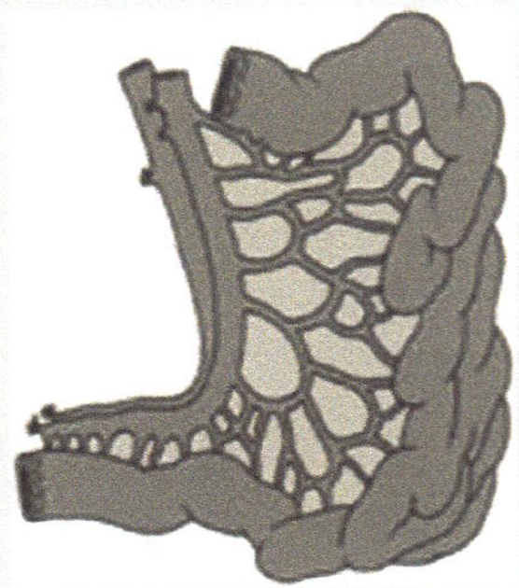 Intestine	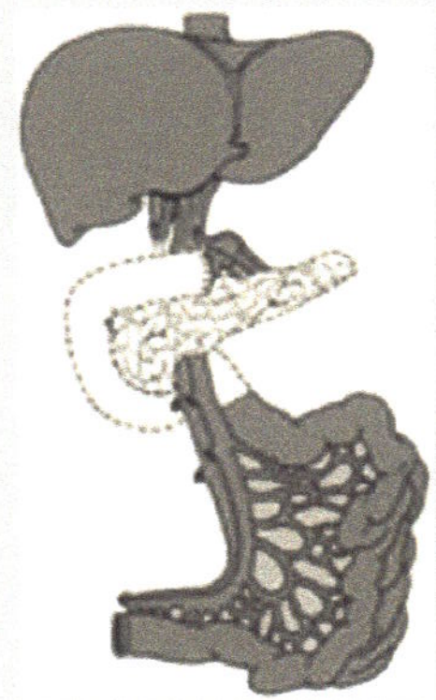 Liver + Intestine[a]	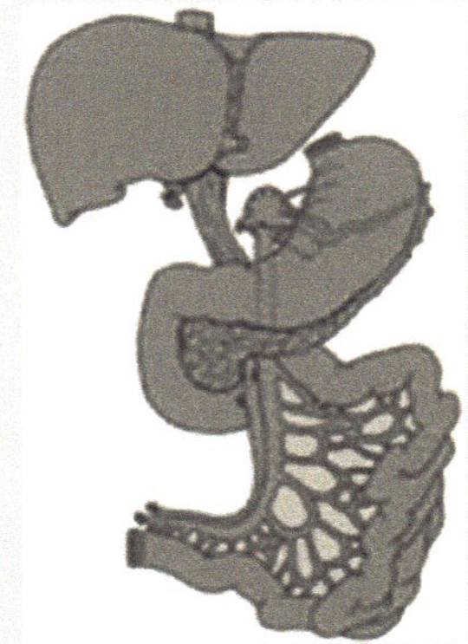 Stomach + Duodenum + Pancreas + Intestine + Liver	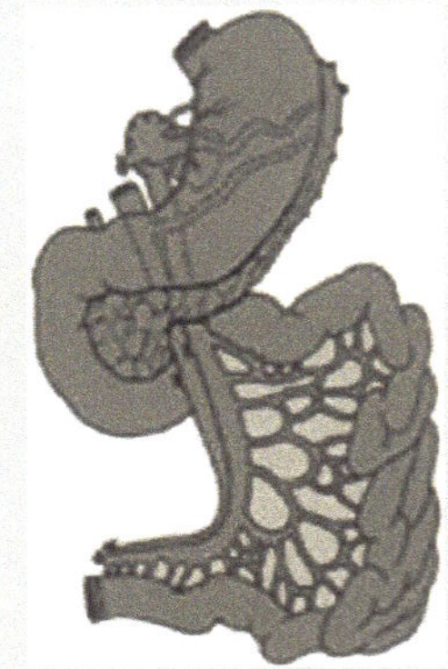 Stomach + Duodenum + Pancreas + Intestine
Subtypes (descriptive)[b]	• Intestine alone • En bloc with colon and/or pancreas	• En bloc with colon and/or kidney	• En bloc with colon and/or kidney • With preserved native pancreaticoduodenal complex and/or spleen	

[a]Inclusion of the pancreaticoduodenal complex (unshaded organs) is optional and commonly used for technical reasons.
[b]Optional or when medically indicated.
Modified from Abu-Elmagd KM. The small bowel contained allografts: existing and proposed nomenclature. Am J Transplant 2011;11(1):184–5.

preserved with forestalling of drastic effects on future reporting metrics and outcome analyses.

Indications

Despite continual improvement in survival, the utilization of the procedure is still limited to patients with combined irreversible intestinal and nutritional failure. The different causes are fully described elsewhere [24]. Nutritional failure is a new term that reflects development of HPN-associated life-threatening complications, presence of an ultrashort gut syndrome, or diagnosis of end-stage gastrointestinal disorders that are not amenable to current medical and surgical rehabilitative measures [15,25]. Vascular thrombosis and Crohn disease are the leading causes of gut failure in adults, and congenital disorders in children. The life-threatening complications associated with HPN are fully defined by the senior author (KAE) in the CMS memorandum that include, and are not limited to, vanishing of the central venous access, frequent catheter-related infection, and presence of significant hepatic injury [15].

Gut rehabilitation

With loss of intrinsic (physiologic) and artificial (HPN) nutritional autonomy being the hallmark of current indication for visceral transplantation, all efforts have been recently made to restore native gut function by using novel medical approaches and innovative surgical techniques [25]. In addition to the standard nutritional measures, enterocyte growth factors have been increasingly used to promote gut adaptation [26]. Teduglutide, a recombinant analog of human glucagon-like peptide-2, has been recently approved in the United States (Gattex) and Europe (Revestive) as the first targeted treatment of short bowel syndrome–associated intestinal failure [27,28].

The technical feasibility of visceral transplantation has fueled the introduction of different nontransplant surgical modalities to treat short bowel syndrome and complex abdominal pathology. Of these are autologous reconstructive and bowel-lengthening procedures [25,29]. With transplantation being used as a rescue therapy, surgical reconstruction has been increasingly applied for patients with multiple enterocutaneous fistulae and residual bowel function (Fig. 2). Creative efforts also have been made to treat abdominal malignancy, including ex vivo tumor resection with gut autotransplantation [30,31].

Bowel lengthening has been increasingly used in both adults and children. Of these are the Bianchi and serial transverse enteroplasty (STEP) procedures (Fig. 3). Both modalities can be successfully performed in patients with dilated bowel loops to reduce transit time, eliminate bacterial overgrowth, and enhance gut absorption. With adjunct comprehensive medical management, nutritional autonomy is possibly achievable within the first few months after surgery. These therapeutic modalities are better offered in a multidisciplinary team approach. The current successful efforts may partially explain the recent reduction in the total number of global visceral transplantations, particularly in children (Fig. 4) [32]. However, failure of such attempts should prompt the need for early transplantation with expected better survival outcome (Fig. 5) [1,2].

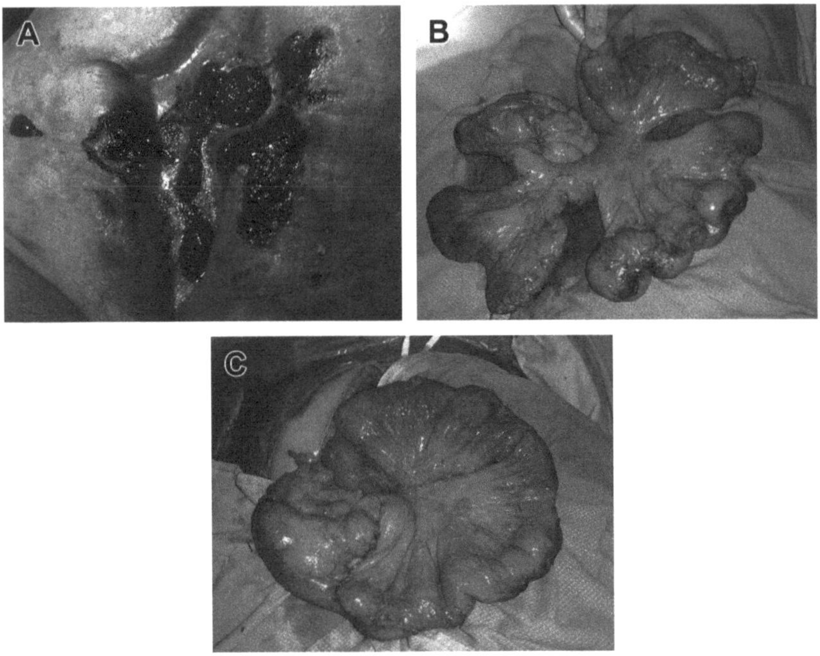

Fig. 2. Surgical rehabilitation of intestinal failure. (*A*) Multiple enterocutaneous fistulae causing intestinal failure. (*B*) Multiple surgical resections. (*C*) Reestablishment of intestinal continuity. Full nutritional autonomy was achieved after 4 weeks.

Equally important is the avoidance of irreversible neurologic and psychosocial impairments that may have a significant impact on the procedure's rehabilitative therapeutic indices [4].

New trends

Recent published data have documented new observations indicative of early referral and evolving indications [1,2,22,24]. With increased awareness, more patients were referred for transplantation before development of HPN-associated liver failure and received liver-free allografts (Fig. 6) [22,32]. Despite its proven immunologic privileges, simultaneous hepatic replacement is indicated only for patients with advanced liver damage and severe cholestasis [1,24]. As a result, more patients underwent isolated intestinal or modified multivisceral transplantation with preservation of native liver, including those with short bowel, pseudo-obstruction, and Gardner syndromes [16,17,24]. In contrast, isolated liver transplantation has been used for liver failure in highly selected patients with short bowel syndrome [33]. Despite current controversies, full multivisceral transplantation with inclusion of the liver has evolved to be an effective therapeutic modality for patients with hepatic failure and

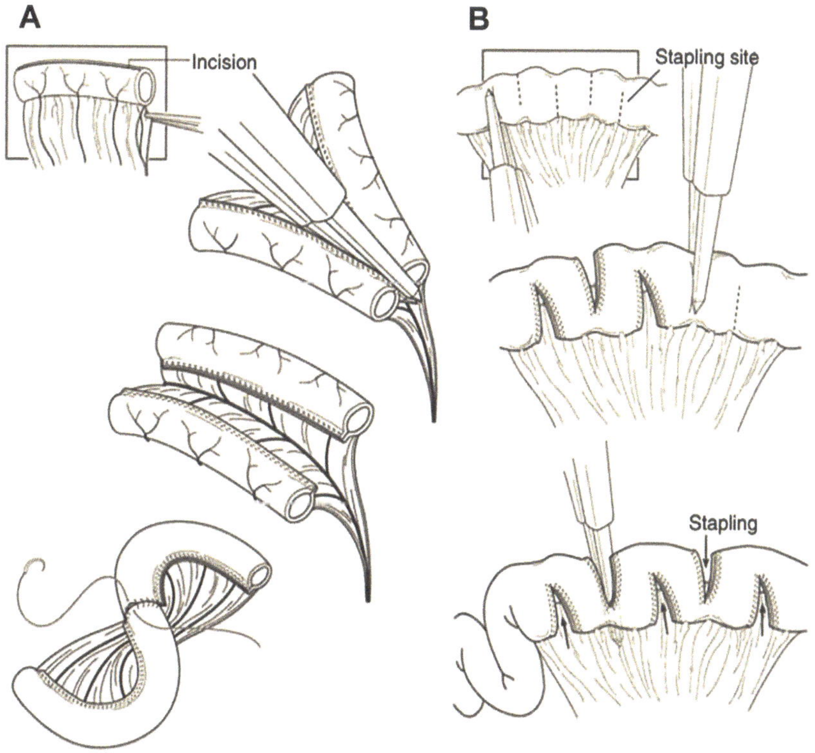

Fig. 3. Bowel-lengthening procedures for short bowel syndrome. (*A*) Bianchi procedure and (*B*) STEP procedure. (*From* Abu-Elmagd KM, Bond G, Matarese L, et al. Gut rehabilitation and intestinal transplantation. Therapy 2005;2(6):855; with permission.)

diffuse portomesenteric venous thrombosis who are not suitable candidates for isolated hepatic replacement [1,34,35]. It is imperative to emphasize that patients with preserved hepatic functions should be considered for portal hypertensive surgery as a permanent therapy or bridge to multivisceral transplantation [35].

Early transplantation

Early consideration for transplantation before development of nutritional failure or progression of a complex abdominal pathology has yet to be the standard of care. However, recently published data favor early transplantation with increased candidacy and better outcome measures [1,2,4,36,37]. Early transplantation is commonly associated with favorable outcome (see Fig. 5) and better QOL [1,2,4]. The native liver can be saved with reduction or elimination of the potential prohibitive risk of dying on the United Network for Organ Sharing (UNOS) waiting list for a liver-contained allograft (Fig. 7) [38]. An additional advantage is the ability to perform allograft enterectomy to rescue the intestine-alone recipients with reinstitution of HPN [1,4].

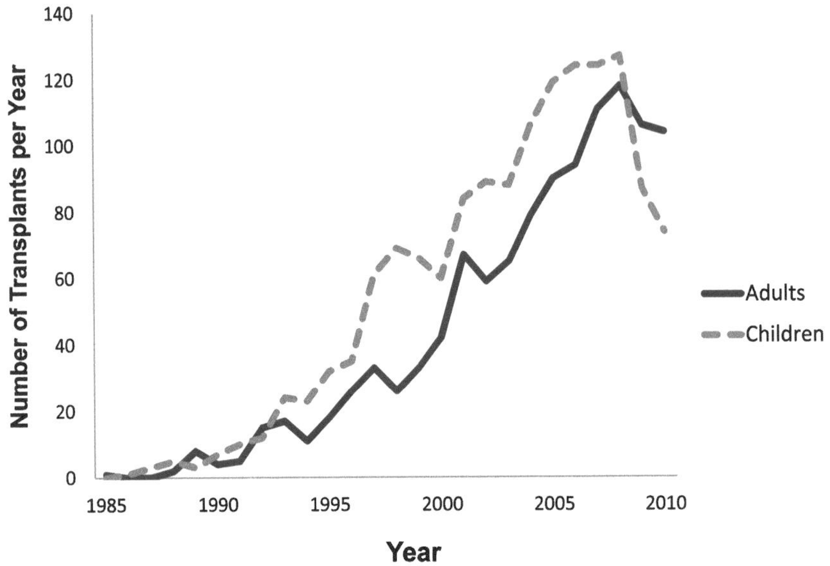

Fig. 4. Worldwide trends in visceral transplant case volumes. After the steady increase of overall case volumes over time, pediatric case volume has decreased since 2008. (*Adapted from* Grant D, Abu-Elmagd K, Mazariegos G, et al. Intestinal Transplant Registry Report: Global Activity and Trends. Am J Transplant 2015;15:210–9; with permission.)

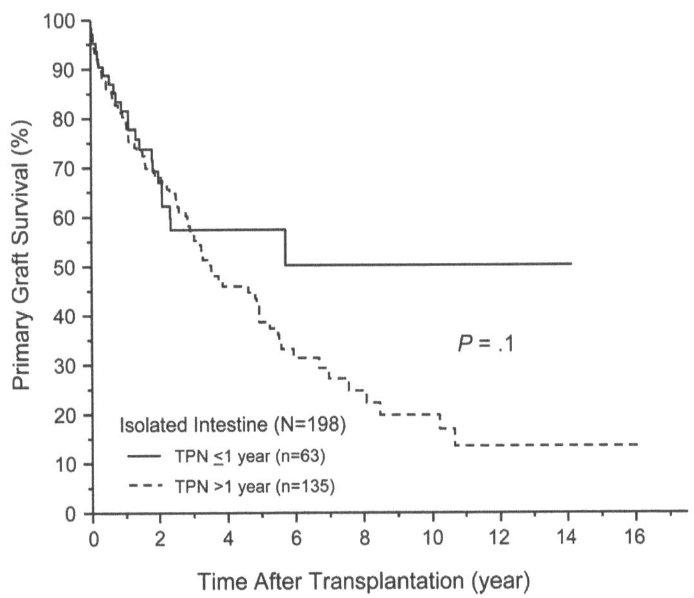

Fig. 5. Graft survival after primary transplantation with isolated intestinal allografts according to duration of parenteral nutrition before transplantation. TPN, total parenteral nutrition. (*From* Abu-Elmagd KM, Costa G, Bond GJ, et al. Five hundred intestinal and multivisceral transplantations at a single center: major advances with new challenges. Ann Surg 2009;250(4):573; with permission.)

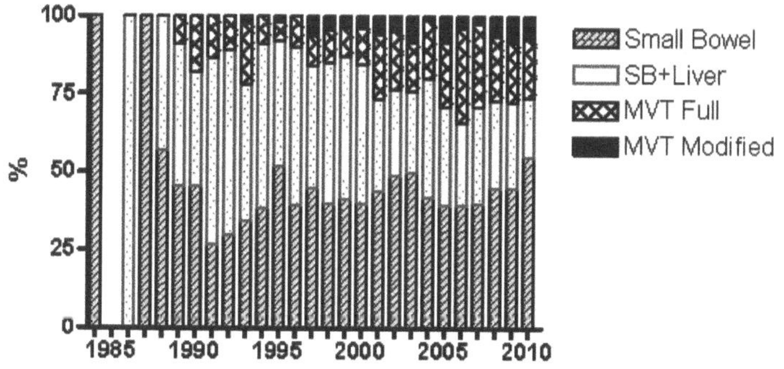

Fig. 6. Changes in the proportion of different types of visceral allografts. Note the proportional decrease in the liver-contained allografts with an increase in the liver-free allografts over time. MVT, multivisceral transplant; SB, small bowel. (*Adapted from* Grant D, Abu-Elmagd K, Mazariegos G, et al. Intestinal Transplant Registry Report: Global Activity and Trends. Am J Transplant 2015;15:210–9; with permission.)

It is imperative to emphasize that the current survival after transplantation is comparable to that of patients with HPN-dependent intestinal failure, despite the use of the procedure as a rescue therapy (Fig. 8) [36]. Equally important is the achievement of nutritional autonomy with better QOL and improved value of health care [1,4,36,39]. Nonetheless, a randomized clinical trial

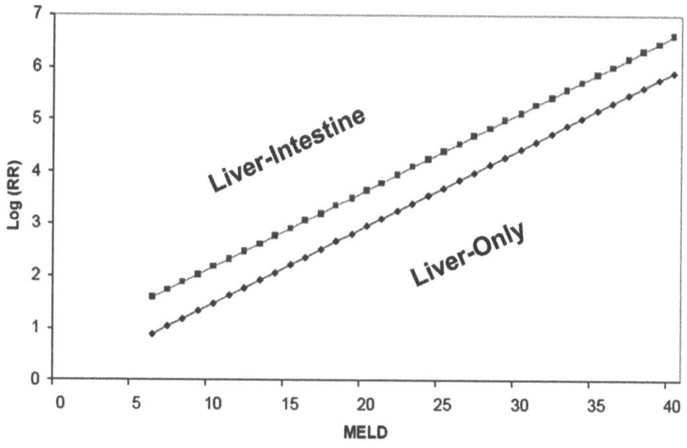

Fig. 7. Relative risk of mortality in transplant candidates for liver-intestine and liver-only allografts on the UNOS/OPTN waiting list. Liver-intestine candidates have a higher risk of mortality compared with liver-only candidates. MELD, Model for End-Stage Liver Disease. (*Adapted from* Abu-Elmagd, K. Intestinal and multivisceral transplant waiting list: Clinical management according to allograft type and current organ allocation system. In: Kirk A, Knechtle S, Larsen C, editors. Textbook of organ transplantation. 1st edition. Oxford, UK: Wiley-Blackwell; 2014. p. 492; with permission.)

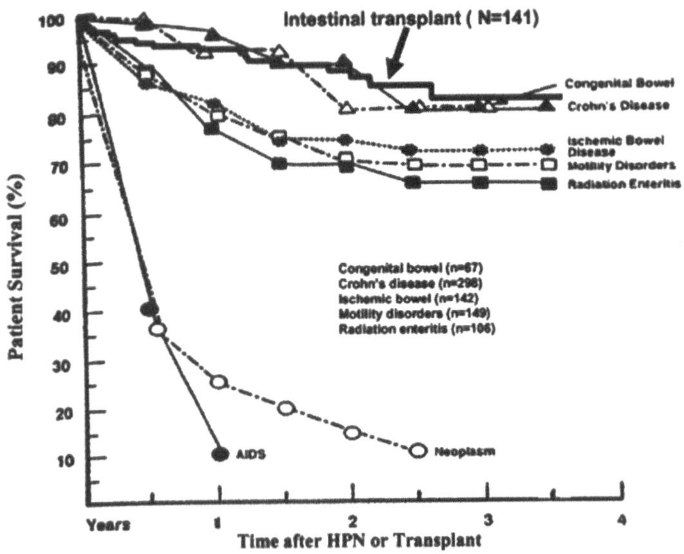

Fig. 8. Comparison of overall patient survival of intestinal transplant recipients and HPN patients without transplant. Despite the use of intestinal transplantation as a rescue therapy for HPN failure, the survival of transplant recipients is favorably comparable to that of HPN patients. (*From* Abu-Elmagd KM. Intestinal transplantation for short bowel syndrome and gastrointestinal failure: current consensus, rewarding outcomes, and practical guidelines. Gastroenterology 2006;130(2):S136; with permission.)

comparing HPN with intestinal transplantation is required to modify the current medical necessity criteria for transplantation candidacy with establishment of new practical guidelines.

Retransplantation

With increased practicality, visceral retransplantation, with the same or more complex composite grafts, is more frequently required as a life-saving procedure [1,4,40,41]. Despite satisfactory outcome (Fig. 9), novel strategies are required to ameliorate the risk of recurrent immune destruction, particularly of the liver-free allograft [1,4,42]. Anti–B-cell therapy, better HLA match, and simultaneous replacement of the native liver by using the domino procedure are novel approaches that could be used to reduce the risk of recurrent rejection-induced graft loss [1,42]. With intestine-alone allografts, a 2-stage surgical strategy with a time interval between allograft enterectomy and retransplantation may achieve a better outcome [4].

Contraindications

The traditional contraindications have been fully addressed in the 2002 *Advances in Surgery* [15]. Since then, a few relevant observations have been recently reported. Poor psychosocial support has been identified as a major risk factor

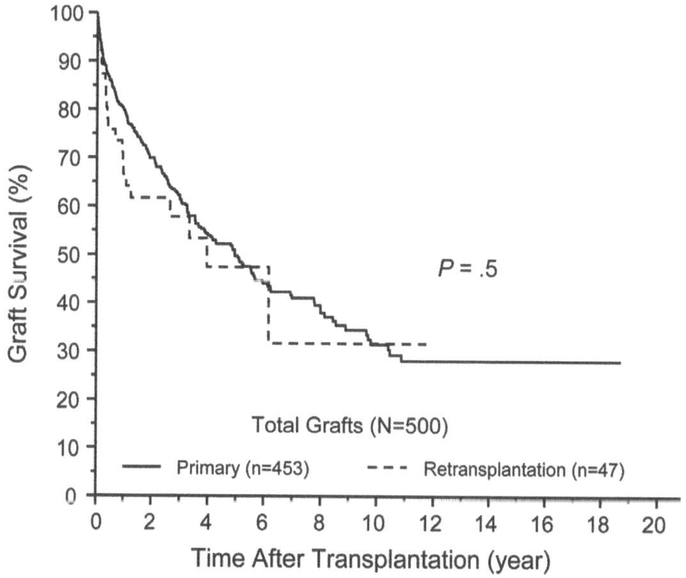

Fig. 9. Allograft survival after primary visceral transplantation and retransplantation. (*From* Abu-Elmagd KM, Costa G, Bond GJ, et al. Five hundred intestinal and multivisceral transplantations at a single center: major advances with new challenges. Ann Surg 2009;250(4):576; with permission.)

for successful outcome [4]. Accordingly, the coexistence of nonfunctional social support should contraindicate transplantation. On the contrary, the presence of controlled neuropsychiatric disorders should not preclude transplantation because successful rehabilitation after surgery has been recently documented [4]. Another evolving barrier is the coexistence of acquired immune deficiencies due to the prohibitive risk of graft-versus-host disease (GVHD) [43,44]. Without innovative immunomodulatory approaches including staged stem cell and visceral transplantation, the procedure should not be considered in the presence of acquired or hereditary immune deficiencies [45,46].

The reported successful survival in patients 50 years of age or older precludes age as a sole contraindication [1]. Chemical dependency, psychosomatic disorders, abdominal infection, and locally advanced desmoid tumors also should be addressed and treated before being considered as a contraindication for transplantation.

Waiting list management

Waiting list management has become the focus of recent efforts to maximize organ utilization, reduce mortality, and improve outcome [38]. Compared with other organs, the visceral transplant candidates are very challenging because of disease complexity. Most of these patients require daily intravenous nutrition associated with life-threatening complications, including line sepsis, central venous thrombosis, and liver failure. Accordingly, judicious monitoring of native organ functions with surveillance protocols for infection, malignancy, and other systemic disorders are required. With the threefold waiting list, and mortality of the liver-intestinal candidates compared with the isolated liver candidates (see Fig. 7), the UNOS/Organ Procurement and Transplantation Network (OPTN) allocation policy has been recently modified to increase the access of the liver-intestine candidates to the national donor pool (http://optn.transplant.hrsa.gov/PoliciesandBylaws2/policies/pdfs/policy_8.pdf).

Global activities

As of May 2011, a total of 2569 transplants have been performed in 2384 patients at 78 centers in all continents but Africa [32]. Increased transplantation activities have been recently witnessed in South America and Asia (Fig. 10). Such an observation reflects the worldwide growing interest in the field and the parallel cumulative increase in the surgical experience with live donor transplant.

Despite the increased practicality, the total yearly activities have decreased over the past few years, particularly among the pediatric population, as shown in Fig. 4 [32]. Such a decline can be partially explained by the growing interest in gut rehabilitation, as described previously, by using comprehensive medical therapy and innovative autologous reconstructive surgery. In addition, there has been a gradual decline in the number of adult liver-contained visceral transplantations in the United States because of previous changes in the UNOS/OPTN policy with limited access to the national donor pool. It is also our expectation that the continual evolution of HPN therapy may further reduce the risk of associated hepatic injury and subsequent need for visceral transplantation [47].

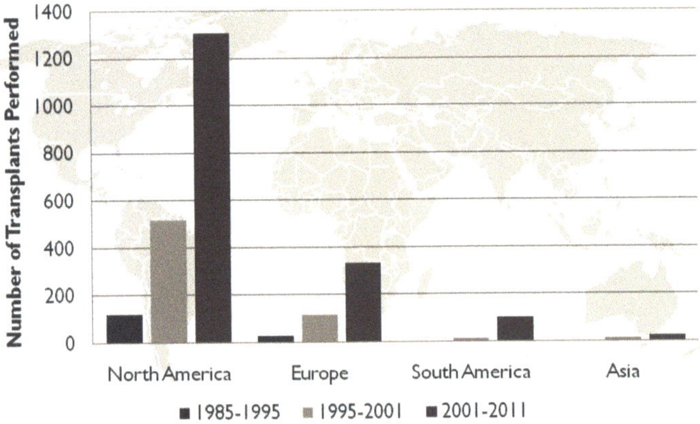

Fig. 10. Geographic distribution of visceral transplantation from 1985 to 2011. (*Adapted from* Grant D, Abu-Elmagd K, Mazariegos G, et al. Intestinal Transplant Registry Report: Global Activity and Trends. Am J Transplant 2015;15:210–9; with permission.)

ADVANCES IN SURGICAL TECHNIQUES

Surgical innovation has been one of the landmarks of the recent evolution of intestinal transplantation. The early challenges experienced with both donor and recipient surgery compiled with organ shortage in the milieu of patients with complex abdominal pathology stimulated relentless efforts toward various technical modifications [1].

Donor techniques

Simultaneous retrieval of both intestine and pancreas from the same donor to be given to 2 different recipients was introduced to overcome the growing demand for both organs [18]. Full preservation of the donor pancreaticoduodenal complex en bloc with the combined liver-intestinal graft was adopted to eliminate biliary complications and maintain continuity of the axial blood supply [1,14]. Retrieval of the colon en bloc with the intestine preserving the ileocecal valve was revisited after its initial introduction at the University of Pittsburgh in 1993 [11,48,49]. Finally, inclusion of the donor spleen as part of the multivisceral graft was applied with the premise to reduce risk of infection and enhance chimerism [50,51]. Unfortunately, such a modification has been associated with increased risk of fatal GVHD and hemolytic anemia [50,51].

Recipient operation

Evisceration of native organs with implantation of the visceral allografts has witnessed several modifications. Modified multivisceral transplantation with preservation of the native liver (Fig. 11A) and spleen with or without the pancreaticoduodenal complex (see Fig. 11B) has been successfully introduced for patients with preserved hepatic functions particularly those with Gardner and pseudo-obstruction syndromes [1,16,17]. The primary objective was to reduce risk of posttransplant lymphoproliferative disorder (PTLD). Other potential advantages included preservation of the portosplenic circulation during allograft implantation, elimination of need for biliary reconstruction, and augmentation of the islet cell mass by retaining native pancreas.

The initial in situ placement of a free donor arterial and venous conduit in the recipient before bringing the visceral allograft to the operative field is introduced by the senior author and later used by others [18]. The technique facilitates a safe vascular reconstruction. The back table Carrel patch arterial reconstruction technique to establish a single arterial conduit for the composite visceral graft has remained the Achilles heel of the donor procedure. However, we have occasionally observed the development of a nonocclusive intraluminal mural clot at the site of reconstruction, most probably due to turbulence of inflow [1,4]. In a few cases, the development of pseudoaneurysms required combined radiologic and surgical approach as a life-saving procedure [52].

Restoration of gastrointestinal continuity also has received various renovations [1]. With modified multivisceral transplantation, the duct-to-duct biliary reconstruction was introduced (see Fig. 11A) and the piggyback duodenoduodenal anastomosis was established in patients with preserved native duodenal sweep [14]. In addition, the native rectosigmoid was preserved in patients with

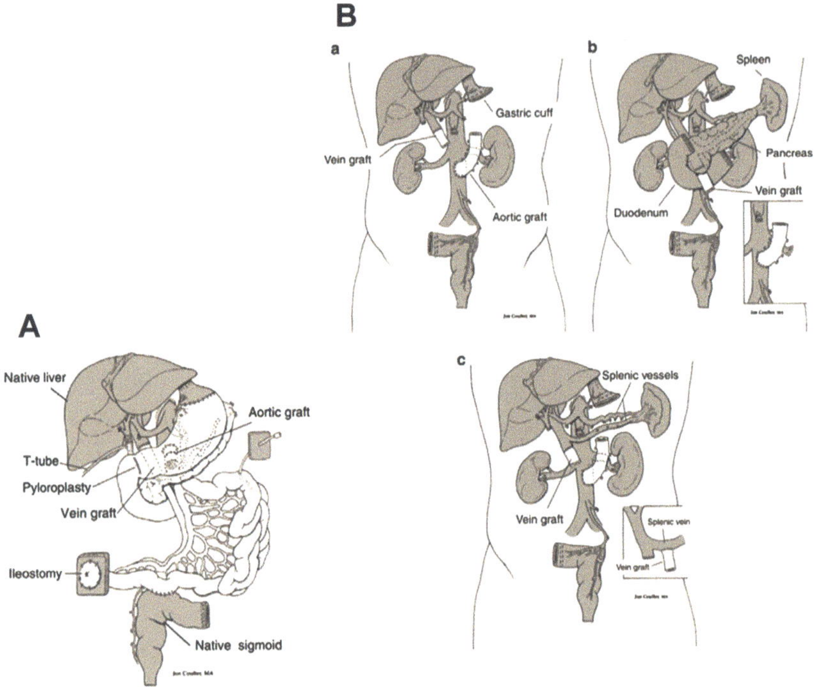

Fig. 11. (*A*) Modified multivisceral transplantation with the preservation of the native liver. Unshaded organs including stomach, duodenum, pancreas, and intestine are transplanted en bloc with a duct-to-duct biliary anastomosis. (*B*) Recipient operation with complete or partial removal of the native left upper abdominal organs for modified multivisceral transplantation. (*a*) Major evisceration with near total gastrectomy, total enterectomy, and pancreaticoduodenectomy. (*b*) Preservation of the splenopancreaticoduodenal complex. (*c*) Pancreaticoduodenectomy with preservation of the native spleen. (*Modified From* Cruz RJ Jr, Costa G, Bond G, et al. Modified "liver-sparing" multivisceral transplant with preserved native spleen, pancreas, and duodenum: technique and long-term outcome. J Gastrointest Surg 2010;14(11):1712–4; with permission.)

pseudo-obstruction and anastomosed to the distal end of the ileal allograft with establishment of successful hind gut reconstruction (Sogawa and colleagues, unpublished data, 2015). An innovative reconstructive surgical procedure also was performed in a patient with Crohn disease with previous total proctocolectomy and preserved anal sphincter using a visceral allograft that contained most of the donor colon. In this recipient, a pull-through operation was successfully performed with excellent long-term functional outcome (Fig. 12) [53].

In recipients with ultrashort gut syndrome and a previous doudenocolonic anastomosis close to the duodenal papilla, a segment of the native colon can be used as a visceral conduit between the native duodenum and proximal end of the allograft jejunum (Fig. 13). The allograft terminal ileum is then anastomosed to the distal end of the remaining native colon.

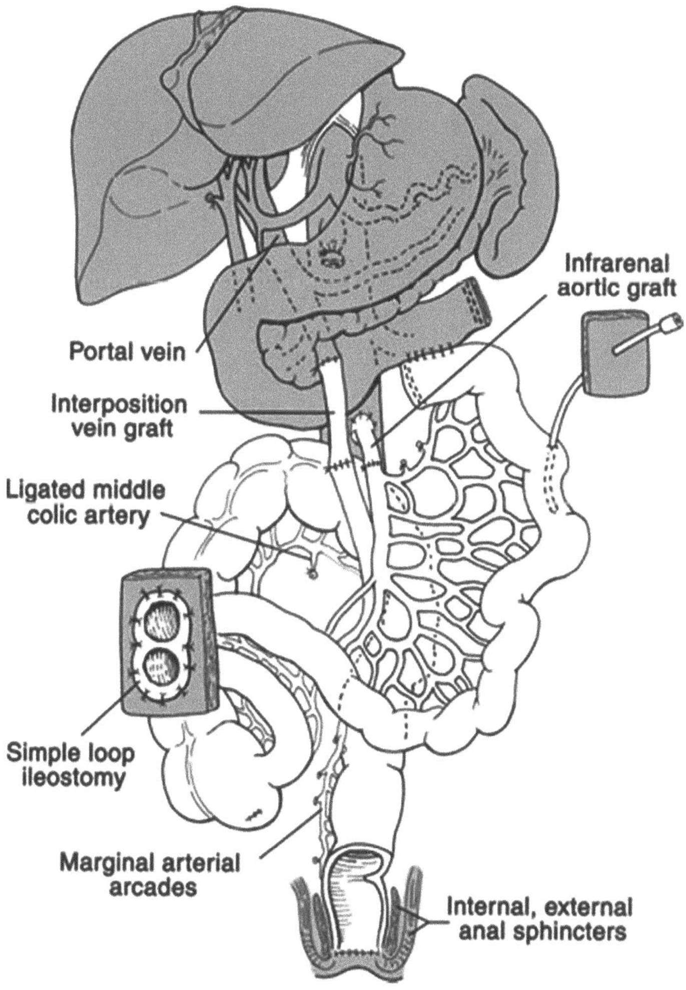

Fig. 12. Hind gut pull-through reconstruction with en bloc colon and intestinal transplantation. (*From* Eid KR, Costa G, Bond GJ, et al. An innovative sphincter preserving pull-through technique with en bloc colon and small bowel transplantation. Am J Transplant 2010;10(8):1941; with permission.)

Abdominal wall reconstruction

One of the challenging problems in the field of visceral transplantation is the loss of the abdominal domain. Such a challenge is due to loss of both volume and abdominal wall tissues [54,55]. The preferred primary abdominal wall closure also could be hampered by the allograft tissue edema following ischemia reperfusion injury. Inadequate abdominal cavity can be addressed before transplantation with implantation of tissue expanders [56]. At time of transplantation, a proportionally smaller organ donor, graft reduction, skin closure with or without

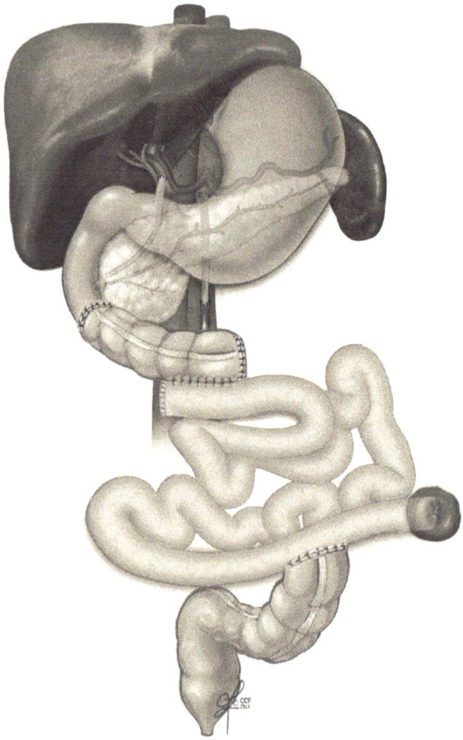

Fig. 13. Colonic interposition and intestinal transplantation. Note that a segment of the native colon is used as a visceral conduit between the native duodenum and the proximal jejunal allograft.

component separation techniques, myocutaneous flap, fascia closure with mesh or other tissue, or simultaneous transplantation of the donor abdominal wall or fascia can be entertained [1,15,54–58]. Abdominal wall complications can be associated with graft loss and patient death, although this association may be a marker only for increased patient complexity. Over the past decade, most of our visceral allograft recipients did not require any major autologous or allo-abdominal wall reconstruction because of the utilization of smaller-size donors and judicious intraoperative intravenous fluid resuscitation with simple abdominal wall skin closure (Kareem Abu-Elmagd, MD, PhD, unpublished data, 2015).

EVOLUTION OF IMMUNOSUPPRESSION

Introduction of novel immunosuppressive and immune modulatory strategies has been one of the seminal contributions that elevated the therapeutic efficacy of visceral transplantation. Although tacrolimus-based immunosuppression has made the procedure clinically feasible in 1990, the prohibitive risk of rejection with the requisite need for chronic high-dose treatment has inhibited its widespread use [13]. With more emphasis on the difficulty of clinical care rather than survival, induction therapy was introduced in 1995 as part of a multiple-drug immunosuppressive cocktail including different cellular and molecular targets [1,2,13]. With better control of rejection, survival was improved at major centers and according to the Intestinal Transplant Registry (ITR) [1,2,59–63]. As expected, the long-term detrimental effect of chronic multiple-drug immunosuppression eroded the observed early survival benefits particularly beyond the 10-year posttransplant landmark (Fig. 14A) [1].

With new insights into the mechanism of allograft acceptance and transplant tolerance, recipient preconditioning combined with posttransplant minimal immunosuppression was introduced at the University of Pittsburgh with the aim to improve allograft stability [3,63,64]. With perioperative partial depletion of the recipient lymphoid cells, amelioration of the initial donor-specific immune response is expected. Jointly, the application of minimal posttransplant immunosuppression has the potential to avoid the possible erosion of the alloengraftment mechanism of clonal exhaustion-deletion without high penalty of destructive immune response [63,64]. With such a novel protocol, further improvement in outcome was achieved with more survival advantage using alemtuzumab (campath-1H) compared with rabbit antithymocyte globulin (Thymoglobulin) (see Fig. 14B) [65]. Reduction in the incidence of intractable rejection, PTLD, and fatal infections partially attributed to better survival along with the ease of postoperative care [1,14,66]. Recent data also have suggested the possible therapeutic benefits of mammalian target of rapamycin inhibitors (sirolimus) as a maintenance therapy [32].

The demonstrated striking ability to further reduce maintenance immunosuppression with recipient pretreatment supports the Pittsburgh hypothesis of successful induction of variable tolerance in these immunologically challenging recipients [1,63–65]. With the unprecedented successful achievement of spaced doses of tacrolimus for up to 8 years in more than 50% of the study recipients, partial tolerance is achievable and drug-free long-term engraftment is within reach as demonstrated in 2 of the Pittsburgh long-term liver-contained visceral allograft survivors [65]. New scientific discoveries, including induction of tolerance with adoptive regulatory T cells or other immune cell therapy along with the introduction of reliable immune assays, will undoubtedly increase safety and further the goal of achieving complete tolerance in this challenging population [3,65,67].

POSTOPERATIVE MANAGEMENT

Enhancement of posttransplant management was the result of cumulative clinical experience, advances in molecular diagnostic techniques, and availability of new antimicrobial drugs [1,66]. In 1994, the clinical availability of the quantitative competitive polymerase chain reaction assay triggered serial monitoring of Epstein-Barr virus (EBV) and cytomegalovirus (CMV) load in peripheral blood [1,13,14,66]. Of the treatment strategies are infectious prophylaxis, preemptive therapy of EBV and CMV viremia, and active treatment of bacterial

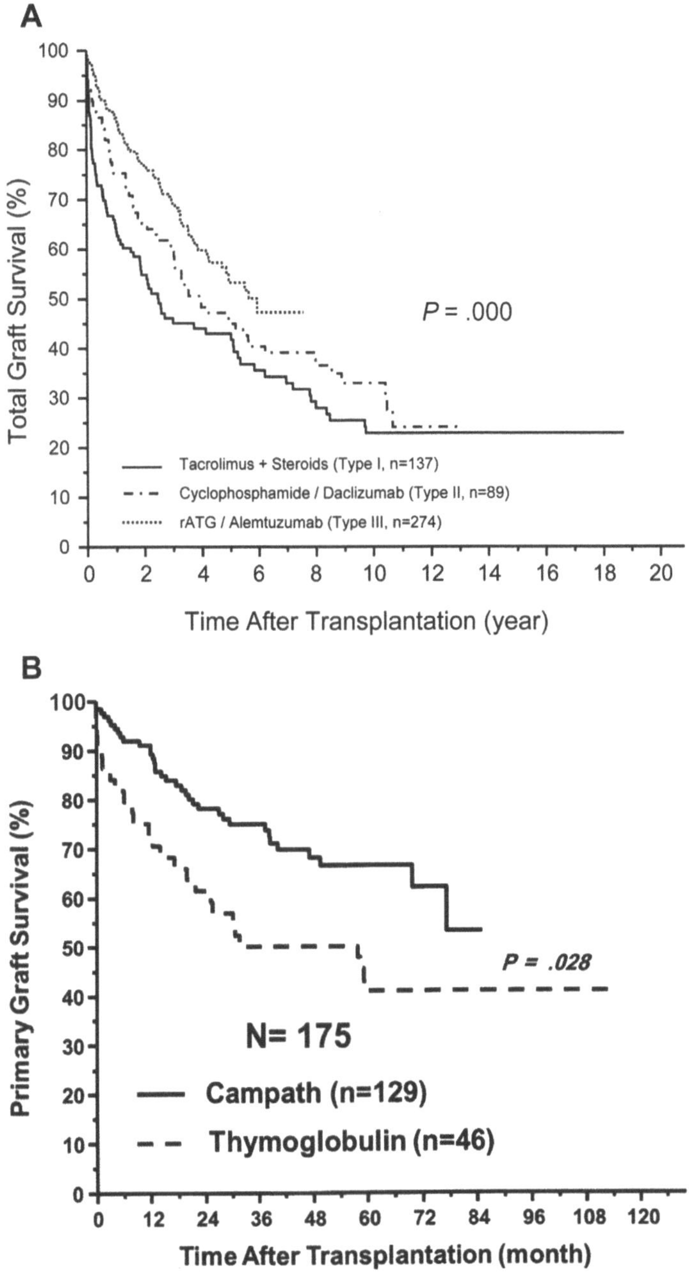

Fig. 14. (*A*) Significant improvement of visceral allograft survival according to type of immunosuppression. (*B*) Better graft survival in patients pretreated with alemtuzumab (Campath-1H) compared with those pretreated with antithymocyte globulin (Thymoglobulin). (*Modified from* Abu-Elmagd KM, Costa G, Bond GJ, et al. Five hundred intestinal and multivisceral transplantations at a single center: major advances with new challenges. Ann Surg 2009;250(4):574, with permission; and Abu-Elmagd KM, Costa G, Bond GJ, et al. A decade of experience with a single dose of rabbit antithymocyte globulin or alemtuzumab pretreatment for intestinal and multivisceral transplantation. Clin Transplant 2012:159, with permission.)

and fungal infections [1]. These management protocols, along with minimization of posttransplant immunosuppression, have significantly reduced risk and mortality of PTLD, CMV, and microbial infections [1,13,14,65,66].

De novo nonlymphoid malignancy also is a potential threat to visceral transplant recipients, particularly long-term survivors, because of the prolonged exposure to different environmental and nonenvironmental oncogenes with foreseeable acquired state of impaired immune surveillance [66]. Regular follow-up with universal and specific tumor surveillance protocols have been effective tools in the early diagnosis, with prompt intervention and satisfactory outcome [66].

With long-term follow-up, close monitoring of the cardiovascular system, glucose homeostasis, skeletal health, and renal functions, along with the standard tumor surveillance protocols, is strongly recommended. Successful interventions have been effective in ameliorating the unwanted impact of the developed long-term morbidities on the health status and QOL of these unique survivors [4].

GRAFT-VERSUS-HOST DISEASE

Despite the high anxiety that was apparent at the 1988 first international small bowel symposium, GVHD has been an unusual complication after visceral transplantation [5]. As part of a very intense 2-way immune interaction, the incidence of GVHD is reported to be less than 10% [1,43,68]. The disease occurs at a relatively higher rate in the composite visceral allograft recipients, particularly children and those who had splenectomy or were pretreated with antilymphocyte-depleting agents [1,43,68]. With detection of circulating or tissue-penetrating donor immunocytes as an essential requirement for the diagnosis of clinically suspected GVHD, our most recent studies documented total repopulation of the recipient immune system with donor-derived multilineage complete chimerism in a few unprecedented cases [1]. Such a potentially fatal phenomenon could be partially induced by a state of hereditary or acquired immune deficiency, including utilization of cytoablation therapy.

LONG-TERM OUTCOME

Survival

The cumulative worldwide clinical experience demonstrated steady improvement in 1-year and 5-year actuarial graft survival with current rates comparable to other solid organ transplantation (Fig. 15A) [32]. However, a time series analysis of conditional 5-year actuarial survival showed only slight improvement over time (see Fig. 15B). Beyond the 5-year milestone, the conditional survival of the largest single-center series showed a patient survival rate of 75% at 10 years and 61% at 15 years, with a graft survival of 59% and 50%, respectively (Fig. 16) [4]. Graft failure and complications of therapy including immunosuppression continued to threaten long-term patient survival with rejection, infection, and renal failure being the leading causes of death [4].

The long-term survival risk factors are summarized in Table 2. Nonfunctional social support and noninclusion of the liver were the most significant risk factors for long-term patient survival and graft failure after the 5-year

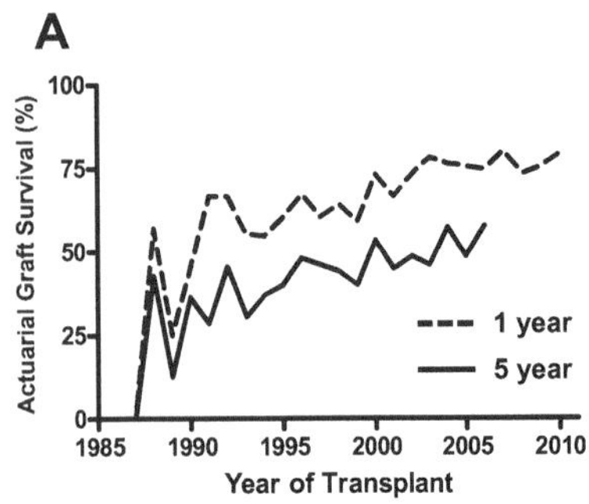

Fig. 15. (*A*) A time series analysis of 1- and 5-year actuarial graft survival showing significant improvement over time (*P*<.001). (*B*) A time series analysis of overall conditional 5-year actuarial graft survival showing only slight improvement over time. Conditional survival over time was similar between adults and children (data not shown). (*Adapted from* Grant D, Abu-Elmagd K, Mazariegos G, et al. Intestinal Transplant Registry Report: Global Activity and Trends. Am J Transplant 2015;15:210–9; with permission.)

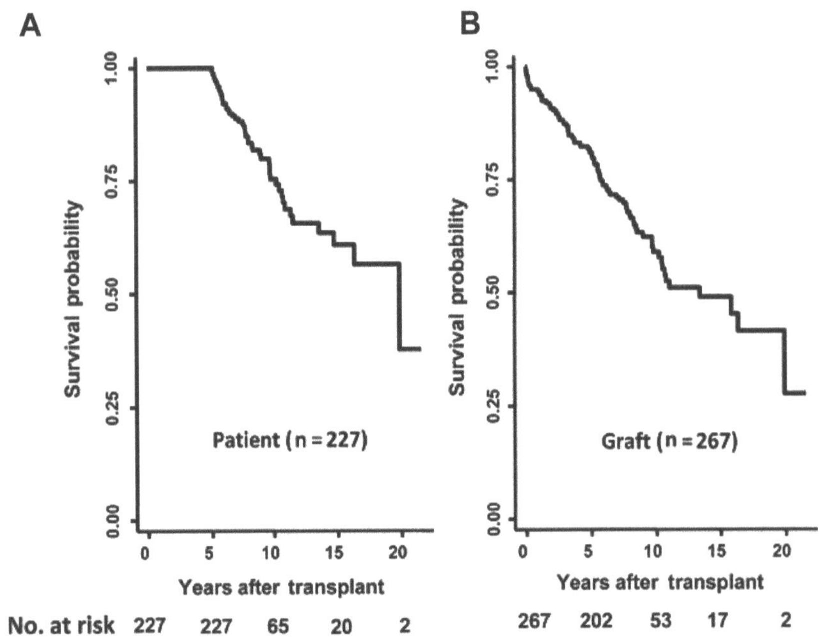

Fig. 16. Kaplan-Meier survival curves for conditional patient (*A*) and graft (*B*) survival after visceral transplantation. The analysis excluded patients who died before the 5-year posttransplant landmark. (*From* Abu-Elmagd KM, Kosmach-Park B, Costa G, et al. Long-term survival, nutritional autonomy, and quality of life after intestinal and multivisceral transplantation. Ann Surg 2012;256(3):494–508; with permission.)

Table 2
Long-term patients and allograft survival risk factors

Variable	*P* value	Hazard ratio	95% confidence interval
Patient			
Lack of social support	.000	6.132	3.370–11.160
Rejection ≤90 d	.016	2.363	1.172–4.765
Female recipient	.025	1.992	1.089–3.646
Recipient age ≥20 y	.025	2.014	1.093–3.711
Retransplantation	.026	2.053	1.089–3.873
No preconditioning	.046	2.013	1.013–4.997
Graft			
Liver-free allograft	.000	3.224	2.026–5.132
Splenectomy	.001	2.212	1.396–3.506
HLA mismatch	.040	1.258	1.011–1.565
Rejection ≤90 d	.046	1.601	1.008–2.541
PTLD	.085	1.638	0.934–2.872

Abbreviations: HLA, human leukocyte antigen; PTLD, posttransplant lymphoproliferative disease.
Modified from Abu-Elmagd KM, Kosmach-Park B, Costa G, et al. Long-term survival, nutritional autonomy, and quality of life after intestinal and multivisceral transplantation. Ann Surg 2012;256(3):494–508.

landmark, respectively (Fig. 17). Other significant predictors include early rejection, recipient sex and age, splenectomy, retransplantation, HLA mismatch, and type of immunosuppression.

Graft function

The ability to restore nutritional autonomy and other graft functions is the second most important metric to assess therapeutic efficacy [4]. The reported high rate of long-term freedom from intravenous nutrition, the improved body mass index (BMI) with higher serum albumin levels than that reported before transplantation, and relative stability of skeletal health, are testimony of sustained excellent allograft function (Fig. 18). Most children showed clinical evidence of normal growth with significant improvement in the pretransplant BMI in adults. The failure to achieve full recovery of gastrointestinal functions, particularly gut motility and fat absorption, is the result of denervation and lymphatic disruption of the intestinal allograft, respectively [69,70].

Quality of life

With the continual improvement in survival outcome, the health-related QOL (HRQOL) issues have become an important primary therapeutic index. The relatively young clinical age of the field with its multifaceted complexity has limited the validity of the currently available tools to assess HRQOL in this unique population. In addition, the utilization of the procedure as a rescue therapy has negatively biased most of the QOL measurements.

A few scattered publications addressed the HRQOL after visceral transplantation among both children and adults by using different study instruments (Table 3) [1,2,4,71–83]. With the use of the child health questionnaire, 2 well-designed studies demonstrated physical and psychosocial functions similar

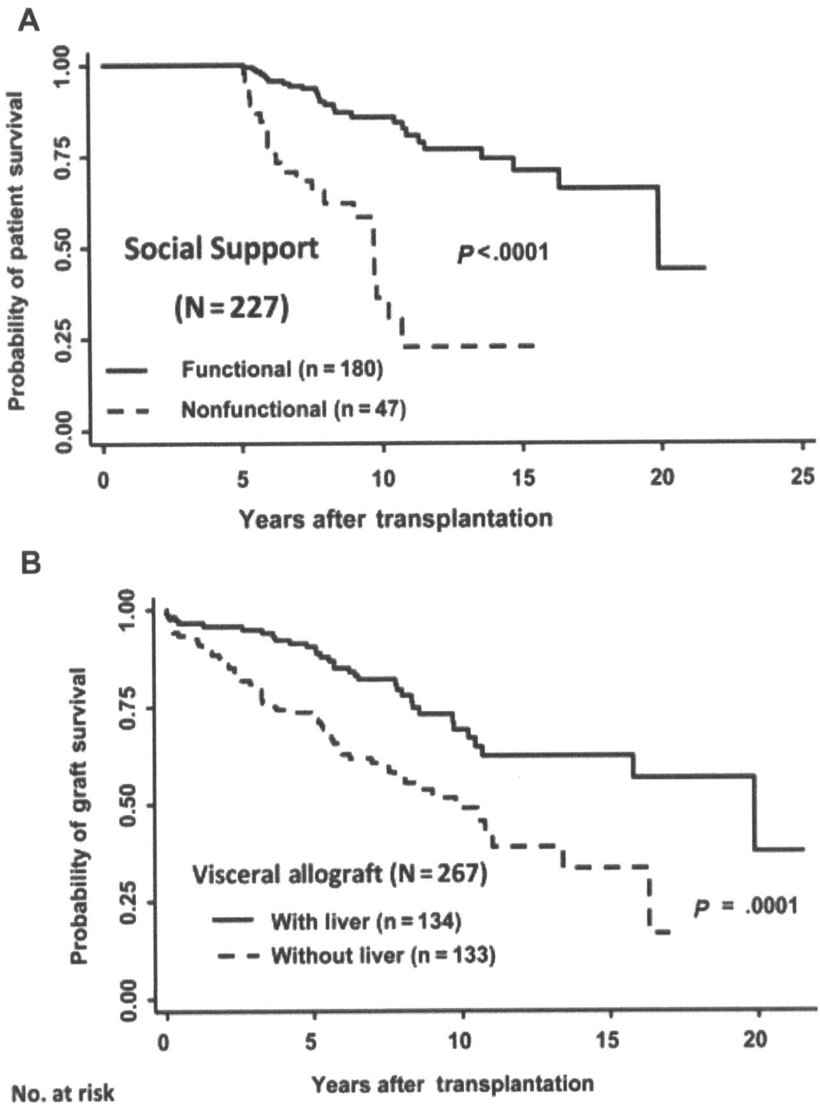

No. at risk					
With liver	134	114	35	15	2
Without liver	133	88	18	2	0

Fig. 17. Long-term conditional survival probability for patients according to social support status (*A*) and overall cumulative graft survival according to allograft type, with special reference to inclusion of the liver (*B*). Both variables were the most significant predictors of long-term patient and graft survival, respectively. (*From* Abu-Elmagd KM, Kosmach-Park B, Costa G, et al. Long-term survival, nutritional autonomy, and quality of life after intestinal and multivisceral transplantation. Ann Surg 2012;256(3):494–508; with permission.)

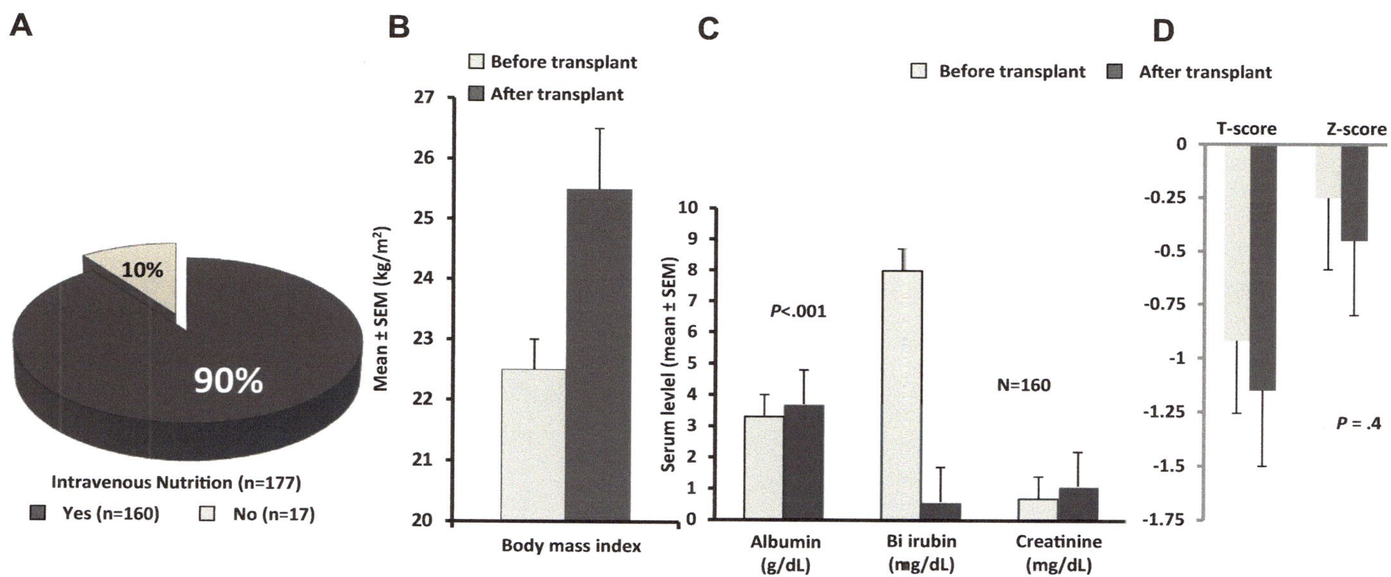

Fig. 18. Assessment of long-term graft function after visceral transplantation according to enteric autonomy defined by freedom from intravenous nutrition and fluid supplement (*A*), BMI (*B*), physiologic biochemical measures (*C*), and skeletal health (*D*). Skeletal health was measured by the dual-energy X-ray absorptiometry (DXA). (*Adapted from* Abu-Elmagd KM, Kosmach-Park B, Costa G, et al. Long-term survival, nutritional autonomy, and quality of life after intestinal and multivisceral transplantation. Ann Surg 2012;256(3):494–508; with permission.)

Table 3
Collected series of quality-of-life assessment in adult and pediatric visceral transplant recipients

				Study design				
				Transplant				
Primary author, year	Center	Age, y	Total no.	vs HPN	Only	Longitudinal follow-up	Follow-up, y	Study instrument
Stenn et al, [77] 1992	Ontario, Canada	>18	5	No	Yes	No	0.3–0.8	Clinical
DiMartini et al, [74] 1998	Pittsburgh, USA	≥18	19	Yes	No	Yes	0.2–4	QOLI
Rovera et al, [75] 1998	Pittsburgh, USA	≥18	20	Yes	No	Yes	0.25–6.5	QOLI
Rovera et al, [76] 1998	Pittsburgh, USA	≥18	9	No	Yes	Yes	0.2–4	QOLI
Sudan et al, [80] 2000	Nebraska, USA	± 18	31	No	Yes	No	>1	Clinical
Cameron et al, [78] 2002	Cambridge, UK	≥18	22	Yes	Yes	Yes	>0.5	NHP, SF-36
Grant et al, [2] 2003	ITR, Worldwide	≥18	406	No	Yes	No	>6	Karnofsky
Sudan et al, [71] 2004[a]	Nebraska, USA	5–18	29	No	Yes	No	>1	CHQ
Pironi et al, [79] 2006	Bologna, Italy	≥18	30	Yes	No	No	0.75	SF-36
O'Keefe et al, [82] 2007	Pittsburgh, USA	≥18	59	Yes	No	Yes	1–2	QOLI
Abu-Elmagd et al, [1] 2009	Pittsburgh, USA	≥18	151	No	Yes	No	>6	Clinical
Golfieri et al, [81] 2010	Bologna, Italy	≥18	24	No	Yes	No	>1	PWB, SQ, WHO
Ngo et al, [72] 2011[a]	UCLA, USA	2–18	24	No	Yes	No	0.5–11.8	CHQ, PedsQL4.0
Abu-Elmagd et al, [4] 2012	Pittsburgh, USA	2–50	227	Yes	Yes	No	5.1–21.6	QOLI
Pironi et al, [83] 2012	Bologna, Italy	18–60	55	Yes	No	No	NA	HPN-QOL

Abbreviations: CHQ, Child Health Questionnaire; HPN, home parenteral nutrition; ITR, Intestinal Transplant Registry; NA, not available; NHP, Nottingham Health Profile; PedsQL4.0, Pediatric Quality of Life; PWB, Psychological Well-Being Scale; QOLI, Quality of Life Inventory; SF-36, Short Form 36; SQ, Symptom Questionnaire; UCLA, University of California Los Angeles; WHO, World Health Organization Quality of Liver-Brief.

[a]Parents were assessed.

Modified from Abu-Elmagd KM, Kosmach-Park B, Costa G, et al. Long-term survival, nutritional autonomy, and quality of life after intestinal and multivisceral transplantation. Ann Surg 2012;256(3):494–508.

to healthy children [71,72]. However, the parental proxy assessments were different from the recipients, with lower response in multiple categories, including physical health and social functioning. In addition, Ngo and colleagues [72] recently revealed lower values among the school-functioning subcategories and psychological health summary score using the Pediatric Quality of Life Inventory instrument.

The HRQOL was addressed in 5 series of adult recipients that were published in peer-reviewed journals with dedicated study design [4,74,75,82,83]. All of these studies demonstrated improvement in many of the QOL domains, with a better overall rehabilitative index than HPN, including the use of treatment-specific questionnaires [83]. With the exception of depression and increased financial demands, successful transplantation offsets the deprived effect of HPN on most of the QOL domains and resolves the chronicity of the primary disease [4,82].

The multidimensional QOL aspects in both adults and children have been recently addressed in a very comprehensive single report reflecting the largest single-center experience with more than 2 decades of follow-up [4]. The study identified, for the first time, a spectrum of different developmental, neurologic, and behavioral disorders among visceral allograft recipients, particularly children, including autism, developmental delay, attention-deficit/hyperactivity disorders, and deafness, at a relatively higher rate than the general population [4]. The investigators attributed these observations to organic brain dysfunctions that occurred due to intestinal failure during the early phases of neuronal, emotional, and physical development. The disease process is also compounded by the pretransplant HPN-associated complications and morbidities that may occur after transplantation. Of the documented pathologic changes are brain atrophy, cerebral vascular insufficiency due to multiple septic emboli, micronutrient deficiencies, trace element toxicities, and liver failure–induced metabolic encephalopathy [84–90]. Accordingly, early consideration for gut rehabilitation, including transplantation, is recommended with the aim to reduce the risk of such devastating irreversible deficits, particularly among the pediatric population.

The long-term rehabilitative efficacy of visceral transplantation was recently accessed by using the socioeconomic milestones [4]. A high education index was reported among all respective age groups with sustained cognitive, psychosocial, and physical functions after all types of visceral transplantation. In addition, the ability to create a nuclear family, having children, and becoming a productive citizen is another valid indicator of a high rehabilitative index after visceral transplantation. Equally important are the high scores of the Lansky and Karnofsky performance scales with normal functional activities in most survivors.

Controversies

Controversies concerning nomenclature and the immunoprotective effect of simultaneously transplanted liver have been assuaged based on historic and recently published data [1,23]. Of the current disputes are the need for gastric replacement in patients with hollow visceral myopathy/neuropathy, medical necessities for full multivisceral transplantation, particularly in patients with diffuse portomesenteric thrombosis, and inclusion of the donor spleen with the multivisceral graft [1,15,50,51]. We believe that simultaneous replacement of the stomach for pseudo-obstruction should be dictated by the severity of gastric involvement [1,91]. We also believe that the premise of splenic allograft inclusion should be carefully reexamined before any further recommendation [1,50,51]. Similarly, the indications for multivisceral transplantation should be better defined to avoid the liberal use of the procedure, particularly for patients with portomesenteric venous thrombosis [1,34,35,92].

Challenges with new insights

With the continual improvement in overall survival, the field of visceral transplantation faces new multifaceted challenges, particularly with postoperative care and sustained long-term outcome. With new insights, the procedure has the potential to be the standard of care for all patients with intestinal failure and complex abdominal pathology.

With endoscopic biopsies being the gold standard for the diagnosis of acute rejection, prediction and early diagnosis continue to be a major challenge in the absence of a reliable serum marker. With the intestine being an unforgivable organ, the discovery of a highly sensitive and specific marker will be a breakthrough in the field. Recently, serum citrulline and fecal calprotectin have been advocated as candidate noninvasive markers [93,94]. Furthermore, the metabolomics of human intestinal transplant rejection have been recently described [95]. Proinflammatory mediator leukotriene E4; vitamins B2, B5, and B6; and taurocholate were identified as reliable markers. In addition, promising novel measures using gene expression profiles and T-cell alloresponses were also identified as viable molecular indicators [96]. These new tools require further studies with a larger population to validate their applicability and reliability in clinical transplantation.

Destructive alloimmunity and complications of long-term immunosuppression continued to be the major threats to visceral allograft longevity [1,2,4]. It is tempting to believe that the visceral allograft high immunogenicity with instability and partial intolerability are the result of a constant dynamic interaction between adaptive and innate immunity [3,97]. In parallel, our most recent published study suggested a strong association between circulating donor-specific anti-HLA antibodies and graft loss due to rejection, particularly chronic arteriopathy (Fig. 19) [42].

Noninclusion of the liver continues to be one of the most significant predictors of late graft loss due to rejection, as shown in Fig. 17 [1,4,13,14]. Hepatic inclusion was associated with better clearance of preformed HLA donor-specific antibodies (DSAs) and lower induction of de novo DSAs [42].

With the continual increase in utilization of liver-free visceral allografts, innovative multifaceted anti-DSA strategies are required to further improve long-term survival. Efforts should be initiated to modify current UNOS regulations

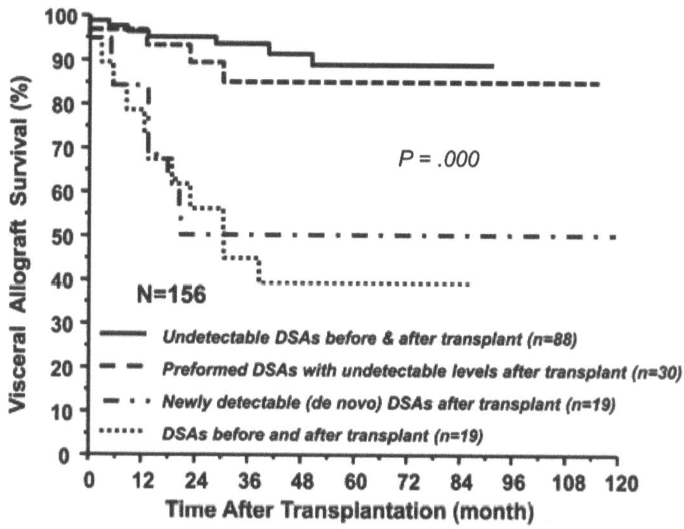

Fig. 19. Cumulative visceral allograft survival according to the status of DSA. De novo and persistent DSA were associated with a significantly lower 5-year survival. (*From* Abu-Elmagd KM, Wu G, Costa G, et al. Preformed and de novo donor-specific antibodies in visceral transplantation: long-term outcome with special reference to the liver. Am J Transplant 2012;12(11):3047–60; with permission.)

to allow national sharing of deceased donor intestine according to favorable HLA and virtual cross-match results. Meanwhile, induction protocols with anti–B-cell proteasome inhibitor "bortezomib" have been recently introduced with initial encouraging results [98]. Other potential approaches include costimulation blockade with belatacept and anticomplement treatment with anti-C5 antibody or a C1-inhibitor [42,99]. Additional innovative therapeutic modalities may emerge from new insights into gut immunity, B-cell homeostasis, and platelet immunologic functions. Another alternative approach is simultaneous replacement of the native liver in a domino transplant procedure, particularly for recipients with recurrent chronic rejection after liver-free visceral retransplantation [1].

It remains to be seen if regulation of innate immunity helps amelioration of chronic allograft injury [42,65]. Mutations of the nucleotide-binding oligomerization domain-containing 2 (NOD2) gene that are associated with Crohn disease have been recently studied and were found to increase the risk of immunologic graft loss [100]. Of the postulated mechanisms is impaired expression of epithelial-derived antimicrobial peptides, which causes disruption of epithelial barrier and subsequent inflammatory cell infiltration into the graft intestinal wall.

The early life-threatening posttransplant morbidities and resultant mortalities are a testimony to the complex postoperative care of these recipients [1]. Despite the potential of disease recurrence and long-term maintenance immunosuppression-related morbidities, the health status of most long-term survivors is sustained with successful interventions to treat hypertension, diabetes, osteoporosis, renal failure, and other associated morbid events. Accordingly, it is imperative to acknowledge the potential negative impact of these morbidities on the complexity of patient care to maintain the overall global health. Therefore, risk adjustment should be considered when quality of care and reimbursement are reviewed by the different stakeholders of health care in comparison with other solid organ transplantation.

SUMMARY

Early seeking for multidisciplinary comprehensive medical and surgical rehabilitative measures including transplantation should always be considered for all HPN-dependent patients. Gut rehabilitation with early restoration of nutritional autonomy has been shown to be associated with better survival and QOL outcomes.

With transplantation and despite the observed improvement in overall survival, further enhancement in long-term outcomes is still needed, particularly of the liver-free allografts. With destructive alloimmunity being the main sinister impediment, innovative tolerogenic strategies are required to enhance allograft longevity particularly in patients who harbor preformed or develop de novo DSA. In addition to further innovations in immunosuppressive and immunomodulatory strategies, other tactics are required, including achievement of better HLA match through modification of the current UNOS allocation policy and simultaneous domino liver transplantation, particularly in patients with failed liver-free visceral allograft due to destructive alloimmunity.

With the status of social support being the most significant predictor of long-term survival, candidacy for visceral transplantation should be carefully assessed and efforts should be directed toward the establishment of multidisciplinary care with skilled psychosocial professionals to reduce the risk and improve social reintegration, particularly in patients with low socioeconomic status and pediatric recipients during transition into adolescence and adulthood.

The current results clearly justify elevating the level of intestinal and multivisceral transplantation to that of other abdominal organs with the privilege to permanently reside in a respected place in the surgical armamentarium.

References

[1] Abu-Elmagd KM, Costa G, Bond GJ, et al. Five hundred intestinal and multivisceral transplantations at a single center: major advances with new challenges. Ann Surg 2009;250(4):567–81.

[2] Grant D, Abu-Elmagd K, Reyes J, et al. 2003 report of the intestine transplant registry: a new era has dawned. Ann Surg 2005;241(4):607–13.

[3] Abu-Elmagd KM, Costa G, Bond GJ, et al. Evolution of the immunosuppressive strategies for the intestinal and multivisceral recipients with special reference to allograft immunity and achievement of partial tolerance. Transpl Int 2009;22(1):96–109.

[4] Abu-Elmagd KM, Kosmach-Park B, Costa G, et al. Long-term survival, nutritional autonomy, and quality of life after intestinal and multivisceral transplantation. Ann Surg 2012;256(3): 494–508.
[5] Abu-Elmagd KM. The history of intestinal transplantation. In: Hakim NS, Papalois VE, editors. History of organ and cell transplantation. London: Imperial College Press; 2003. p. 171–93.
[6] Starzl TE, Todo S, Fung J, et al. FK 506 for human liver, kidney, and pancreas transplantation. Lancet 1989;2(8670):1000–4.
[7] Grant D, Wall W, Mimeault R, et al. Successful small-bowel/liver transplantation. Lancet 1990;335(8683):181–4.
[8] Todo S, Tzakis AG, Abu-Elmagd K, et al. Intestinal transplantation in composite visceral grafts or alone. Ann Surg 1992;216(3):223–34.
[9] Grant D. International intestinal transplant registry: current results of intestinal transplantation. Lancet 1996;347(9018):1801–3.
[10] Abu-Elmagd K, Todo S, Tzakis A, et al. Three years clinical experience with intestinal transplantation. J Am Coll Surg 1994;179(4):385–400.
[11] Todo S, Reyes J, Furukawa H, et al. Outcome analysis of 71 clinical intestinal transplantations. Ann Surg 1995;222(3):270–80.
[12] Grant D. Intestinal transplantation: 1997 report of the international registry: intestinal transplant registry. Transplantation 1999;67(7):1061–4.
[13] Abu-Elmagd K, Reyes J, Todo S, et al. Clinical intestinal transplantation: new perspectives and immunologic considerations. J Am Coll Surg 1998;186(5):512–25.
[14] Abu-Elmagd K, Reyes J, Bond G, et al. Clinical intestinal transplantation: a decade of experience at a single center. Ann Surg 2001;234(3):404–16.
[15] Abu-Elmagd K, Bond G, Reyes J, et al. Intestinal transplantation: a coming of age. Adv Surg 2002;36:65–101.
[16] Cruz RJ Jr, Costa G, Bond G, et al. Modified "liver-sparing" multivisceral transplant with preserved native spleen, pancreas, and duodenum: technique and long-term outcome. J Gastrointest Surg 2010;14(11):1709–21.
[17] Cruz RJ Jr, Costa G, Bond GJ, et al. Modified multivisceral transplantation with spleen-preserving pancreaticoduodenectomy for patients with familial adenomatous polyposis "Gardner's Syndrome". Transplantation 2011;91(12):1417–23.
[18] Abu-Elmagd K, Fung J, Bueno J, et al. Logistics and technique for procurement of intestinal, pancreatic, and hepatic grafts from the same donor. Ann Surg 2000;232(5):680–7.
[19] Matsumoto C, Fishbein TM. Modified multivisceral transplantation with splenopancreatic preservation. Transplantation 2007;83(2):234–6.
[20] Abu-Elmagd KM. Preservation of the native spleen, duodenum, and pancreas in patients with multivisceral transplantation: nomenclature, dispute of origin, and proof of premise. Transplantation 2007;84(9):1208–9.
[21] Hernandez F, Andres AM, Encinas JL, et al. Preservation of the native spleen in multivisceral transplantation. Pediatr Transplant 2013;17(6):556–60.
[22] Mazariegos GV, Steffick DE, Horslen S, et al. Intestine transplantation in the United States, 1999-2008. Am J Transplant 2010;10(4):1020–34.
[23] Abu-Elmagd KM. The small bowel contained allografts: existing and proposed nomenclature. Am J Transplant 2011;11(1):184–5.
[24] Abu-Elmagd KM. Intestinal transplantation: indications and patient selection. In: Langnas AN, Goulet O, Quigley EM, et al, editors. Intestinal failure: diagnosis, management and transplantation. Oxford, UK: Wiley-Blackwell; 2008. p. 245–53.
[25] Abu-Elmagd KM, Bond G, Matarese L, et al. Gut rehabilitation and intestinal transplantation. Therapy 2005;2(6):853–64.
[26] Byrne TA, Wilmore DW, Iyer K, et al. Growth hormone, glutamine, and an optimal diet reduces parenteral nutrition in patients with short bowel syndrome: a prospective, randomized, placebo-controlled, double-blind clinical trial. Ann Surg 2005;242(5):655–61.

[27] Vipperla K, O'Keefe SJ. Study of teduglutide effectiveness in parenteral nutrition-dependent short-bowel syndrome subjects. Expert Rev Gastroenterol Hepatol 2013;7(8):683–7.
[28] Jeppesen PB. New approaches to the treatments of short bowel syndrome-associated intestinal failure. Curr Opin Gastroenterol 2014;30(2):182–8.
[29] Sudan D, Thompson J, Botha J, et al. Comparison of intestinal lengthening procedures for patients with short bowel syndrome. Ann Surg 2007;246(4):593–601.
[30] Kato T, Lobritto SJ, Tzakis A, et al. Multivisceral ex vivo surgery for tumors involving celiac and superior mesenteric arteries. Am J Transplant 2012;12(5):1323–8.
[31] Tzakis AG, Pararas NB, Tekin A, et al. Intestinal and multivisceral autotransplantation for tumors of the root of the mesentery: long-term follow-up. Surgery 2012;152(1):82–9.
[32] Grant D, Abu-Elmagd K, Mazariegos G, et al. Intestinal Transplant Registry Report: Global Activity and Trends. AJT 2015;15:201–19.
[33] Lawrence JP, Dunn SP, Billmire DF, et al. Isolated liver transplantation for liver failure in patients with short bowel syndrome. J Pediatr Surg 1994;29(6):751–3.
[34] Vianna RM, Mangus RS, Kubal C, et al. Multivisceral transplantation for diffuse portomesenteric thrombosis. Ann Surg 2012;255(6):1144–50.
[35] Costa G, Cruz R, Abu-Elmagd KM, et al. Surgical shunt versus TIPS for treatment of variceal hemorrhage in the current era of liver and multivisceral transplantation. In: Geller D, editor. Surgical Clinics of North America. Philadelphia: Elesevier Saunders; 2010. p. 891–905.
[36] Abu-Elmagd KM. Intestinal transplantation for short bowel syndrome and gastrointestinal failure: current consensus, rewarding outcomes, and practical guidelines. Gastroenterology 2006;130(2):S132–7.
[37] Quintini C, Ward G, Shatnawei A, et al. Mortality of intra-abdominal desmoid tumors in patients with familial adenomatous polyposis: a single center review of 154 patients. Ann Surg 2012;255(3):511–6.
[38] Abu-Elmagd K. Intestinal and multivisceral transplant waiting list: Clinical management according to allograft type and current organ allocation system. In: Kirk A, Knechtle S, Larsen C, editors. Textbook of organ transplantation. 1st edition. Oxford, UK: Wiley-Blackwell; 2014.
[39] Abu-Elmagd KM, Reyes J, Fung JJ, et al. Evolution of clinical intestinal transplantation: improved outcome and cost effectiveness. Transplant Proc 1999;31(1–2):582–4.
[40] Mazariegos GV, Soltys K, Bond G, et al. Pediatric intestinal retransplantation: techniques, management, and outcomes. Transplantation 2008;86(12):1777–82.
[41] Desai CS, Khan KM, Gruessner AC, et al. Intestinal retransplantation: analysis of organ procurement and transplantation network database. Transplantation 2012;93(1):120–5.
[42] Abu-Elmagd KM, Wu G, Costa G, et al. Preformed and de novo donor specific antibodies in visceral transplantation: long-term outcome with special reference to the liver. Am J Transplant 2012;12(11):3047–60.
[43] Mazariegos GV, Abu-Elmagd K, Jaffe R, et al. Graft versus host disease in intestinal transplantation. Am J Transplant 2004;4(9):1459–65.
[44] Reyes J, Todo S, Green M, et al. Graft-versus-host disease after liver and small bowel transplantation in a child. Clin Transplant 1997;11(5):345–8.
[45] Gilroy RK, Coccia PF, Talmadge JE, et al. Donor immune reconstitution after liver-small bowel transplantation for multiple intestinal atresia with immunodeficiency. Blood 2004;103(3):1171–4.
[46] Rizzi M, Neumann C, Fielding AK, et al. Outcome of allogeneic stem cell transplantation in adults with common variable immunodeficiency. J Allergy Clin Immunol 2011;128(6):1371–4.
[47] Venick RS, Calkins K. The impact of intravenous fish oil emulsions on pediatric intestinal failure-associated liver disease. Curr Opin Organ Transplant 2011;16(3):306–11.

[48] Todo S, Tzakis A, Reyes J, et al. Small intestinal transplantation in humans with or without the colon. Transplantation 1994;57(6):840–8.
[49] Kato T, Selvaggi G, Gaynor JJ, et al. Inclusion of donor colon and ileocecal valve in intestinal transplantation. Transplantation 2008;86(2):293–7.
[50] Tzakis AG, Kato T, Levi DM, et al. 100 multivisceral transplants at a single center. Ann Surg 2005;242(4):480–90.
[51] Kato T, Tzakis AG, Selvaggi G, et al. Transplantation of the spleen: effect of splenic allograft in human multivisceral transplantation. Ann Surg 2007;246(3):436–44.
[52] Amesur NB, Zajko AB, Costa G, et al. Combined surgical and interventional radiologic management strategies in patients with arterial pseudo-aneurysms after multivisceral transplantation. Transplantation 2014;97(2):235–44.
[53] Eid KR, Costa G, Bond GJ, et al. An innovative sphincter preserving pull-through technique with en bloc colon and small bowel transplantation. Am J Transplant 2010;10(8):1940–6.
[54] Carlsen BT, Farmer DG, Busuttil RW, et al. Incidence and management of abdominal wall defects after intestinal and multivisceral transplantation. Plast Reconstr Surg 2007;119(4):1247–55.
[55] Mangus RS, Kubal CA, Tector AJ, et al. Closure of the abdominal wall with acellular dermal allograft in intestinal transplantation. Am J Transplant 2012;12:S55–9.
[56] Watson MJ, Kundu N, Coppa C, et al. Role of tissue expanders in patients with loss of abdominal domain awaiting intestinal transplantation. Transpl Int 2013;26(12):1184–90.
[57] Gondolesi G, Selvaggi G, Tzakis A, et al. Use of the abdominal rectus fascia as a nonvascularized allograft for abdominal wall closure after liver, intestinal, and multivisceral transplantation. Transplantation 2009;87(12):1884–8.
[58] Levi DM, Tzakis AG, Kato T, et al. Transplantation of the abdominal wall. Lancet 2003;361(9376):2173–6.
[59] Fishbein TM, Kaufman SS, Florman SS, et al. Isolated intestinal transplantation: proof of clinical efficacy. Transplantation 2003;76(4):636–40.
[60] Farmer DG, McDiarmid SV, Yersiz H, et al. Outcomes after intestinal transplantation: a single-center experience over a decade. Transplant Proc 2002;34(3):896–7.
[61] Abu-Elmagd K, Fung J, McGhee W, et al. The efficacy of daclizumab for intestinal transplantation: preliminary report. Transplant Proc 2000;32(6):1195–6.
[62] Tzakis AG, Kato T, Nishida S, et al. Preliminary experience with campath 1H (C1H) in intestinal and liver transplantation. Transplantation 2003;75(8):1227–31.
[63] Starzl TE, Zinkernagel RM. Transplantation tolerance from a historical perspective. Nat Rev Immunol 2001;1(3):233–9.
[64] Starzl TE, Murase N, Abu-Elmagd K, et al. Tolerogenic immunosuppression for organ transplantation. Lancet 2003;361(9368):1502–10.
[65] Abu-Elmagd KM, Costa G, Bond GJ, et al. A decade of experience with a single dose of rabbit antithymocyte globulin or alemtuzumab pretreatment for intestinal and multivisceral transplantation. Clin Transplant 2012;155–66.
[66] Abu-Elmagd KM, Mazariegos G, Costa G, et al. Lymphoproliferative disorders and de novo malignancies in intestinal and multivisceral recipients: improved outcomes with new outlooks. Transplantation 2009;88(7):926–34.
[67] Bradley JA. Transplant tolerance by Treg therapy. Am J Transplant 2014;14(1):5–6.
[68] Wu G, Selvaggi G, Nishida S, et al. Graft-versus-host disease after intestinal and multivisceral transplantation. Transplantation 2011;91(2):219–24.
[69] Abu-Elmagd K, Reyes J, Fung J. Transplantation of the human intestine: the forbidden organ. Curr Opin Organ Transplant 1998;3(4):286–92.
[70] Rovera GM, Schoen RE, Goldbach B, et al. Intestinal and multivisceral transplantation: dynamics of nutritional management and functional autonomy. JPEN J Parenter Enteral Nutr 2003;27(4):252–9.

[71] Sudan D, Iyer K, Horslen S, et al. Assessment of quality of life after pediatric intestinal transplantation by parents and pediatric recipients using the child health questionnaire. Transplant Proc 2002;34(3):963–4.
[72] Ngo KD, Farmer DG, McDiarmid SV, et al. Pediatric health-related quality of life after intestinal transplantation. Pediatr Transplant 2011;15(8):849–54.
[73] Matarese LE, Costa G, Bond G, et al. Therapeutic efficacy of intestinal and multivisceral transplantation: survival and nutrition outcome. Nutr Clin Pract 2007;22(5):474–81.
[74] DiMartini A, Rovera GM, Graham TO, et al. Quality of life after small intestinal transplantation and among home parenteral nutrition patients. JPEN J Parenter Enteral Nutr 1998;22(6):357–62.
[75] Rovera GM, DiMartini A, Schoen RE, et al. Quality of life of patients after intestinal transplantation. Transplantation 1998;66(9):1141–5.
[76] Rovera GM, DiMartini A, Graham TO, et al. Quality of life after intestinal transplantation and on total parenteral nutrition. Transplant Proc 1998;30(6):2513–4.
[77] Stenn PG, Lammens P, Houle L, et al. Psychiatric psychosocial and ethical aspects of small bowel transplantation. Transplant Proc 1992;24(3):1251–2.
[78] Cameron EA, Binnie JA, Jamieson NV, et al. Quality of life in adults following small bowel transplantation. Transplant Proc 2002;34(3):965–6.
[79] Pironi L, Paganelli F, Lauro A, et al. Quality of life on home parenteral nutrition or after intestinal transplantation. Transplant Proc 2006;38(6):1673–5.
[80] Sudan DL, Iverson A, Weseman RA, et al. Assessment of function, growth and development, and long-term quality of life after small bowel transplantation. Transplant Proc 2000;32(6):1211–2.
[81] Golfieri L, Lauro A, Tossani E, et al. Psychological adaptation and quality of life of adult intestinal transplant recipients: University of Bologna experience. Transplant Proc 2010;42(1):42–4.
[82] O'Keefe SJ, Emerling M, Koritsky D, et al. Nutrition and quality of life following small intestinal transplantation. Am J Gastroenterol 2007;102(5):1093–100.
[83] Pironi L, Baxter JP, Lauro A, et al. Assessment of quality of life on home parenteral nutrition and after intestinal transplantation using treatment-specific questionnaires. Am J Transplant 2012;12:S60–6.
[84] Idoate MA, Martinez AJ, Bueno J, et al. The neuropathology of intestinal failure and small bowel transplantation. Acta Neuropathol 1999;97(5):502–8.
[85] Dekaban AS. Changes in brain weights during the span of human life: relation of brain weights to body heights and body weights. Ann Neurol 1978;4(4):345–56.
[86] El-Tatawy S, Badrawi N, El Bishlawy A. Cerebral atrophy in infants with protein energy malnutrition. AJNR Am J Neuroradiol 1983;4(3):434–6.
[87] Kawakubo K, Iida M, Matsumoto T, et al. Progressive encephalopathy in a Crohn's disease patient on long-term total parenteral nutrition: possible relationship to selenium deficiency. Postgrad Med J 1994;70(821):215–9.
[88] Martínez AJ. The neuropathology of organ transplantation: comparison and contrast in 500 patients. Pathol Res Pract 1998;194(7):473–86.
[89] Small SL, Fukui MB, Bramblett GT, et al. Immunosuppression-induced leukoencephalopathy from tacrolimus. Ann Neurol 1996;40(4):575–80.
[90] Kulick D, Deen D. Specialized nutrition support. Am Fam Physician 2011;83(2):173–83.
[91] Lauro A, Zanfi C, Pellegrini S, et al. Isolated intestinal transplant for chronic intestinal pseudo-obstruction in adults: long-term outcome. Transplant Proc 2013;45(9):3351–5.
[92] Selvaggi G, Weppler D, Nishida S, et al. Ten-year experience in porto-caval hemitransposition for liver transplantation in the presence of portal vein thrombosis. Am J Transplant 2007;7(2):454–60.

[93] Hibi T, Nishida S, Garcia J, et al. Citrulline level is a potent indicator of acute rejection in the long term following pediatric intestinal/multivisceral transplantation. Am J Transplant 2012;12:S27–32.
[94] Sudan D, Vargas L, Sun Y, et al. Calprotectin: a novel noninvasive marker for intestinal allograft monitoring. Ann Surg 2007;246(2):311–5.
[95] Girlanda R, Cheema AK, Kaur P, et al. Metabolomics of human intestinal transplant rejection. Am J Transplant 2012;12:S18–26.
[96] Sindhi R, Ashokkumar C, Higgs BW, et al. Allospecific CD154+ T-cytotoxic memory cells as potential surrogate for rejection risk in pediatric intestine transplantation. Pediatr Transplant 2012;16(1):83–91.
[97] Fishbein TM. Intestinal transplantation. N Engl J Med 2009;361(10):998–1008.
[98] Abu-Elmagd K. The concept of gut rehabilitation and the future of visceral transplantation. Nat Rev Gastroenterol Hepatol 2015;12:108–20.
[99] Stegall MD, Diwan T, Raghavaiah S, et al. Terminal complement inhibition decreases antibody-mediated rejection in sensitized renal transplant recipients. Am J Transplant 2011;11(11):2405–13.
[100] Fishbein T, Novitskiy G, Mishra L, et al. NOD2-expressing bone marrow-derived cells appear to regulate epithelial innate immunity of the transplanted human small intestine. Gut 2008;57(3):323–30.

Advances in Surgery 49 (2015) 65–77
ADVANCES IN SURGERY

Which Is Best for Abdominal Aortic Aneurysms Treatment with Chronic Renal Insufficiency

Endovascular Aneurysm Repair or Open Repair?

Bao-Ngoc Nguyen, MD*, Anton N. Sidawy, MD, MPH

Department of Surgery, George Washington University, 2150 Pennsylvania Avenue, Washington, DC 20037, USA

Keywords

• Endovascular repair • Open repair • Abdominal aortic aneurysm
• Chronic renal insufficiency • Intra-vascular ultrasound • CO_2 arteriogram
• Duplex ultrasound

Key points

- Endovascular aneurysm repair (EVAR) should be the first-line therapy for abdominal aortic aneurysm (AAA) in patients with moderate renal dysfunction (30 mL/min < estimated glomerular filtration rate [eGFR] <60 mL/min) because of better outcomes compared with open repair.
- Elective repair of AAA in patients with severe renal dysfunction (eGFR <30 mL/min) should be avoided because of significant risk of postoperative renal failure/dialysis with either EVAR or open repair.
- Intravascular ultrasound (IVUS) and CO_2 arteriograms should be used for the initial EVAR procedure to minimize contrast nephrotoxicity.
- Follow-up protocols after EVAR should include color duplex ultrasound and abdominal radiograph to prevent further decline of renal function due to multiple CT angiograms (CTAs).

INTRODUCTION

Endovascular aneurysm repair (EVAR) has become the first-line treatment of infrarenal AAAs in patients with appropriate anatomy because of superior early outcomes and equivalent long-term results compared with standard

The authors have nothing to disclose.

*Corresponding author. 2150 Pennsylvania Avenue #6B-411, Washington, DC 20037.
E-mail address: bnnguyen@mfa.gwu.edu

0065-3411/15/$ – see front matter
http://dx.doi.org/10.1016/j.yasu.2015.03.014

open repair [1]. Nevertheless, despite its minimally invasive nature, EVAR is not an entirely benign procedure. The use of intra-arterial contrast during and after the procedure to monitor for endoleaks is a potential source of nephropathy, which could cause up to 10% decrease in creatinine clearance after the first year [2]. Likewise, up to 20% of patients with open AAA repair (OPEN) had decreased renal function postoperatively [3]. These statistics referred to all patients with AAAs; for patients with impaired renal function at baseline, any further decline in renal function could be catastrophic because that could push them toward dialysis. More importantly, chronic renal insufficiency (CRI) has been identified as an independent predictor of early and late mortalities in both OPEN and EVAR [3–7].

This high-risk patient population presents a real dilemma for the vascular surgeons regarding which approach should be used to treat patients with infrarenal aneurysms who have suitable anatomy for both endovascular and open repair. EVAR is less invasive but requires the use of contrast during implantation, whereas OPEN is known to have higher operative mortality than EVAR. In addition, the hemodynamic shifts associated with OPEN are not favorable to a fragile renal function either. This article reviews the current data in the literature regarding these 2 treatment modalities for this challenging patient population.

THE MECHANISMS OF POSTOPERATIVE DECLINE IN RENAL FUNCTION AFTER ABDOMINAL AORTIC ANEURYSM REPAIR

Acute renal failure could complicate the outcomes of up to 12% of patients undergoing OPEN, resulting in a significant increase in hospital mortality (25%–66%) [8–10]. Even in the cases of infrarenal clamping, renal perfusion could be altered due to any technical difficulty, such as dissection or atheroemboli to the renal arteries due to the proximity of clamping site to the aortic origin of these arteries. In addition, the ischemia/reperfusion effect of the lower extremities and the overall hemodynamic shift during the operation could lead to postoperative renal dysfunction. Nevertheless, most renal function impairment after OPEN occurs in the immediate postoperative and slowly recovers with time.

On the other hand, although EVAR spares patients the perioperative hemodynamic shift, the continuing exposure to contrast during the procedure from angiogram used to deliver the endovascular device and after the procedure from multiple follow-up CT scans could be detrimental to both short-term and long-term renal function. Atheroemboli from manipulation of the catheters/wires in shaggy aortas and stent graft migration are other causes of impaired renal perfusion after EVAR. Regardless of the type of stent grafts used, there is an average 10% decrease in creatinine clearance after the first year of EVAR [2,11,12]; but does contrast nephropathy during the initial procedure play a major role or is the cumulative effect of multiple follow-up CT angiograms the real culprit?

Contrast-induced nephropathy typically causes a peak of serum creatinine approximately 2 to 3 days after the procedure and frequently recovers afterward. Although theoretically, the risk of contrast nephropathy is higher in patients with chronic renal dysfunction, it turns out that as much as 90 mL of contrast could be used for EVAR in patients with CRI without an increase in serum creatinine [13]. Even when there was an increase in serum creatinine, it was only a transient phenomenon which occurs approximately on the second or third post-operative day and quickly returned to baseline at postoperative day 4 [14]. Therefore, elevated creatinine is not an absolute contraindication to the use of contrast for the initial EVAR procedure. This emphasizes the importance of minimizing subsequent contrast exposure during follow-up.

Another risk factor of long-term renal dysfunction in EVAR is the issue of whether bare-metal suprarenal fixation of the endografts could cause emboli and stenosis of the renal arteries and impede perfusion. Unfortunately, the definitive answer to this question is still elusive. There are as many studies in the literature that showed no difference between infrarenal and suprarenal fixation of stent grafts [2,11,12] as there are those that insisted suprarenal fixation increased the risk of renal dysfunction [15,16].

THE COMPARISON BETWEEN OPEN REPAIR AND ENDOVASCULAR ANEURYSM REPAIR IN PATIENTS WITH CHRONIC RENAL INSUFFICIENCY

The incidence of worsening renal function in AAA repair for patients with normal preoperative renal function is 5.4% [17]. For this patient population, there was no significant difference in change of renal function between EVAR and OPEN either in the immediate postoperative period, at 30 days, or at 1 year after the procedure [18–20]. The risk of postoperative renal dysfunction increases 2- to 3-fold in patients with preexisting CRI [17]. Although there are many studies reporting postoperative outcomes of OPEN and EVAR for infrarenal aortic aneurysms in patients with chronic renal dysfunction, there are only a few studies specifically comparing these 2 approaches. The first study was an analysis of a single-institution experience, wherein 100 patients with chronic renal dysfunction underwent AAA repair–half of the cohort received OPEN and the other half underwent EVAR [21]. The investigators defined CRI as serum creatinine greater than 1.5. There was no difference in the magnitude of change in serum creatinine or creatinine clearance between OPEN and EVAR at postoperative period or during follow-up [21].

The second study came from the University of Arizona Health Sciences Center and was published in 2008 [22]. The outcomes of 100 patients with renal dysfunction undergoing EVAR were compared with another 100 patients with OPEN. Although renal function was worse at 30 days for OPEN, it recovered with time whereas the opposite applied to EVAR. Renal function was better at 30 days for EVAR but it continued to decline slowly. As a result, there was no difference in renal function between OPEN and EVAR at 24 months [22]. The investigators attributed the continuing decline of renal function in EVAR to the exposure to contrast from serial follow-up CTAs [22].

Recently, the authors analyzed the American College of Surgeons National Surgical Quality Improvement Program (ACS NSQIP) database to investigate the 30-day outcomes of AAA repair in patients with CRI, specifically comparing OPEN and EVAR [23]. Preoperative renal function was assessed by eGFR calculated by the Chronic Kidney Disease Epidemiology Collaboration equation and CRI was defined as pretreatment eGFR less than 60 mL/min/1.73 m^2. To analyze with more granularity whether the degree of severity of preoperative renal dysfunction affects outcomes, the authors subdivided the patients into moderate renal dysfunction (30mL/min/1.73 m^2 < eGFR <60 mL/min/1.73 m^2) and severe renal dysfunction (eGFR <30 mL/min/1.73 m^2). The main postoperative outcomes were 30-day mortality, renal dysfunction, pulmonary complications, cardiovascular events, and combined outcomes. There were more than 14,000 patients identified between 2005 and 2010; 36% of the patients had CRI. Among these patients with CRI, approximately 90% had moderate renal dysfunction and 10% had severe renal dysfunction. Patients with preoperative dialysis were not included (Fig. 1). EVAR patients had significantly lower 30-day mortality and were less likely to have renal, pulmonary, cardiovascular, and combined postoperative events (Table 1). Multivariate analysis confirmed the superiority of EVAR over OPEN for significantly lower 30-day mortality, renal dysfunction, pulmonary complications, and cardiovascular events (see Table 1).

Regarding the effect of the severity of preoperative renal function on postoperative complications, when patients were stratified based on the degree of preoperative renal dysfunction (moderate or severe), similar results were observed for patients with moderate renal dysfunction in terms of superiority of EVAR compared with OPEN. Specifically, OPEN had 3.6 times higher risk of postoperative renal impairment and 5.1 times higher risk of dialysis compared with EVAR. In contrast, there was no benefit of EVAR over OPEN in patients with severe renal dysfunction because the complication rates were equally

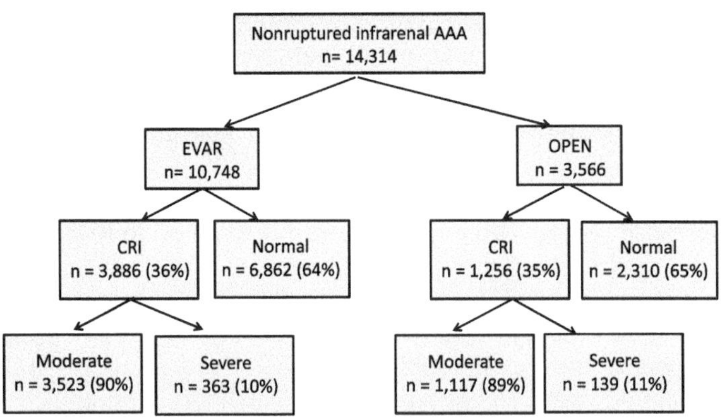

Fig. 1. Distribution of patients who underwent infrarenal AAA repair in the NSQIP database from 2005 to 2010.

Table 1
Intraoperative and postoperative outcomes of all patients with chronic renal insufficiency (eGFR <60 mL/min/1.73 m^2)

	Treatment group			
Outcomes	Endovascular aneurysm repair (n = 3886) n (%) or mean ± SD	Open repair (n = 1256) n (%) or mean ± SD	Odds ratio (95% CI)	P^a
Intraoperative				
General anesthesia	3249 (83.6%)	1237 (98.5%)	—	<.0001
Operation time (min)	156.2 ± 68.6	220.4 ± 89.7	—	<.0001
Blood transfusion (U)	0.34 ± 1.2	2.87 ± 3.6	—	<.0001
Postoperative				
Mortality	70 (1.8%)	74 (5.9%)	3.7 (2.6–5.3)	<.0001
Renal impairment	103 (2.7%)	102 (8.1%)	3.0 (2.2–4.0)	<.0001
Pulmonary complications	145 (3.7%)	239 (19.0%)	5.5 (4.4–7.0)	<.0001
Cardiovascular events	69 (1.8%)	42 (3.3%)	2.0 (1.3–3.0)	.0008
Combined events	273 (7.0%)	314 (25.0%)	4.3 (3.6–5.2)	<.0001
Hospital length of stay (d)	3.6 ± 5.6	10.7 ± 11.7	—	<.0001

[a]Multivariate *P* value, corrected for all significant differences in preoperative variables.

high in both types of repair, much higher than in those patients with moderate renal dysfunction. The only benefit of EVAR over OPEN in the subset of patients with severe preoperative renal dysfunction was fewer pulmonary complications (Fig. 2, Table 2) [23].

STRATEGIES TO AVOID SHORT-TERM NEPHROTOXICITY AND LONG-TERM DECLINE IN RENAL FUNCTION AFTER ENDOVASCULAR ANEURYSM REPAIR

Although all 3 studies discussed previously have consistently shown better renal function in the immediate postoperative period after EVAR even in the

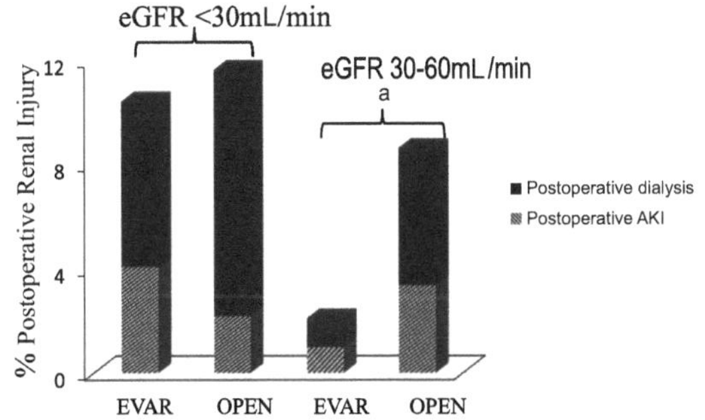

Fig. 2. EVAR is most beneficial in preserving postoperative renal function in patients with moderate renal dysfunction. AKI, acute kidney injury. [a]$P<.05$.

Table 2
Postoperative outcomes stratified by severity of preoperative renal dysfunction

	Severity of preoperative renal dysfunction							
	Moderate (30 mL/min < eGFR <60 mL/min)				Severe (eGFR <30 mL/min)			
Outcomes	Endovascular aneurysm repair (n = 3523)	Open repair (n = 1117)	Odds ratio	P[a]	Endovascular aneurysm repair (n = 363)	Open repair (n = 139)	Odds ratio	P[a]
Mortality	55 (1.6%)	66 (5.9%)	4.1	<.0001	15 (4.1%)	8 (5.8%)	1.35	.53
Cardiovascular events	57 (1.6%)	37 (3.3%)	2.19	.0004	12 (3.3%)	5 (3.6%)	0.9	.85
Renal	66 (1.9%)	87 (7.8%)	4.17	<.0001	37 (10.2%)	15 (10.85)	1.01	.99
Acute kidney injury	34 (1.0%)	38 (3.4%)	3.61	<.0001	15 (4.1%)	3 (2.2%)	0.51	.29
Dialysis	37 (1.1%)	58 (5.2%)	5.16	<.0001	23 (6.3%)	13 (9.4%)	1.52	.24
Pulmonary	120 (3.4%)	201 (18.0%)	5.50	<.0001	25 (6.95)	38 (27.3%)	4.98	<.0001
All combined	212 (6.0%)	269 (24.1%)	4.73	<.0001	61 (16.8%)	45 (42.5%)	2.55	<.01

[a]Multivariate *P* value, corrected for all significant differences in preoperative variables.

setting of intra-arterial contrast usage, the short-term nephrotoxicity of contrast usage should not be taken lightly. Every effort should be made to minimize the volume of contrast used during the initial EVAR procedure. IVUS has been shown to be a useful tool for localizing the positions of the renal arteries and iliac bifurcations for accurate graft deployment and generally reduced the volume of contrast by 50%, from 123 mL to 67 mL (Fig. 3) [24]. As a result, there was less renal deterioration when IVUS was used [25]. Although there are data suggesting that IVUS could achieve equivalent results to conventional aortogram with approximately 10% early endoleaks [24,26,27], it lacks the ability

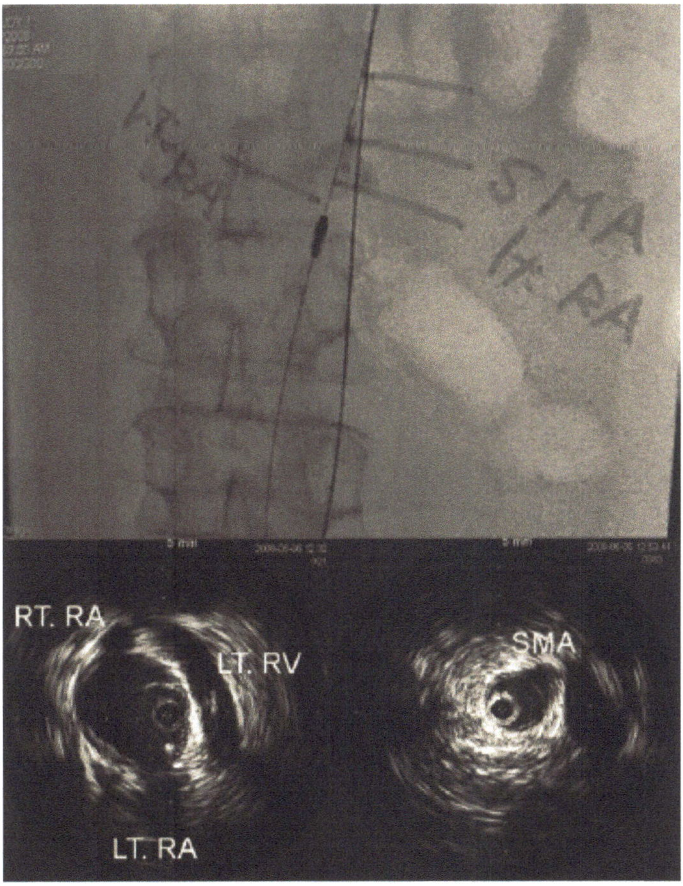

Fig. 3. IVUS is used to identify the origin of the superior mesenteric artery (SMA) and bilateral right and left renal arteries (RT.RA; LT.RA) adjacent to the left renal vain (LT.RV). The exact location of these abdominal branches (celiac artery, superior mesenteric artery, and bilateral renal arteries) are marked on the monitor under fluoroscopy. (*From* Handa N, Tomita S, Kato M, et al. Endovascular stent-graft repair for abdominal aortic aneurysm in a patient with cardiac and renal dysfunction. Gen Thorac Cardiovasc Surg 2009;57:204; with permission.)

to detect endoleaks intraoperatively. Therefore, a completion arteriogram is recommended with either intra-arterial contrast or CO_2.

CO_2 angiogram was first discovered by Hawkins in 1982 [28] when he inadvertently injected air in the celiac artery and observed the negative contrast effect of it. CO_2 angiogram was subsequently discovered. It dissolves almost instantaneously after displacement and is rapidly eliminated by the lungs. It is not nephrotoxic and nonallergenic. For these reasons, CO_2 has been chosen as the agent of choice for patients with preexisting renal dysfunction (Fig. 4). In patients with moderate renal dysfunction (30< glomerular filtration rate [GFR] <60 mL/min), the exclusive use of contrast resulted in a 12.7% greater decrease in eGFR compared with EVAR done with CO_2 arteriogram [29]. Although CO_2 is not as sensitive as contrast in detecting type II endoleaks, its ability to detect type I endoleaks is acceptable (Figs. 5 and 6) [30]. At 12 months, CO_2 EVAR imaging had a similar endoleak rate compared with iodinated contrast EVAR imaging [29].

Minimizing the use of intra-arterial contrast during the initial EVAR procedure is only the first step toward preserving renal function because multiple follow-up CTAs contribute significantly to the continuing decline of renal function after EVAR [1,31]. Duplex ultrasound has been the proposed alternative. In the hands of an experienced vascular technologist, this technology is accurate at measuring the sac size and serves as an excellent test for monitoring the evolution of the post-EVAR aneurysm sacs (Fig. 7). It could better characterize the localization of the endoleaks than CTA because of its dynamic nature

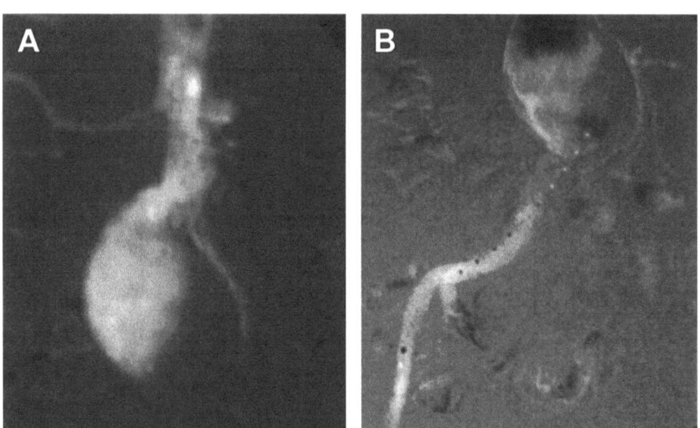

Fig. 4. Preoperative CO_2 angiogram performed of the (*A*) abdominal aorta and (*B*) pelvis. The proximal aortic neck demonstrates an adequate proximal fixation site and the iliac arteries are of sufficient length and caliber for endovascular access. (*From* Bush RL, Lin PH, Bianco CC, et al. Endovascular aortic aneurysm repair in patients with renal dysfunction or severe contrast allergy: utility of imaging modalities without iodinated contrast. Ann Vasc Surg 2002;16:541; with permission.)

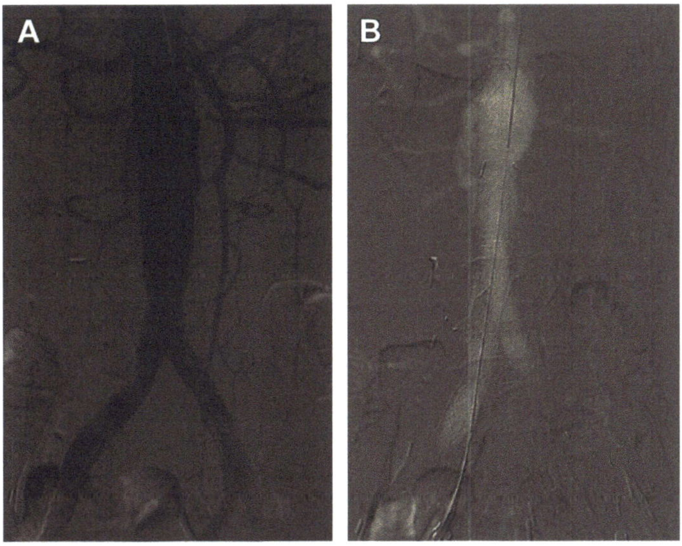

Fig. 5. (*A*) Contrast aortogram showed a type I endoleak, which was also clearly visualized by (*B*) CO_2 digital subtraction aortogram. (*From* Huang SG, Woo K, Moos JM, et al. A Prospective study of carbon dioxide digital subtraction versus standard contrast arteriography in the detection of endoleaks in endovascular abdominal aortic aneurysm repairs. Ann Vasc Surg 2013;27:43; with permission.)

[32]. Although there is suggestion that duplex alone is safe and equally good as CTA in monitoring endoleaks [33], another imaging modality to complement duplex, such as abdominal radiograph, should be considered [34]. Whereas duplex can measure aneurysm size, identify and characterize endoleak, and visualize limb kinking, abdominal radiograph could detect stent graft migration

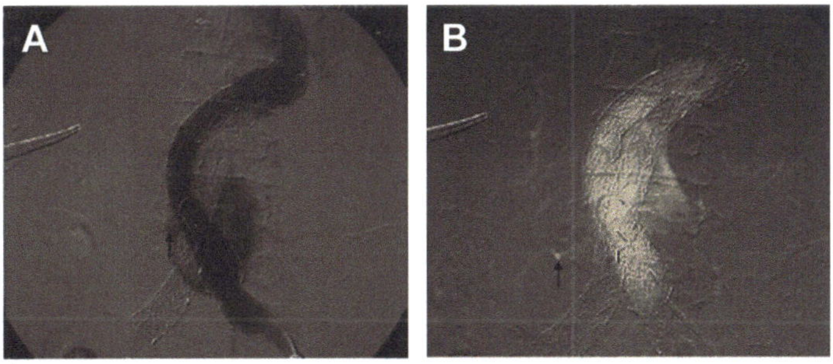

Fig. 6. Type II endoleak intraoperatively documented by (*A*) contrast and (*B*) CO_2 digital subtraction aortogram. Arrows point to feeding lumbar arteries. (*From* Chao A, Major K, Kumar SR, et al. Carbon dioxide digital subtraction angiography-assisted endovascular aortic aneurysm repair in the azotemic patient. J Vasc Surg 2007;45:456; with permission.)

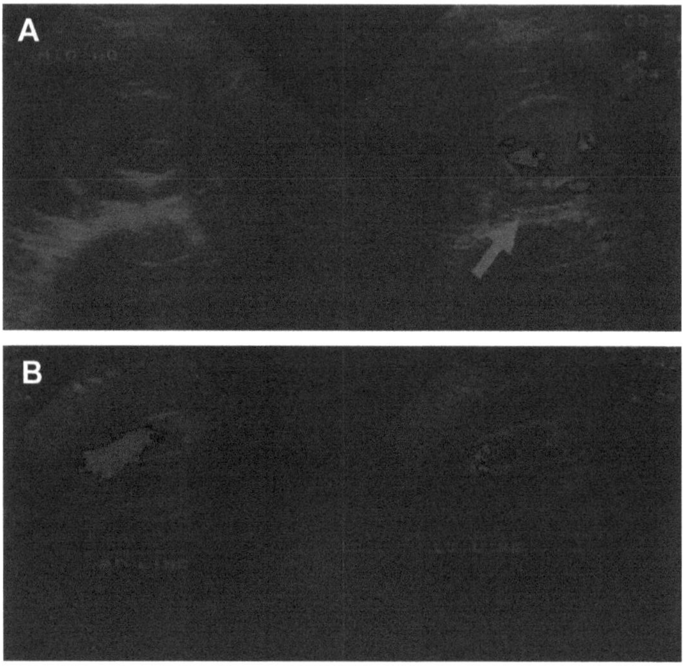

Fig. 7. B-mode (gray-scale) and color duplex images of the main trunk of a modular endograft within the (*A*) native aortic sac and (*B*) iliac limbs. The arrow demonstrates flow within the endograft, thus representing an endoleak is present. The presence of a presistent arterial (pulsative) signal confirms the presence of an endoleak. (*From* Bush RL, Lin PH, Bianco CC, et al. Endovascular aortic aneurysm repair in patients with renal dysfunction or severe contrast allergy: utility of imaging modalities without iodinated contrast. Ann Vasc Surg 2002;16:543; with permission.)

and structural disintegration [34]. When Harrison and colleagues [34] applied a protocol to perform routine annual duplex and abdominal radiograph together to monitor post-EVAR patients and only use CTA if abnormalities identified or the duplex was undiagnostic, they found that CTA was required in only 17% of the time.

SUMMARY

CRI is found in 30% to 40% of patients with aortic aneurysms [23,35]. Because operative outcomes for patients with renal dysfunction are known to be significantly worse compared with those with normal renal function [4], it is critical that the approach offered to these already disadvantaged patients should provide the best possible outcomes.

Although many surgeons prefer OPEN for these patients to avoid the use of contrast for the initial procedure and multiple follow-up CTAs, data from the ACS NSQIP demonstrated that EVAR was the preferred option for patients with moderate renal dysfunction because of better 30-day outcomes and thus should be first-line therapy for patients with the appropriate anatomy. Intraoperative contrast should be minimized with the use of IVUS or CO_2 arteriograms because these techniques have been shown safe and significantly decrease the risk of postoperative renal dysfunction compared with conventional contrast.

The differential findings the authors detected between moderate and severe renal insufficiency are important to the management of AAA patients in everyday practice. The finding that patients with moderate renal insufficiency fare better with EVAR compared with OPEN is contrary to current and common understanding. The fact that the mortality of EVAR is just as high as OPEN in patients with severe renal dysfunction should caution against any elective repair, OPEN or EVAR, unless the risk of impending rupture is high enough to justify the repair. According to a study in Veterans Affairs patients with large aneurysms who were managed nonoperatively because of high surgical risks, 1-year rupture rates were 9.4% for AAAs of 5.5 to 5.9 cm, 20% for 6.5 to 6.9 cm, and 32.5% for greater than or equal to 7 cm [36,37]. The authors' study reported a mortality rate of 4%, renal dysfunction of 10%, and all-combined mortality/morbidity of 17% in EVAR for patients with severe renal dysfunction [23]. When the risk of rupture is balanced against the risk of major complications with AAA repair in this patient population, the risk/benefit ratio in asymptomatic aneurysms of 5.5 cm in diameter or lower does not favor repair.

Even after a decision to proceed with treatment is made and the best approach is chosen for this challenging patient population, renal function continues to decline if the follow-up process is not carefully considered. The combination of duplex ultrasound/abdominal radiograph should be used to monitor aneurysm sac size, the integrity of the endograft, and the presence of endoleaks. In the setting of type II endoleaks without aneurysm sac enlargement, expectant management is a reasonable option. If type I endoleak is suspected, however, the approach of diagnostic CO_2 arteriograms with possible intervention rather than CTA with contrast is preferable.

References

[1] EVAR Trial Participants. Endovascular aneurysm repair versus open repair in patients with abdominal aortic aneurysm (EVAR trial 1): randomised controlled trial. Lancet 2005;365:2179–86.

[2] Alsac JM, Zarins CK, Heikkinen MA, et al. The impact of aortic endografts on renal function. J Vasc Surg 2005;41:926–30.

[3] Nathan DP, Brinster CJ, Jackson BM, et al. Predictors of decreased short- and long-term survival following open abdominal aortic aneurysm repair. J Vasc Surg 2011;54:1237–43.

[4] Patel VI, Lancaster RT, Mukhopadhyay S, et al. Impact of chronic kidney disease on outcomes after abdominal aortic aneurysm repair. J Vasc Surg 2012;56:1206–13.

[5] Lomazzi C, Mariscalco G, Piffaretti G, et al. Endovascular treatment of elective abdominal aortic aneurysms: independent predictors of early and late mortality. Ann Vasc Surg 2011;25:299–305.

[6] Ohrlander T, Dencker M, Dias NV, et al. Cardiovascular predictors for long-term mortality after EVAR for AAA. Vasc Med 2011;16:422–7.

[7] Azizzadeh A, Sanchez LA, Miller CC 3rd, et al. Glomerular filtration rate is a predictor of mortality after endovascular abdominal aortic aneurysm repair. J Vasc Surg 2006;43:14–8.
[8] Hertzer NR, Mascha EJ, Karafa MT, et al. Open infrarenal abdominal aortic aneurysm repair: the Cleveland Clinic experience from 1989 to 1998. J Vasc Surg 2002;35:1145–54.
[9] Braams R, Vossen V, Lisman BA, et al. Outcome in patients requiring renal replacement therapy after surgery for ruptured and non-ruptured aneurysm of the abdominal aorta. Eur J Vasc Endovasc Surg 1999;18:323–7.
[10] Olsen PS, Schroeder T, Perko M, et al. Renal failure after operation for abdominal aortic aneurysm. Ann Vasc Surg 1990;4:580–3.
[11] Pisimisis GT, Bechara CF, Barshes NR, et al. Risk factors and impact of proximal fixation on acute and chronic renal dysfunction after endovascular aortic aneurysm repair using glomerular filtration rate criteria. Ann Vasc Surg 2013;27:16–22.
[12] Maclerewicz J, Walker SR, Vincent R, et al. Vascular surgical society of great britain and ireland: perioperative renal function following endovascular repair of abdominal aortic aneurysm with suprarenal and infrarenal stents. Br J Surg 1999;86:696.
[13] Guntani A, Okadome J, Kawakubo E, et al. Clinical results of endovascular abdominal aortic aneurysm repair in patients with renal insufficiency without hemodialysis. Ann Vasc Dis 2012;5:166–71.
[14] Mehta M, Veith FJ, Lipsitz EC, et al. Is elevated creatinine level a contraindication to endovascular aneurysm repair? J Vasc Surg 2004;39:118–23.
[15] Grego F, Frigatti P, Antonello M, et al. Suprarenal fixation of endograft in abdominal aortic aneurysm treatment: focus on renal function. Ann Surg 2004;240:169–78.
[16] Bockler D, Krauss M, Mansmann U, et al. Incidence of renal infarctions after endovascular AAA repair: relationship to infrarenal versus suprarenal fixation. J Endovasc Ther 2003;10: 1054–60.
[17] Joseph MG, McCollum PT, Lusby RJ. Abnormal pre-operative creatinine levels and renal failure following abdominal aortic aneurysm repair. Aust N Z J Surg 1989;59:539–41.
[18] Brown LC, Brown EA, Greenhalgh RM, et al. Renal function and abdominal aortic aneurysm (AAA): the impact of different management strategies on long-term renal function in the UK EndoVascular Aneurysm Repair (EVAR) Trials. Ann Surg 2010;251:966–75.
[19] Gawenda M, Brunkwall J. Renal response to open and endovascular repair of abdominal aortic aneurysm: a prospective study. Ann Vasc Surg 2008;22:1–4.
[20] Greenberg RK, Chuter TA, Lawrence-Brown M, et al. Analysis of renal function after aneurysm repair with a device using suprarenal fixation (Zenith AAA Endovascular Graft) in contrast to open surgical repair. J Vasc Surg 2004;39:1219–28.
[21] Parmer SS, Fairman RM, Karmacharya J, et al. A comparison of renal function between open and endovascular aneurysm repair in patients with baseline chronic renal insufficiency. J Vasc Surg 2006;44:706–11.
[22] Mills JL Sr, Duong ST, Leon LR Jr, et al. Comparison of the effects of open and endovascular aortic aneurysm repair on long-term renal function using chronic kidney disease staging based on glomerular filtration rate. J Vasc Surg 2008;47:1141–9.
[23] Nguyen BN, Neville RF, Rahbar R, et al. Comparison of outcomes for open abdominal aortic aneurysm repair and endovascular repair in patients with chronic renal insufficiency. Ann Surg 2013;258:394–9.
[24] Bush RL, Lin PH, Bianco CC, et al. Endovascular aortic aneurysm repair in patients with renal dysfunction or severe contrast allergy: utility of imaging modalities without iodinated contrast. Ann Vasc Surg 2002;16:537–44.
[25] Hoshina K, Kato M, Miyahara T, et al. A retrospective study of intravascular ultrasound use in patients undergoing endovascular aneurysm repair: its usefulness and a description of the procedure. Eur J Vasc Endovasc Surg 2010;40:559–63.
[26] von Segesser LK, Marty B, Ruchat P, et al. Routine use of intravascular ultrasound for endovascular aneurysm repair: angiography is not necessary. Eur J Vasc Endovasc Surg 2002;23:537–42.

[27] Pearce BJ, Jordan WD Jr. Using IVUS during EVAR and TEVAR: improving patient outcomes. Semin Vasc Surg 2009;22:172–80.
[28] Hawkins IF, Caridi JG. Carbon dioxide (CO2) digital subtraction angiography: 26-year experience at the University of Florida. Eur Radiol 1998;8:391–402.
[29] Criado E, Upchurch GR Jr, Young K, et al. Endovascular aortic aneurysm repair with carbon dioxide-guided angiography in patients with renal insufficiency. J Vasc Surg 2012;55:1570–5.
[30] Huang SG, Woo K, Moos JM, et al. A prospective study of carbon dioxide digital subtraction versus standard contrast arteriography in the detection of endoleaks in endovascular abdominal aortic aneurysm repairs. Ann Vasc Surg 2013;27:38–44.
[31] Parfrey PS, Griffiths SM, Barrett BJ, et al. Contrast material-induced renal failure in patients with diabetes mellitus, renal insufficiency, or both. A prospective controlled study. N Engl J Med 1989;320:143–9.
[32] Bakken AM, Illig KA. Long-term follow-up after endovascular aneurysm repair: is ultrasound alone enough? Perspect Vasc Surg Endovasc Ther 2010;22:145–51.
[33] Beeman BR, Doctor LM, Doerr K, et al. Duplex ultrasound imaging alone is sufficient for midterm endovascular aneurysm repair surveillance: a cost analysis study and prospective comparison with computed tomography scan. J Vasc Surg 2009;50:1019–24.
[34] Harrison GJ, Oshin OA, Vallabhaneni SR, et al. Surveillance after EVAR based on duplex ultrasound and abdominal radiography. Eur J Vasc Endovasc Surg 2011;42:187–92.
[35] Walsh SR, Tang T, Sadat U, et al. Preoperative glomerular filtration rate and outcome following open abdominal aortic aneurysm repair. Vasc Endovascular Surg 2007;41:225–9.
[36] Lederle FA. A summary of the contributions of the VA cooperative studies on abdominal aortic aneurysms. Ann N Y Acad Sci 2006;1085:29–38.
[37] Lederle FA, Johnson GR, Wilson SE, et al. Rupture rate of large abdominal aortic aneurysms in patients refusing or unfit for elective repair. JAMA 2002;287:2968–72.

Advances in Surgery 49 (2015) 79–93

ADVANCES IN SURGERY

What Is the Optimal Treatment of Papillary Thyroid Cancer?

Christa L. Jillard, MD, Randall P. Scheri, MD, Julie Ann Sosa, MD, MA*

Section of Endocrine Surgery, Department of Surgery, Duke University School of Medicine, DUMC 2945, Durham, NC 27710, USA

Keywords

• Papillary thyroid cancer • Thyroid surgery • Thyroidectomy
• Small molecule therapy

Key points

- Cervical ultrasound should be used for preoperative evaluation of the primary papillary thyroid cancer tumor as well as regional lymph node basins; cross-sectional imaging can sometimes be an important adjunct for surgical planning.
- For low-risk papillary thyroid cancer, surgical options include total thyroidectomy and thyroid lobectomy; patient preference is an important factor in surgical decision-making.
- Compartmental lymph node dissection should be performed for clinically and radiographically positive lymph nodes.
- The role of radioactive iodine is evolving and should be used selectively for tumors that are at intermediate and high risk for recurrence.
- Advances in small molecule therapies offer promise for the management of locally advanced and metastatic iodine-refractory disease.

BACKGROUND

Thyroid cancer has increased in incidence by 5.4% to 6.5% per year between 2006 and 2010, which represents a more rapid increase than that for any other malignancy in the United States [1]. It is the most common malignancy among women less than 35 years of age, and it is anticipated to become the third most common cancer among American women by 2019, surpassing uterine and

The authors have nothing to disclose.

*Corresponding author. *E-mail address*: Julie.Sosa@duke.edu

0065-3411/15/$ – see front matter
http://dx.doi.org/10.1016/j.yasu.2015.03.007

colon and rectal cancers. Papillary thyroid cancer (PTC) is the most common histologic type, representing approximately 90% of all thyroid cancers. According to the American Cancer Society, more than 62,980 patients will be diagnosed with thyroid cancer in 2014 [1]. Although half of this increase is attributed to the identification of tumors less than 1 cm in size (papillary thyroid microcarcinomas) through increased use of radiologic imaging, the observed increase in incidence of PTC across all tumor sizes suggests that the causes of the epidemic are manifold [2,3].

The overall prognosis of PTC is excellent, with an estimated 5-year survival rate of 98% [1]. The evolving epidemiology of PTC underscores the importance of continuous assessment of practice guidelines to assure contemporary evidence-based management of patients.

PREOPERATIVE EVALUATION

A detailed patient history should evaluate for compressive symptoms of dysphagia, dyspnea, and globus sensation, any of which can raise concern for locally advanced disease. Dysphonia is concerning for tumor involving the recurrent laryngeal nerve. Rapid increase in size of thyroid nodules or onset of symptoms concerning for local invasion suggests an aggressive disease process. Physical examination should include a focused evaluation of the neck, with particular attention directed to the thyroid gland and regional lymph nodes in the central and lateral neck compartments. Thyroid cancers are frequently firm to hard on palpation and may have irregular borders. Nodules that are fixed or immobile are concerning for locally advanced disease. Enlarged cervical lymph nodes are concerning for metastases. Patients with subjective or objective voice change or evidence for locally advanced disease should be evaluated with laryngoscopy to assess vocal cord function; cross-sectional imaging with computed tomography (CT) can be helpful in this setting and when retropharyngeal and mediastinal involvement is suspected.

Preoperative cervical ultrasound should be performed for all patients with PTC or a suspicion for PTC to assess the extent of the primary tumor, regional lymph nodes, and their relationship to surrounding structures. Furthermore, studies have demonstrated an advantage to surgeon-directed ultrasonography, such that operative management may be directly altered, highlighting its utility as an important practice adjunct [4]. Specific features of thyroid nodules suspicious for PTC include microcalcifications, irregular borders, hypoechoic appearance, taller than wide dimensions, and increased vascularity (Fig. 1) [5]. Imaging features of lymph nodes suspicious for containing metastases include size greater than 1 cm (except for size >1.5 cm in level II in the lateral neck where normal lymph nodes can be larger), loss of fatty hilum, presence of microcalcifications, cystic appearance, increased vascularity, and round rather than oval shape [6,7]. Although ultrasound features of lymph nodes may suggest malignancy, the accuracy of ultrasound varies greatly based on imaging features and operator experience. The sensitivity of ultrasound for lymph node metastases ranges from 10% to 90%, and specificity

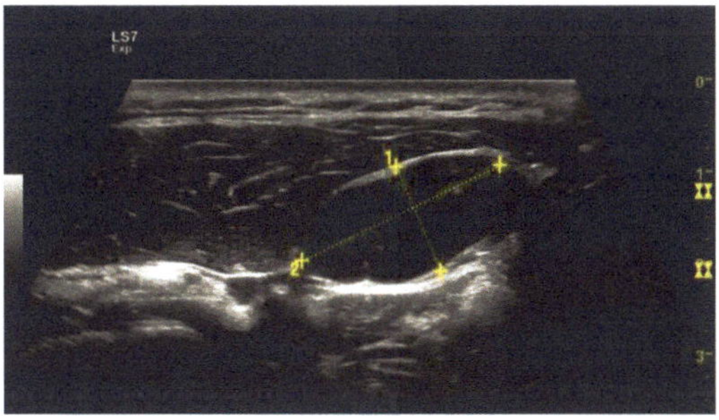

Fig. 1. Ultrasound of suspicious thyroid nodule with hypoechoic appearance, irregular borders, and microcalcifications.

ranges from 89% to 99% [8]. Accordingly, fine-needle aspiration should be performed for all suspicious-appearing lymph nodes. Thyroglobulin (Tg) washout of the fine-needle aspirate of cervical lymph nodes may increase the accuracy of cytology from a sensitivity and specificity of 83% and 98% to 98% and 94%, respectively [9].

Cross-sectional imaging with CT is not routinely used but can be helpful to facilitate surgical planning for cancers that are suspected to be locally advanced (particularly with posterior extension), associated with bulky central or lateral compartment lymphadenopathy with potential vascular involvement (Fig. 2A), or associated with retropharyngeal or mediastinal extension (see Fig. 2B). This

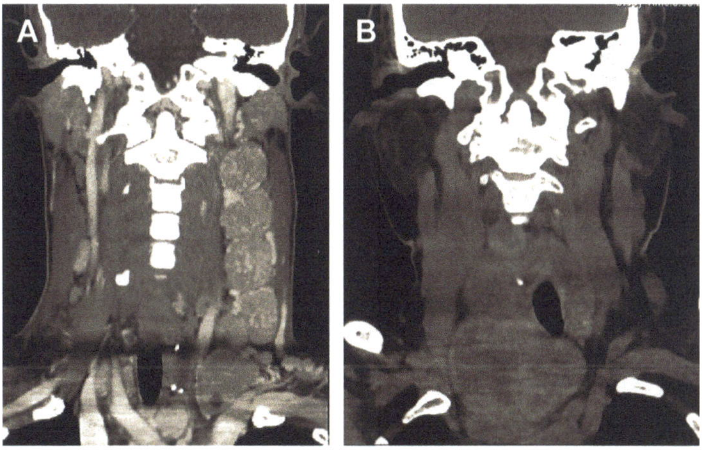

Fig. 2. (*A*) CT demonstrating significant lateral lymphadenopathy. (*B*) CT demonstrating substernal thyroid extension.

imaging can assess for invasion into surrounding structures, including the trachea, esophagus, larynx, and major vascular structures. Intravenous contrast can facilitate visualization, and recent data suggest that the iodine-containing contrast usually does not significantly delay radioactive iodine administration in patients with intact renal function [10].

EXTENT OF SURGERY

The mainstay of treatment of PTC is surgical resection; however, there is a long-standing debate regarding whether total thyroidectomy or thyroid lobectomy is better. Advocates of total thyroidectomy argue that surgery can be performed safely, and that complete thyroid resection facilitates more efficient postoperative radioactive iodine therapy, addresses the risk of multifocal and bilateral disease, and facilitates both oncologic surveillance via utilization of serial serum Tg levels and imaging with ultrasonography and nuclear uptake scans (Table 1) [11]. Recurrence is reduced, and survival might be extended. Proponents of lobectomy counter by arguing that PTC is an indolent disease with an excellent prognosis, and exposure of patients to the increased risks of hypoparathyroidism and recurrent laryngeal nerve injury that are associated with total thyroidectomy is unjustified, because there is not a clear survival or recurrence benefit [12–15]. A prospective randomized trial comparing total thyroidectomy to lobectomy with regard to complications, recurrence rates, and disease-specific mortality would be needed to definitively resolve this debate. Udelsman and colleagues [16] demonstrated that approximately 12,000 patients would need to be enrolled because of the relative scarcity of events, and the costs of such a trial are thought to be prohibitive. As a result, treatment algorithms continue to be informed largely by retrospective analyses.

The 2009 American Thyroid Association (ATA) guidelines for the management of thyroid nodules and differentiated thyroid cancer recommended total thyroidectomy for all PTCs measuring greater than 1 cm in size [17]. A study by Bilimoria and colleagues [18] using the National Cancer Database (NCDB) included 52,173 patients with PTC and showed a higher risk of mortality

Table 1
Extent of surgery: reasons for/against total thyroidectomy

For	Against
Tumor size >1 cm	Tumor size <1 cm
Regional or distant metastases	Localized tumor
Multifocal and/or bilateral disease	Increased risk of RLN injury, hypoparathyroidism
Need for postoperative RAI	Indolent disease that does not imply a significant risk of mortality or recurrence
Facilitates surveillance with Tg or imaging	—

Abbreviations: RAI, radioactive iodine; RLN, recurrent laryngeal nerve.

(relative risk [RR] 1.31, $P = .009$) and recurrence (RR 1.15, $P = .04$) at 10 years for patients with tumors greater than 1 cm who underwent thyroid lobectomy compared with total thyroidectomy. More recent studies have revealed different results, challenging this ATA recommendation. Subsequently, a study by Mendelsohn and colleagues [19] using the Surveillance, Epidemiology, and End Results (SEER) database that included 22,724 patients with PTC failed to show any survival difference between thyroid lobectomy and total thyroidectomy. A more contemporary study by Adam and colleagues [15] using the NCDB included 61,775 patients with PTC and found no survival advantage associated with total thyroidectomy compared with thyroid lobectomy for patients with tumors 1 to 4 cm in size. This analysis used sophisticated statistical methodology and adjusted for patient comorbidities, tumor multifocality, extrathyroidal extension, nodal disease, distant metastases, and completeness of resection, which are variables that were not addressed in the Bilimoria study.

As a result of these studies, experts have begun to advocate for a more individualized approach to the extent of surgery for patients with low-risk PTC. It is important to note that the ATA guidelines serve as a generalized construct on which clinical decision-making should be based. Surgeons must continue to weigh the risks versus the benefits for the individual patient, and the operation selected must be consistent with the overall treatment plan that optimally is formulated by a multidisciplinary team. Transdisciplinary communication, particularly during transitions of care, is essential for assuring an integrated and expedited management approach to the patient with complex thyroid cancer [20]. Intermediate- and high-risk tumor features (including extrathyroidal extension/locally advanced disease, multifocality, aggressive histologies, vascular invasion, nodal and distant metastatic disease) and patient-specific factors (eg, history of familial thyroid cancer, head and neck irradiation) warrant consideration of total thyroidectomy regardless of tumor size, because they imply stronger consideration of adjuvant radioactive iodine therapy and close surveillance because of an increased risk of recurrence. In addition, a surgeon's experience in thyroid surgery is important to consider when formulating surgical planning and level of aggressive treatment, because patients of high-volume surgeons on average have fewer complications and shorter length of stay than patients of low-volume surgeons [21]. Although the risks of complications are muted following thyroid lobectomy and total thyroidectomy when surgery is performed by high-volume surgeons, risks of total thyroidectomy on average are higher compared with thyroid lobectomy due to the greater extent of dissection regardless of the experience of the surgeon [12].

The extent of surgery for papillary thyroid microcarcinoma (PTMC) is another topic of significant debate. PTMC is defined as a tumor less than or equal to 1 cm in size. These tumors have increased in incidence and now represent 49% of all newly diagnosed thyroid cancers in the United States [2]. The clinical significance of these PTMCs is unclear; as a result, there is widespread variation in management, which ranges from careful surveillance to thyroid lobectomy to total thyroidectomy with or without radioactive iodine. PTMC is traditionally viewed as a low-risk cancer associated with an excellent prognosis. The 2009 ATA guidelines stated that thyroid lobectomy alone is sufficient for PTMC that occurs in the absence of other risk factors, such as extrathyroidal extension, a family history of thyroid cancer, or a history of head and neck radiation. A study by Wang and colleagues [22] using the SEER database included 29,512 patients with PTMC and analyzed treatment patterns and patient outcomes. Mean tumor size was 0.53 ± 3.1 cm, and 27.8% of the tumors were multifocal. Overall, 73.4% of patients were treated with total thyroidectomy, and 31.3% received radioactive iodine. The 5- and 10-year disease-specific survival rates were 99.6% and 99.3%, respectively. There was no difference in overall survival between patients treated with thyroid lobectomy or total thyroidectomy. Furthermore, overall survival of patients who underwent any thyroid surgery was similar to that of the general population in the United States.

A study from Japan by Ito and colleagues [23] evaluated the potential role of nonoperative management for PTMC among 1235 patients with active ultrasound surveillance over the course of 18 to 227 (average 75) months of follow-up. Progression to clinically significant disease was defined as either an increase in tumor size to 12 mm or the development of lymph node metastases. Patients who developed clinically significant disease were subsequently treated with surgical resection. At 10-year follow-up, only 6.8% of patients progressed to clinically significant disease. In a subgroup analysis, progression at 10 years was observed in 22.5%, 4.5%, and 2.5% of patients who were less than 40, 40–60, and greater than 60 years, respectively. None of the patients in the study developed distant metastases or died of PTC. These 2 studies demonstrate in a compelling fashion that PTMC is an indolent disease; they support the recommendation of a limited surgical approach for patients with PTMC, and they suggest consideration of surveillance for a subgroup of older patients. More aggressive interventions may be appropriate for younger patients and for those tumors that have worrisome features.

MANAGEMENT OF REGIONAL LYMPH NODES

The cervical lymph nodes are divided into anatomic levels I–VI, and they are segregated into the central (level VI) and lateral (level I–V) neck compartments. Level VII lymph nodes refer to the pretracheal and paratracheal superior mediastinal lymph nodes between the innominate vein and sternal notch. Lymph node metastases from PTC occur most frequently in the central compartment (level VI). Lateral compartment metastases are infrequent without central compartment involvement; these "skip" metastases are thought to constitute approximately 12% of all metastases to this location [8]. The ATA Consensus Statement on the Terminology and Classification of Central Neck Dissection was published in 2009 [24], and the Consensus Review and Statement Regarding the Anatomy, Terminology, and Rationale for Lateral Neck Dissection in Differentiated Thyroid Cancer was published in 2012 (Fig. 3) [7]. A therapeutic central neck dissection should be performed for clinically

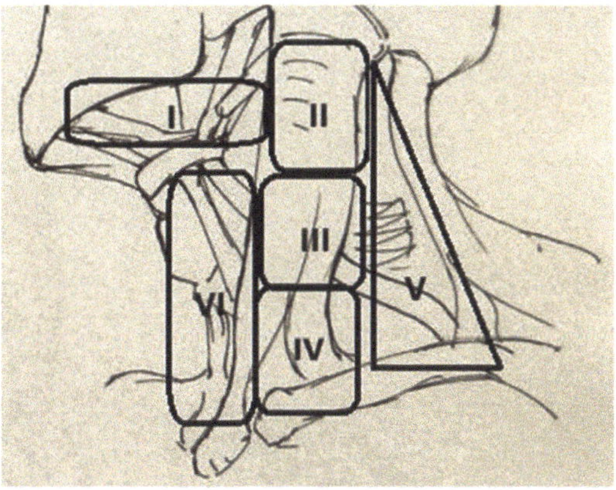

Fig. 3. Lymph node compartments in the neck.

and radiographically evident central lymph node metastases, and complete compartmental extirpation should be performed; "berry-picking" has no role at the time of primary operation. Central neck dissection should encompass removal of all prelaryngeal, pretracheal, and either unilateral or bilateral paratracheal lymph nodes [25]. This dissection may be extended if needed to include the retropharyngeal, retroesophageal, paralargyngopharyngeal, and superior mediastinal lymph node basins. The anatomic boundaries of the central (level VI) compartment are the hyoid superiorly, the innominate artery inferiorly, and the carotid artery laterally. In cases of biopsy-proven lateral cervical lymph node metastases, compartmental neck dissection of levels IIa, III, IV, and Vb should be performed routinely with preservation of the internal jugular vein, sternocleidomastoid muscle, and spinal accessory nerve [17]. PTC rarely metastasizes to levels I, IIb, and Va, so dissection in those areas should generally only be performed for biopsy-proven metastases to these additional lateral compartment locations.

The role of prophylactic central lymph node dissection (pCLND) for PTC is controversial. Although regional lymph node metastases are common in PTC and may be as high as 80% [26], the significance of clinically occult (micro)metastases is unclear. Proponents of pCLND state that excision of the central lymph nodes can lend staging information for planning of adjuvant therapy, decreases postoperative Tg levels, and may decrease recurrence rates [27]. However, opponents of pCLND argue that the increased risk of at least transient recurrent laryngeal nerve injury and hypoparathyroidism associated with the addition of pCLND [28,29] without any demonstrable survival benefit is not warranted (Table 2).

No randomized clinical trial has been performed to adequately address this issue, because it would require a very large sample size to achieve statistical significance in patient outcomes [30]. In a meta-analysis of studies evaluating

Table 2
Arguments for/against prophylactic central neck dissection for papillary thyroid cancer

For	Against
Improved accuracy in staging	May lead to higher rates of RLN injury and hypoparathyroidism
May lead to lower recurrence and mortality rates	No level 1 data to support that recurrence and mortality rates are reduced
Decreased need for remedial surgery	Most thyroidectomies in the United States are performed by low-volume thyroid surgeons
Decreased postoperative Tg levels	—

Abbreviation: RLN, recurrent laryngeal nerve.

pCLND performed by Wang and colleagues [27], no difference was shown in recurrence or long-term complication rates between patients who underwent total thyroidectomy alone and those who underwent total thyroidectomy with pCLND. A trend toward lower recurrence rates was observed with pCLND; however, it was estimated that 31 patients would need to be treated with pCLND to avoid just one recurrence. This finding suggests that any benefit of pCLND may be small, and if performed, should be done by high-volume, experienced thyroid surgeons to minimize the risk of complications. The 2009 ATA guidelines stated that pCLND may be beneficial in a select group of patients that are at high risk for lymph node metastases and recurrence, that is, tumors greater than 4 cm or those with extrathyroidal extension [17].

Another hotly debated issue is the relevance of the BRAF V600E mutation, which is present in just less than 50% of Americans with PTC. The debate centers on whether the BRAF V600E mutation portends a higher risk of metastatic disease in the central compartment, and whether it should be used as a criterion for pCLND. Data are conflicting, because some studies have found BRAF V600E to be an independent predictor of central lymph node metastases [31], whereas others have not [32]. More data are likely needed here [33].

RADIOACTIVE IODINE ABLATION

After total thyroidectomy, treatment with I-131 can be used to ablate residual thyroid tissue or treat presumed occult or clinically apparent metastatic disease. Ablation of remnant tissues allows for improved surveillance and detection of recurrence using serial serum Tg levels. Radioactive iodine in the adjuvant setting is dosed according to tumor characteristics and risk stratification. Postoperative risk stratification is essential to optimize disease surveillance and therapeutic management. Extrapolated from multiple validated staging systems, including the American Joint Committee on Cancer [34], TNM Classification of Malignant Tumors [35], and the Metastases, Age, Completeness of Resection, Invasion, Size system [36], the 2009 ATA Initial Risk Stratification System is recommended for PTC patients treated with thyroidectomy to predict the risk of disease recurrence and provide guidance for adjuvant treatment. Although additional prognostic factors such as lymph node involvement and mutational status can be used to individualize treatment, the 3-tiered system classifies patients as having low, intermediate, or high risk of recurrence [17].

Factoring in patients' risk stratification, the 2009 ATA guidelines recommended I-131 ablation therapy for patients with evidence of extrathyroidal extension or distant metastasis, regardless of tumor size. It is recommended that radioactive iodine be considered for patients with tumor size 1 to 4 cm who have regional lymph node involvement or a combination of other high-risk features, such as larger tumor size, metastatic lymph nodes, and aggressive subtypes of PTC that suggest intermediate to high risk of recurrence or mortality. I-131 ablation is not recommended in patients with tumor size less than 1 cm without other high-risk features [17]. The dose of I-131 administered varies according to both the clinical intent and the disease burden. A dose of 30 to 50 mCi may be reserved for thyroid remnant ablation, whereas a larger dose of 100 to 200 mCi may be used for treatment of occult and clinically apparent metastatic disease.

Radioactive iodine ablation can be achieved with either thyroid hormone withdrawal or preparation with recombinant human thyroid-stimulating hormone (rhTSH). Two randomized trials have demonstrated comparable efficiency of thyroid remnant ablation in patients with low-risk PTC when treated with rhTSH or thyroid hormone withdrawal using either 30 or 100 mCi of I-131 [37,38]. Although cost for patients treated with rhTSH was greater, quality of life was significantly improved because the side effects of thyroid hormone withdrawal were avoided.

SURVEILLANCE

Surveillance following thyroidectomy and adjuvant therapy permits early identification of disease recurrence. Frequency and intensity of surveillance are dependent on the patient's perceived recurrence risk. The ATA recommends checking serum Tg levels and cervical ultrasound at 6 to 12 months following initial treatment. Initial Tg levels should be TSH-suppressed, followed by stimulated Tg if TSH-suppressed Tg is undetectable. Those patients at low risk for recurrence with elevated Tg, and those patients at intermediate risk and high risk, should also have a diagnostic whole-body radioactive iodine scan [17,25]. Patients with undetectable Tg levels and negative ultrasounds can be followed annually with repeat Tg testing and sonographic imaging. Those patients with increasing Tg levels but negative cervical ultrasonography and uptake scans should undergo PET/CT, which can detect tumors that have undergone dedifferentiation or who are no longer iodine-avid. PET/CT is less accurate than ultrasound and intravenous contrast-enhanced CT for detection of persistent and recurrent PTC [39], so PET/CT should be used selectively for patients with iodine-refractory disease.

MANAGEMENT OF RECURRENT DISEASE

More than 30% of patients with PTC develop tumor recurrence, with greater than 60% occurring in the first decade after diagnosis [40]. PTC can recur locally in the thyroid bed, regionally in the cervical lymph nodes, or distantly. The site of recurrence is prognostic of survival. Patients with cervical lymph node recurrence have the best survival, whereas patients with local recurrence in the extranodal soft tissues of the neck have intermediate survival, and patients with distant metastases have the most compromised survival [41].

Once a patient is diagnosed with recurrent PTC, a thorough evaluation to determine the extent of disease is critical for appropriate management of the patient. Pertinent medical records, prior operative reports, and pathology slides should be obtained for all patients. Traditional treatment of recurrent PTC includes surgery, observation, I-131 therapy, or external beam radiation therapy. As most patients have disease localized to the neck, the favored treatment is complete surgical resection of the tumor. A decision for surgery is best derived after multidisciplinary evaluation and requires a thoughtful assessment of the risks of surgery and the extent of disease, taking into consideration patient preference and surgeon experience. The presence of distant metastatic disease and the rate of progression also should be taken into consideration. In select cases, resection of cervical recurrences in patients with distant disease may be performed for palliation of symptoms and airway protection and to permit more efficient delivery of adjuvant I-131 to extracervical disease. Before surgical intervention, fine-needle aspiration biopsy of the tumor is recommended to definitively confirm recurrent disease. Preoperative evaluation with laryngoscopy to evaluate vocal cord function in addition to radiological evaluation with cervical ultrasound and selective use of contrast-enhanced CT is also recommended to assess the extent of disease and facilitate surgical planning.

The risks of remedial surgery in the central neck and lateral neck include injury to the recurrent laryngeal nerve, thoracic duct, hypoparathyroidism, and injury to other major nerve structures, including the spinal accessory nerve, hypoglossal nerve, marginal branch of the facial nerve, phrenic nerve, brachial plexus, or sympathetic trunk. The frequency of recurrent laryngeal nerve injury ranges from 0% to 4.7%, and hypoparathyroidism ranges from 0% to 7% for remedial surgery in recently published studies [42]. Intraoperative recurrent (and superior) laryngeal nerve stimulation and monitoring may be considered in these high-risk patients. An observational study by Chan and colleagues [43] included 1000 nerves at risk for patients who had thyroidectomy using either recurrent laryngeal nerve monitoring or nerve visualization alone. In a subgroup analysis, the authors found that patients undergoing remedial surgery had lower recurrent laryngeal nerve injury rates when nerve monitoring was used as an intraoperative adjunct, suggesting that nerve monitoring may be associated with improved outcomes for patients requiring remedial thyroid surgery. Additional studies are needed to further evaluate the benefit of intraoperative nerve monitoring for remedial thyroid surgery.

Surgical resection should be a compartment-oriented central or lateral neck dissection as long as the compartment has not been previously cleared in a thorough fashion. If the recurrence is in a field that has previously undergone a compartment-oriented dissection by an experienced surgeon, then a more directed approach incorporating surgeon-directed ultrasound or wire localization can help identify residual tumor and direct surgery in more treacherous operative fields. For patients with low-volume or low-risk disease, observation is a viable option, particularly in reoperative surgical fields where surgery may be difficult and associated with significant risk. In a study by Robenshtok and colleagues [44], 166 postthyroidectomy PTC patients with suspicious cervical lymph nodes (median size 1.3 cm [0.5–2.7 cm]) were observed with serial ultrasounds. Although some patients did not have biopsy-proven lymph node metastases, only 20% of the lymph nodes increased in size by greater than 3 mm at 3.5 years follow-up, and no patients developed complications. More studies are needed to determine the ideal management of patients with limited, low risk lymph node metastases.

Patients who are not candidates for remedial surgery due to significant comorbidities, challenging disease location, microscopic disease, or a treacherous reoperative field may be treated with radioactive iodine if they are still iodine-avid. Dosimetry can be considered, particularly in young patients and patients with extensive pulmonary disease, because it will permit optimal I-131 dosing to tumor while minimizing risk for patients who may require multiple treatments with radioactive iodine. For iodine-refractory disease, alternative modalities such as external beam radiation or ethanol ablation may be helpful. Prior external beam radiation to the neck makes remedial surgery more challenging, but it should not preclude re-resection if gross disease is identified. Ethanol ablation or other ablative therapies are most useful for patients with limited cervical nodal metastases who are at unacceptably high risk for surgical complications to obtain locoregional disease control [17]. In a study by Hay and colleagues [45], 25 PTC patients with 37 nodal neck recurrences in previously dissected surgical fields were treated with ethanol ablation in 1 to 5 outpatient sessions. After ablation, 35 of 37 tumors decreased in size, and 17 disappeared. None of the patients developed permanent hoarseness, required surgical resection, or died of PTC after an average 5.4 years follow-up. These alternative modalities provide a treatment option before initiation of systemic therapy for the rare patient with unresectable, locally advanced disease.

SYSTEMIC THERAPY

For distant recurrent disease, iodine-avid disease should be treated with I-131 therapy. The treatment of iodine-refractory disease is challenging, and until recently, there were few options for treatment. Traditional chemotherapy agents such as doxorubicin have not demonstrated a therapeutic benefit in the setting of metastatic PTC [46,47]. Small molecule therapy with tyrosine kinase inhibitors is a growing area of research in iodine-refractory locally advanced and metastatic PTC. Recent trials have demonstrated partial response rates and stabilization of disease in 50% to 60% of patients for approximately 1 to 2 years [48–50]. However, tyrosine kinase inhibitors are marked by significant side effects and should be reserved for unresectable, non-iodine-avid progressive or symptomatic disease [51–53]. Currently, sorafenib is the only tyrosine kinase inhibitor approved by the US Food and Drug Administration for this indication based on the results of the DECISION trial; however, results from a phase 3 trial evaluating the tyrosine kinase inhibitor lenvatinib are promising, and many anticipate additional approvals in the near future, with the hope that more small molecule therapies will become available to treat these challenging patients [54,55].

SUMMARY

Surgery continues to be the mainstay of treatment of patients with PTC. Extent of surgery, lymph node management, and adjunctive therapy need to be tailored for each patient using a personalized approach based on evidence-based guidelines and increasingly sophisticated risk-stratification systems to optimize patient outcomes. More parsimonious use of radioactive iodine is evolving. Advances in the development of additional small molecule therapies offer promise for patients with locally advanced and distant metastatic iodine-refractory disease. It is important that surgeons be involved in clinical trials and developing guidelines for the management of advanced PTC. It has yet to be determined whether these novel small molecule therapies could provide benefit in the neoadjuvant setting, and in what order and combination they should be delivered if there comes a time when more than one drug is approved.

References

[1] American Cancer Society. Cancer facts & figures. Atlanta (GA): American Cancer Society; 2014.

[2] Davies L, Welch HG. Increasing incidence of thyroid cancer in the United States, 1973-2002. JAMA 2006;295:2164–7.

[3] Cramer JD, Fu P, Harth KC, et al. Analysis of the rising incidence of thyroid cancer using the Surveillance, Epidemiology and End Results national cancer data registry. Surgery 2010;148:1147–52 [discussion: 1152–3].

[4] Carneiro-Pla D, Amin S. Comparison between preconsultation ultrasonography and office surgeon-performed ultrasound in patients with thyroid cancer. World J Surg 2014;38: 622–7.

[5] Koike E, Noguchi S, Yamashita H, et al. Ultrasonographic characteristics of thyroid nodules: prediction of malignancy. Arch Surg 2001;136:334–7.

[6] Shin LK, Olcott EW, Jeffrey RB, et al. Sonographic evaluation of cervical lymph nodes in papillary thyroid cancer. Ultrasound Q 2013;29:25–32.

[7] Stack BC Jr, Ferris RL, Goldenberg D, et al. American Thyroid Association consensus review and statement regarding the anatomy, terminology, and rationale for lateral neck dissection in differentiated thyroid cancer. Thyroid 2012;22:501–8.

[8] Fritze D, Doherty GM. Surgical management of cervical lymph nodes in differentiated thyroid cancer. Otolaryngol Clin North Am 2010;43:285–300, viii.

[9] Moon JH, Kim YI, Lim JA, et al. Thyroglobulin in washout fluid from lymph node fine-needle aspiration biopsy in papillary thyroid cancer: large-scale validation of the cutoff value to

determine malignancy and evaluation of discrepant results. J Clin Endocrinol Metab 2013;98:1061–8.
[10] Nimmons GL, Funk GF, Graham MM, et al. Urinary iodine excretion after contrast computed tomography scan: implications for radioactive iodine use. JAMA Otolaryngol Head Neck Surg 2013;139:479–82.
[11] Kebebew E, Clark OH. Differentiated thyroid cancer: "complete" rational approach. World J Surg 2000;24:942–51.
[12] Hauch A, Al-Qurayshi Z, Randolph G, et al. Total thyroidectomy is associated with increased risk of complications for low- and high-volume surgeons. Ann Surg Oncol 2014;21:3844–52.
[13] Nixon IJ, Ganly I, Patel SG, et al. Thyroid lobectomy for treatment of well differentiated intrathyroid malignancy. Surgery 2012;151:571–9.
[14] Matsuzu K, Sugino K, Masudo K, et al. Thyroid lobectomy for papillary thyroid cancer: long-term follow-up study of 1,088 cases. World J Surg 2014;38:68–79.
[15] Adam MA, Pura J, Gu L, et al. Extent of surgery for papillary thyroid cancer is not associated with survival: an analysis of 61,775 patients. Ann Surg 2014;260:601–5 [discussion: 605–7].
[16] Udelsman R, Lakatos E, Ladenson P. Optimal surgery for papillary thyroid carcinoma. World J Surg 1996;20:88–93.
[17] Cooper DS, Doherty GM, Haugen BR, et al. Revised American Thyroid Association management guidelines for patients with thyroid nodules and differentiated thyroid cancer. Thyroid 2009;19:1167–214.
[18] Bilimoria KY, Bentrem DJ, Ko CY, et al. Extent of surgery affects survival for papillary thyroid cancer. Ann Surg 2007;246:375–81 [discussion: 381–4].
[19] Mendelsohn AH, Elashoff DA, Abemayor E, et al. Surgery for papillary thyroid carcinoma: is lobectomy enough? Arch Otolaryngol Head Neck Surg 2010;136:1055–61.
[20] Carty SE, Doherty GM, Inabnet WB 3rd, et al. American Thyroid Association statement on the essential elements of interdisciplinary communication of perioperative information for patients undergoing thyroid cancer surgery. Thyroid 2012;22:395–9.
[21] Sosa JA, Bowman HM, Tielsch JM, et al. The importance of surgeon experience for clinical and economic outcomes from thyroidectomy. Ann Surg 1998;228:320–30.
[22] Wang TS, Goffredo P, Sosa JA, et al. Papillary thyroid microcarcinoma: an over-treated malignancy? World J Surg 2014;38:2297–303.
[23] Ito Y, Miyauchi A, Kihara M, et al. Patient age is significantly related to the progression of papillary microcarcinoma of the thyroid under observation. Thyroid 2014;24:27–34.
[24] Carty SE, Cooper DS, Doherty GM, et al. Consensus statement on the terminology and classification of central neck dissection for thyroid cancer. Thyroid 2009;19:1153–8.
[25] Elfenbein DM, Scheri RP, Roman S, et al. Detection and management of cervical lymph nodes in papillary thyroid cancer. Expert Rev Endocrinol Metab 2013;8:365–78.
[26] Watkinson JC, Franklyn JA, Olliff JF. Detection and surgical treatment of cervical lymph nodes in differentiated thyroid cancer. Thyroid 2006;16:187–94.
[27] Wang TS, Cheung K, Farrokhyar F, et al. A meta-analysis of the effect of prophylactic central compartment neck dissection on locoregional recurrence rates in patients with papillary thyroid cancer. Ann Surg Oncol 2013;20:3477–83.
[28] Giordano D, Valcavi R, Thompson GB, et al. Complications of central neck dissection in patients with papillary thyroid carcinoma: results of a study on 1087 patients and review of the literature. Thyroid 2012;22:911–7.
[29] White ML, Gauger PG, Doherty GM. Central lymph node dissection in differentiated thyroid cancer. World J Surg 2007;31:895–904.
[30] Carling T, Carty SE, Ciarleglio MM, et al. American Thyroid Association design and feasibility of a prospective randomized controlled trial of prophylactic central lymph node dissection for papillary thyroid carcinoma. Thyroid 2012;22:237–44.

[31] Howell GM, Nikiforova MN, Carty SE, et al. BRAF V600E mutation independently predicts central compartment lymph node metastasis in patients with papillary thyroid cancer. Ann Surg Oncol 2013;20:47–52.
[32] Lee KC, Li C, Schneider EB, et al. Is BRAF mutation associated with lymph node metastasis in patients with papillary thyroid cancer? Surgery 2012;152:977–83.
[33] Tufano RP, Teixeira GV, Bishop J, et al. BRAF mutation in papillary thyroid cancer and its value in tailoring initial treatment: a systematic review and meta-analysis. Medicine 2012;91:274–86.
[34] Edge SB. American Joint Committee on Cancer. AJCC cancer staging manual. 7th edition. New York; London: Springer; 2010.
[35] Gospodarowicz MK, Sobin LH, Wittekind C, International Union against Cancer. TNM classification of malignant tumours. 7th edition. Chichester, West Sussex (United Kingdom); Hoboken (NJ): Wiley-Blackwell; 2009.
[36] Hay ID, Bergstralh EJ, Goellner JR, et al. Predicting outcome in papillary thyroid carcinoma: development of a reliable prognostic scoring system in a cohort of 1779 patients surgically treated at one institution during 1940 through 1989. Surgery 1993;114:1050–7 [discussion: 1057–8].
[37] Schlumberger M, Catargi B, Borget I, et al. Strategies of radioiodine ablation in patients with low-risk thyroid cancer. N Engl J Med 2012;366:1663–73.
[38] Mallick U, Harmer C, Yap B, et al. Ablation with low-dose radioiodine and thyrotropin alfa in thyroid cancer. N Engl J Med 2012;366:1674–85.
[39] Seo YL, Yoon DY, Baek S, et al. Detection of neck recurrence in patients with differentiated thyroid cancer: comparison of ultrasound, contrast-enhanced CT and (18)F-FDG PET/CT using surgical pathology as a reference standard: (ultrasound vs. CT vs. (18)F-FDG PET/CT in recurrent thyroid cancer). Eur Radiol 2012;22:2246–54.
[40] Mazzaferri EL, Jhiang SM. Long-term impact of initial surgical and medical therapy on papillary and follicular thyroid cancer. Am J Med 1994;97:418–28.
[41] Mazzaferri EL, Kloos RT. Current approaches to primary therapy for papillary and follicular thyroid cancer. J Clin Endocrinol Metab 2001;86:1447–63.
[42] Magarey MJ, Freeman JL. Recurrent well-differentiated thyroid carcinoma. Oral Oncol 2013;49:689–94.
[43] Chan WF, Lang BH, Lo CY. The role of intraoperative neuromonitoring of recurrent laryngeal nerve during thyroidectomy: a comparative study on 1000 nerves at risk. Surgery 2006;140:866–72 [discussion: 872–3].
[44] Robenshtok E, Fish S, Bach A, et al. Suspicious cervical lymph nodes detected after thyroidectomy for papillary thyroid cancer usually remain stable over years in properly selected patients. J Clin Endocrinol Metab 2012;97:2706–13.
[45] Hay ID, Lee RA, Davidge-Pitts C, et al. Long-term outcome of ultrasound-guided percutaneous ethanol ablation of selected "recurrent" neck nodal metastases in 25 patients with TNM stages III or IVA papillary thyroid carcinoma previously treated by surgery and 131I therapy. Surgery 2013;154:1448–54 [discussion: 1454–5].
[46] Sherman SI. Cytotoxic chemotherapy for differentiated thyroid carcinoma. Clin Oncol (R Coll Radiol) 2010;22:464–8.
[47] Spano JP, Vano Y, Vignot S, et al. GEMOX regimen in the treatment of metastatic differentiated refractory thyroid carcinoma. Med Oncol 2012;29:1421–8.
[48] Anderson RT, Linnehan JE, Tongbram V, et al. Clinical, safety, and economic evidence in radioactive iodine-refractory differentiated thyroid cancer: a systematic literature review. Thyroid 2013;23:392–407.
[49] Cabanillas ME, Waguespack SG, Bronstein Y, et al. Treatment with tyrosine kinase inhibitors for patients with differentiated thyroid cancer: the M. D. Anderson experience. J Clin Endocrinol Metab 2010;95:2588–95.
[50] Sherman SI. Targeted therapies for thyroid tumors. Mod Pathol 2011;24(Suppl 2):S44–52.

[51] Sacks W, Braunstein GD. Evolving approaches in managing radioactive iodine-refractory differentiated thyroid cancer. Endocr Pract 2014;20:263–75.
[52] Schlumberger M, Brose M, Elisei R, et al. Definition and management of radioactive iodine-refractory differentiated thyroid cancer. Lancet Diabetes Endocrinol 2014;2: 356–8.
[53] Thomas L, Lai SY, Dong W, et al. Sorafenib in metastatic thyroid cancer: a systematic review. Oncologist 2014;19:251–8.
[54] Brose MS, Nutting CM, Jarzab B, et al. Sorafenib in radioactive iodine-refractory, locally advanced or metastatic differentiated thyroid cancer: a randomised, double-blind, phase 3 trial. Lancet 2014;384:319–28.
[55] Schlumberger M, Makoto T, Wirth LJ, et al. A phase 3, multicenter, double-blind, placebo-controlled trial of lenvatinib (E7080) in patients with 131I-refractory differentiated thyroid cancer (SELECT). J Clin Oncol 2014;32(5suppl):LBA6008.

Advances in Surgery 49 (2015) 95–105
ADVANCES IN SURGERY

Does Diet Make a Difference Following Colon Surgery?

Cheryl Lau, MD, FRCS(Edin)[a], Edward Phillips, MD[b,*]

[a]Jurong Health Services, 38 Dakota Crescent, Suite 07-09, Singapore 399938, Singapore; [b]Division of General Surgery, Department of Surgery, Cedars-Sinai Medical Center, 8700 Beverly Boulevard, Suite 8215NT, Los Angeles, CA 90048, USA

Keywords

• Diet • Colon and rectum surgery • Postoperative • Metabolism

Key points

- There is little justification for the continuation of the outdated practice of keeping colorectal surgery patients NPO (nothing by mouth) from day 1 after surgery.
- Early enteral feeding has a direct positive effect on the gut by preserving the mucosal integrity and the gut-associated lymphoid tissues.
- Postoperative bowel function itself also normalizes more rapidly when early enteral nutrition is offered, leading to earlier bowel movements.
- Given the overwhelming evidence supporting its safety, early diet can, and should be, adopted with confidence as part of standard postoperative care.

INTRODUCTION

Over the past 2 decades, research has improved our understanding on the importance of early enteral diet following colorectal surgery. We have steadily transitioned from the historical practice of routine nasogastric tube decompression, to allowing oral diet only after passage of first flatus, to the present time when level 1 evidence shows early enteral nutrition improves postoperative intestinal recovery.

Few subjects generate as much controversy as the type and timing of enteral nutrition to be given in the postoperative period. Adoption of early feeding has been slow, in part because of fear of postoperative morbidity, including vomiting, aspiration, and anastomotic complications [1].

The authors have nothing to disclose.

*Corresponding author. *E-mail address*: edward.phillips@cshs.org

0065-3411/15/$ – see front matter
http://dx.doi.org/10.1016/j.yasu.2015.03.008

Malnutrition in colorectal surgical patients

There is considerable evidence to show that major postoperative complications are related to nutritional status. After abdominal surgery, well-nourished patients experience significantly lower morbidity (29% and 72%) and mortality (4% and 23%) compared with malnourished patients [2]. Patients are often malnourished preoperatively in part because of their disease state and side effects of medical therapies, such as chemotherapy.

Cancer cachexia also can be present and is a multifactorial syndrome in which an ongoing loss of skeletal muscle mass cannot be fully reversed by conventional nutritional support. This leads to progressive functional impairment [3]. It is due to reduced food intake and abnormal metabolism that is driven by low-grade tumor-induced activation of proinflammatory cytokines, including interleukin (IL)-1, IL-6, and tumor necrosis factor (TNF)-α. The incidence of malnutrition in patients with colorectal cancer can be as high as 30% to 40% [4,5].

Patients with inflammatory bowel disease are at increased risk of protein-deficit malnutrition due to reduced caloric intake, increased energy expenditure from inflammation, and gastrointestinal protein loss from inflamed intestinal mucosa [6,7].

Surgery itself also contributes to the nutritional shortfall. Surgical stress creates a catabolic state, increasing protein and energy requirements that may compromise immune function, diminish muscle strength, delay wound healing, and increase morbidity [8]. Macronutrients (fat, protein, and glycogen) from fat tissue and skeletal muscle reserves are redistributed to more metabolically active tissues, such as the liver and visceral organs. The total nitrogen losses after major elective abdominal surgery range between 40 and 80 g (approximately 1–2 kg of lean body mass) and can increase to 150 g when limited support is provided [9]. This can lead to the onset of protein calorie malnutrition (defined as a negative balance of 100 g of nitrogen and 10,000 kcal) within a few days [10].

Traditions and dogmas

Classic teaching states that due to reflex inhibition, the gastrointestinal system will be inactive for a while after abdominal surgery [11]. It was deemed reasonable to subject the patient to "bowel rest" by fasting or routine gastric decompression, followed by progressive reintroduction of feeds once the gastrointestinal tract was "working." Usually only intravenous fluids were administered until bowel function returned, this return being perceived as the passing of flatus, or a bowel movement, or the presence of bowel sounds. The reasons for this were to "rest" the bowel to decrease the risks of nausea, vomiting, ileus, aspiration, and anastomotic breakdown. Even when oral feeds were started, a conservative daily progression was adhered to, which consisted of sips of water, a clear liquid diet, a full liquid diet, and only then advancing to a soft diet [12].

However, the concept of bowel rest after colorectal surgery is flawed. Starvation does not inhibit bowel function. Moreover, prolonged starvation decreases splanchnic blood flow and results in profound structural and functional changes to the gastrointestinal tract. Recent data suggest that enteral nutrition, particularly with a lipid-rich and protein-rich formula has a beneficial anti-inflammatory effect on the gastrointestinal mucosa [13,14]. Lipid-rich and protein-rich nutrition within gut lumen triggers a vagal reflex via peripheral cholecystokinin-1 receptors and this reduces local and systemic activation of peripheral nicotinic acetylcholine receptors on inflammatory cells. These data suggest that prolonged bowel rest is harmful, not beneficial.

The concept that bowel sounds are a reliable marker of return of normal bowel function also is flawed. Before resumption of coordinated motility after surgery, there are random electrical impulses followed by random muscle contractions [15]. In this situation, bowel sounds can indicate antegrade movement of bowel contents. Furthermore, bowel sounds may or may not be present with normal bowel activity [16]. As early as 50 years ago, motility studies have demonstrated that small bowel peristalsis occurs within 4 hours after surgery [17]. Waldhausen and colleagues [18] measured gastrointestinal myoelectric and clinical patterns of recovery after laparotomy. Small bowel myoelectric activity returned immediately after surgery, whereas it took on average 2.4 days for the return of bowel sounds and 5 days for the passage of flatus. The investigators were unable to find any relationship between bowel myoelectric activity and bowel sounds. Bowel sounds should not be used to guide the initiation of enteral nutrition.

Moss [19] also provided physiologic evidence that diet could be given immediately after laparotomy and colorectal excision. In this study, a full-strength elemental diet was delivered into the duodenum immediately postoperatively. Using radiolabeled albumin, he demonstrated that 94% of the albumin was absorbed with achievement of a positive protein balance by 5 hours postoperatively. Furthermore, barium motility studies performed on the first postoperative day demonstrated clinically sufficient peristalsis. Gastric and small-intestinal activity returns within hours of surgery and colonic activity returns by postoperative day 2 or 3 [18,20,21].

What about providing nutrition in the form of total parenteral nutrition?

Opponents against early enteral feeds may argue that provision of nutrients in the form of total parenteral nutrition (TPN) can mitigate the caloric deficit while the patient is kept NPO (nothing by mouth).

Simply providing the nutrients is not enough. The route of administration is important as well. Studies in healthy human volunteers demonstrated impaired neutrophil function and an exaggerated glucagon and epinephrine production after endotoxin challenge in subjects receiving TPN and complete bowel rest for 7 days, compared with subjects receiving enteral feedings [22]. The human volunteers fed parenterally also manifested a prolonged acute-phase protein response, increased peripheral amino acid mobilization, and increased peripheral lactate production. It appears that TPN may exacerbate the physiologic derangements seen in the catabolic phase through an enhancement of cytokine production, as well as through an exaggerated metabolic response mediated by the counterregulatory hormones. Furthermore, because TPN is less effective in maintaining the gut barrier and host immune function than enteral feeding, the indiscriminate use of TPN in the face of a functioning gastrointestinal tract is not justified [23]. There is an ever-enlarging body of clinical and experimental evidence demonstrating that TPN may impair host immune defenses [24,25]. In contrast to TPN, enteral nutrition appears to preserve host immune function [26].

Surgical stress leads to splanchnic ischemia. The gastrointestinal (GI) tract, being a proinflammatory and cytokine-producing organ, thus perpetuates the systemic inflammatory and hypermetabolic responses. This evidence, plus the observation that parenteral nutrition is associated with gut atrophy and increased gut permeability, shows enteral feeding is superior to parenteral nutrition and should be provided whenever possible.

Safety concerns with early enteral feeds

Some surgeons worry that early enteral feeding may increase the risk of postoperative ileus and disrupt the newly constructed intestinal anastomosis.

Postoperative ileus (POI) is common after colorectal surgery. In an observational study involving 17,000 patients undergoing colectomy, POI occurred in approximately 18% [27]. Three major mechanisms contribute to POI: opioids, neural sympathetic inhibitory reflexes, and intestinal inflammatory responses [28].

The inflammatory cascade that results from intestinal manipulation and surgical stress contributes to POI [29]. Animal studies show that the severity of intestinal manipulation is directly related to the degree of neutrophil infiltration into the intestinal muscularis and the severity of postoperative intestinal dysmotility [30,31]. Intestinal manipulation also increases cyclooxygenase-2 expression and elevates prostaglandin levels, which, in turn, decreases jejunal contractility [32]. Moreover, this effect is not just limited to the manipulated bowel segment, but also the entire GI tract [33,34]. The mechanism for this is largely unknown, but it is hypothesized to be due to reduction in intestinal blood perfusion and translocation of endogenous cellular danger molecules and cytokines from the distant site of surgical trauma.

The inhibited motility of the postsurgical GI tract is also related to disorganized electrical activity and lack of coordinated propulsions [21,35]. The migrating motor complex (MMC), which propels intraluminal contents during the fasting state, is shortened and may produce retrograde contractions in the small bowel [36]. This MMC activity is believed to be the only stimulus to bowel contractions if patients are not being fed enterally after surgery.

In a canine model, Kawasaki and colleagues [37] compared the effects of enteral nutrition on GI motility after open abdominal surgery. They demonstrated that enteral nutrition hastened recovery of gut motility. Therefore, early postoperative enteral feeding may be an effective way to decrease the duration of postoperative ileus. This is based on the fact that enteral feeding stimulates reflexes that produce coordinated propulsive bowel activity and increases the secretion of GI hormones that increase bowel motility [35]. Food intake also stimulates colonic motility (via the gastro-colic reflex) in postoperative patients as it does in healthy controls [38].

Fear of anastomotic dehiscence caused by food boluses is ostensibly a key reason for avoidance of early feeding in colorectal surgery. This concept of protecting the anastomosis overlooks that endogenous GI secretions of up to 6 L per day continue to be secreted and reabsorbed, irrespective of volume of enteral intake [39]. Furthermore, wound healing is critically dependent on capillary perfusion and microcirculation that provides oxygen and substrates for healing. An adequate supply of protein to the anastomosis is important; starvation and protein catabolism is likely to increase the risk of wound and anastomotic dehiscence. In an animal model, Moss and colleagues [40] demonstrated that early enteral feeding doubled the bursting pressure of the colorectal anastomosis, with the anastomoses containing significantly higher concentration of collagen and collagen precursors than those of the unfed controls. Multiple experimental studies have demonstrated that early enteral feeding after bowel surgery is associated with improved wound healing, greater wound strength, and higher wound hydroxyproline and collagen accumulation [41,42].

The current clinical evidence on early enteral feeding

Before the widespread adoption of enhanced recovery after surgery (ERAS) programs, a 2001 meta-analysis looked at the outcomes of 837 patients who received elective GI surgery from 11 prospective randomized controlled trials (RCT) that compared early enteral feeding to NPO after surgery [43]. It showed that there was no advantage to keeping patients NPO after elective GI surgery and early feeding may be of benefit in decreasing infections and shortening postoperative length of stay. Importantly, there was no difference in the incidence of anastomotic dehiscence, wound infections, pneumonia, intra-abdominal abscess, or mortality. A Cochrane review also dispelled the traditional concept of keeping postoperative patients NPO [44]. This review included 1224 patients who underwent predominantly colorectal surgery and found no significant differences in intra-abdominal abscess and anastomotic dehiscence in oral nutrition initiated within 24 hours, compared with oral nutrition only when tolerated. Boelens and colleagues [45] looked at early enteral nutrition versus early TPN in patients who received rectal surgery and found that the early enteral nutrition group had significantly less ileus and anastomotic leakage.

In a 2011 meta-analysis of 15 RCTs and 1240 patients (most patients were undergoing colorectal surgery, either with laparoscopy or open), early feeding within 24 hours led to a statistically significant reduction in postoperative complications. There was also a nonsignificant trend favoring early enteral nutrition with respect to mortality, anastomoses integrity, days to flatus, days to first bowel movement, and length of stay [46].

In particular, despite long-held concerns that early feeding would increase the likelihood of anastomotic dehiscence, this finding was not significantly associated with the early nutrition in any individual study that reported on this outcome [44,47].

Most early enteral feeding in colorectal surgery studies have been done in patients undergoing elective surgery. What about early oral feeding after emergency colorectal surgery? Compared with elective surgery, emergency surgery carries higher risks of postoperative morbidity because of higher rates of intestinal ischemia, the hostile peritoneal environment (infection) and the more precarious intestinal anastomoses.

A retrospective study on 84 patients who had emergency bowel resection and/or anastomosis reported that early enteral feeding was feasible in hemodynamically stable patients [48]. A randomized trial compared early oral feeding (within 24 hours) to traditional postoperative feeds advancement and found no differences in complication rates, postoperative ileus, or length of hospital stay. These results cannot be extrapolated to emergency colorectal surgery because most patients recruited had surgery for appendicitis and only approximately 9% had intestinal resections [49]. Well-designed RCTs are needed to address the safety of early enteral feeding in emergency colorectal surgery [50].

Providing early solids from day 1

The next logical step in our paradigm shift to early feeds is to study the safety of solids started on postoperative day 1. There is no physiologic reason why a surgical patient with an intact swallowing mechanism cannot be started on solids as the first-line diet. The clear-fluid diet includes clear juices, carbonated beverages, broths, and gelatin. This provides approximately 500 to 600 kilocalories and only 5 to 10 g of protein per day and is unquestionably inadequate for meeting energy, protein, and micronutrient needs [51].

In fact, patients do find the solid diet more appetizing than bland clear feeds. A survey was conducted on 145 patients who received elective colorectal surgery about their preferred first postoperative meal within 72 hours of surgery and preferred solid foods as early as the first postoperative day [52].

As early as 1994, a small RCT was conducted on patients receiving open colorectal surgery to address this question [53]. This underpowered study compared a regular diet on the first postoperative day to traditional feedings and found no differences in tolerance and a trend toward a shorter length of stay.

In the study by Han-Geurts and colleagues [54], 128 patients undergoing abdominal surgery (either colon resection or vascular surgery) were randomized to 2 groups: conventional postoperative dietary approach (increasing amounts of liquids for the first 3 days, then to diet from day 4), or patients were allowed to choose what they wanted to eat and when they wanted to eat it. Need for nasogastric tube reinsertion and postoperative morbidity did not differ between the 2 groups. Significantly, the time to tolerating solid food was 2 days for patients on the self-selected dietary regime and 5 days for patients assigned to the conventional postoperative dietary approach.

One of the criticisms of the study was small sample size and lack of documenting what the ad-lib diet group actually consumed.

Another colorectal surgery study involved patients randomized to receive liquids on the first postoperative day followed by a regular diet after 1000 mL had been tolerated versus a traditional postoperative feeding course. It was concluded that the early feeding was safe and tolerated [55].

Finally, a recent RCT addressed this issue by specifically comparing solid diet with liquid diet from postoperative day 1 in patients who received elective colorectal surgery. Those with early solid diet had a statistically significant reduction in length of stay and better patient tolerance, with no differences in morbidity [56].

Does immunonutrition enteral supplementation make a difference?

Recent research has focused on the composition of nutritional regimens. The potential for specific nutrients to exert beneficial physiologic effects beyond that of a normal diet have led to immune-enhancing diets in patients after surgery.

These immune-enhancing diets contain factors (glutamine, fiber, omega-3 fatty acids, nucleosides, and high levels of arginine) that support immune function, as well as enterocyte growth and function. Immunonutrition therapy can potentially result in fewer infectious complications and reduced length of hospital stay [57,58].

A recent meta-analysis of 21 RCTs including 2730 patients presented the literature evaluating immune-nutrition after major elective GI surgery [59]. Immunonutrition decreased overall complications when delivered before surgery and after surgery. In particular, there were fewer infectious complications and shorter hospital stay but had no influence on mortality. The heterogeneity of the studies made it difficult to comment on the specific role of immune-nutrients on outcomes. What is apparent is that if the immune-modifying nutrition support is provided early in the course of the surgical patient's illness and is given in rather large amounts, its benefits are more easily detected. Two immune-nutrients are studied in detail. Glutamine is an essential amino acid that plays a vital role in nitrogen transport and acid-base homeostasis and is also involved in antioxidant defense mechanisms by influencing glutathione synthesis. It is rapidly depleted from muscle stores in catabolic states. Glutamine has been shown to maintain intestinal permeability in postoperative patients [60]. Glutamine supplementation, especially high-dose parenteral supplementation, in elective surgical patients is documented to reduce infectious complications and length of stay [61,62]. In addition to glutamine supplementation itself, a recent study conducted found that an arginine-supplemented immune-enhancing diet increased plasma glutamine levels [63]. Arginine, an amino acid required for multiple metabolic processes and lymphocyte development, becomes depleted during surgical stress. Lowered arginine circulating levels and increased arginase activity have been observed in surgical trauma [64,65]. A recent meta-analysis on the evidence for specifically supplementing arginine in surgical patients reported that it resulted in a considerable reduction in infectious complications and shorter length of hospital stay without having an overall significant effect on mortality when compared with standard care. Limitations of the meta-analysis include the time span over which the studies included were conducted (2 decades) and the heterogeneity and small sample size of the included studies. In subgroup analysis, no substantial reduction in hospital stay was observed in patients with lower GI surgery [65]. Animal data by Sato and colleagues [66] showed in an in vivo ischemic model of superior mesenteric artery occlusion that free enteral arginine delivered to the lumen was toxic to the mucosal surface. As such, hemodynamically unstable surgical patients with poor gut perfusion are not candidates for supplemental arginine [67].

SUMMARY

There is little justification for the continuation of the outdated practice of keeping colorectal surgery patients NPO from day 1 after surgery. Early enteral feeding has a direct positive effect on the gut by preserving the mucosal integrity and the gut-associated lymphoid tissues. Postoperative bowel function itself also normalizes more rapidly when early enteral nutrition is offered, leading to earlier bowel movements. Furthermore, it appears to confer significant benefits to the postoperative course, especially when incorporated into a multimodal ERAS program. Promising research showed that starting a solid diet from day 1 also is feasible and safe. Given the overwhelming evidence supporting its safety, early diet can, and should, be adopted with confidence as part of standard postoperative care.

References

[1] Rohatiner T, Wend J, Rhodes S, et al. A prospective evaluation of current practices of early postoperative feeding after elective intestinal surgery. Am Surg 2012;10:1147–50.
[2] Meguid MM, Debonis D, Meguid V, et al. Complications of abdominal operations for malignant disease. Am J Surg 1988;156:341–5.
[3] Fearon K, Strasser F, Anker SD, et al. Definition and classification of cancer cachexia: an international consensus. Lancet Oncol 2011;12(5):489–95.
[4] Schwegler I, von Holzen A, Gutzwiller JP, et al. Nutritional risk is a clinical predictor of postoperative mortality and morbidity in surgery for colorectal cancer. Br J Surg 2010;97:92–7.
[5] Bozzetti F, Mariani L, Lo Vullo S, et al. The nutritional risk in oncology: a study of 1,453 cancer outpatients. Support Care Cancer 2012;20:1919–28.
[6] Mijac DD, Jankovic GL, Jorga J. Nutritional status in patients with active inflammatory bowel disease: prevalence of malnutrition and methods for routine nutritional assessment. Eur J Intern Med 2010;21:315–9.
[7] Nguyen GC, Munsell M, Harris ML. Nationwide prevalence and prognostic significance of clinically diagnosable protein-calorie malnutrition in hospitalized inflammatory bowel disease patients. Inflamm Bowel Dis 2008;14(8):1105–11.
[8] Wilmore DW. Metabolic response to severe surgical illness: overview. World J Surg 2000;24:705.
[9] Kinney JM, Elwyn DH. Protein metabolism and injury. Annu Rev Nutr 1983;3:433.

[10] Babineau TJ, Borlase BC, Blackburn GL. Applied total parental nutrition in the critically ill. In: Rippe JM, Irwin RS, Alpert JS, et al, editors. Intensive care medicine. Boston: Little, Brown and Co; 1991. p. 1675.
[11] Rothnie NG, Harper RA, Catchpole BN. Early postoperative gastrointestinal activity. Lancet 1963;2:64–7.
[12] Waters JM. Postoperative nutrition: past, present, and future. Support Line 2011;32(5):2–7.
[13] Lubbers T, de Haan JJ, Luyer MD, et al. Cholecystokinin/Cholecystokinin-1 receptor-mediated peripheral activation of the afferent vagus by enteral nutrients attenuates inflammation in rats. Ann Surg 2010;252:376–82.
[14] Li J, Kudsk KA, Gocinski B, et al. Effects of parenteral and enteral nutrition on gut-associated lymphoid tissue. J Trauma 1995;39:44–51.
[15] Livingston EH, Passaro EP Jr. Postoperative ileus. Dig Dis Sci 1990;35(1):121–32.
[16] Toumadre JP, Barclay M, Fraser R. Small intestinal motor patterns in critically ill patients after major abdominal surgery. Am J Gastroenterol 2001;96(8):2418–26.
[17] Nachlas MM, Younis MT, Roda CP, et al. Gastrointestinal motility studies as a guide to postoperative management. Ann Surg 1972;175:510–22.
[18] Waldhausen JH, Shaffrey ME, Skenderis BS 2nd, et al. Gastrointestinal myoelectric and clinical patterns of recovery after laparotomy. Ann Surg 1990;211:777–84 [discussion: 785].
[19] Moss G. Maintenance of gastrointestinal function after bowel surgery and immediate enteral full nutrition. II. Clinical experience, with objective demonstration of intestinal absorption and motility. JPEN J Parenter Enteral Nutr 1981;5:215–20.
[20] Böhm B, Milsom JW, Fazio VW. Postoperative intestinal motility following conventional and laparoscopic intestinal surgery. Arch Surg 1995;130:415.
[21] Clevers GJ, Smout AJ, van der Schee EJ, et al. Myo-electrical and motor activity of the stomach in the first days after abdominal surgery: evaluation by electrogastrography and impedance gastrography. J Gastroenterol Hepatol 1991;6:253.
[22] Meyer J, Yurt RW, Duhaney R, et al. Differential neutrophil activation before and after endotoxin infusion in enterally versus parenterally fed human volunteers. Surg Gynecol Obstet 1988;167:501–9.
[23] Fong Y, Marano MA, Barber A, et al. Total parenteral nutrition and bowel rest modify the response to endotoxin in humans. Ann Surg 1989;210:449–56.
[24] The Veterans Affairs Total Parenteral Nutrition Cooperative Study Group. Perioperative total parenteral nutrition in surgical patients. N Engl J Med 1991;325:525–32.
[25] Moore FA, Feliciano DF, Andrassy JR. Early enteral feeding compared with parenteral, reduces postoperative septic complications: the result of a meta-analysis. Ann Surg 1991;216:172–83.
[26] Wilmore DW, Smith RJ, O'Dwyer ST. The gut: a central organ after surgical stress. Surgery 1988;104:917–23.
[27] Lyer S, Saunders WB, Stemkowski S. Economic burden of postoperative ileus associated with colectomy in the United States. J Manag Care Pharm 2009;15:485.
[28] Delaney CP, Kehlet H, Senagore AJ, et al. Postoperative ileus: profiles, risk factors, and definitions—a framework for optimizing surgical outcomes in patients undergoing major abdominal and colorectal surgery. 2006. Available at: http://www.or-live.com/cmeducation/1720/cme/cme_eula.cfm. Accessed August 29, 2014.
[29] Kalff JC, Turler A, Schwarz NT. Intra-abdominal activation of a local inflammatory response within the human muscularis externa during laparotomy. Ann Surg 2003;237:301–15.
[30] Wehner S, Behrendt FF, Lyutenski BN. Inhibition of macrophage function prevents intestinal inflammation and postoperative ileus in rodents. Gut 2007;56:176.
[31] Türler A, Moore BA, Pezzone MA. Colonic postoperative inflammatory ileus in the rat. Ann Surg 2002;236:56.
[32] Schwarz NT, Kalff JC, Türler A. Prostanoid production via COX-2 as a causative mechanism of rodent postoperative ileus. Gastroenterology 2001;121:1354.

[33] de Jonge WJ, van den Wijngaard RM, The FO. Postoperative ileus is maintained by intestinal immune infiltrates that activate inhibitory neural pathways in mice. Gastroenterology 2003;125:1137.
[34] Schwarz NT, Kalff JC, Türler A. Selective jejunal manipulation causes postoperative panenteric inflammation and dysmotility. Gastroenterology 2004;126:159.
[35] Luckey A, Livingston E, Tache Y. Mechanisms and treatment of postoperative ileus. Arch Surg 2003;138(2):206–14.
[36] Behm B, Stollman N. Postoperative ileus: etiologies and interventions. Clin Gastroenterol Hepatol 2003;1(2):71–80.
[37] Kawasaki N, Suzuki Y, Nakayoshi T. Early postoperative enteral nutrition is useful for recovering gastrointestinal motility and maintaining the nutritional status. Surg Today 2009;39: 225–30.
[38] Kasparek MS, Mueller MH, Glatzle J. Postoperative colonic motility increases after early food intake in patients undergoing colorectal surgery. Surgery 2004;136:1019–27.
[39] Boron WF, Boulpaep EL, editors. Medical physiology. Philadelphia: Saunders; 2003.
[40] Moss G, Greenstein A, Levy S. Maintenance of GI function after bowel surgery and immediate enteral full nutrition. I. Doubling of canine colorectal anastomotic bursting pressure and intestinal wound mature collagen content. JPEN J Parenter Enteral Nutr 1980;4: 535–8.
[41] Kiyama T, Efron DT, Tantry U. Effect of nutritional route on colonic anastomotic healing in the rat. J Gastrointest Surg 1999;3:441–6.
[42] Khalili TM, Navarro RA, Middleton Y. Early postoperative enteral feeding increases anastomotic strength in a peritonitis model. Am J Surg 2001;182:621–4.
[43] Lewis SJ, Egger M, Sylvester PA, et al. Early enteral feeding versus "nil by mouth" after gastrointestinal surgery: systematic review and meta-analysis of controlled trials. BMJ 2001;323(7316):773–6.
[44] Andersen HK, Lewis SJ, Thomas S. Early enteral nutrition within 24h of colorectal surgery versus later commencement of feeding for postoperative complications. Cochrane Database Syst Rev 2006;(4):CD004080.
[45] Boelens PG, Heesakkers FF, Luyer MD. Reduction of postoperative ileus by early enteral nutrition in patients undergoing major rectal surgery: prospective, randomized, controlled trial. Ann Surg 2014;259(4):649–55.
[46] Osland E, Yunus RM, Khan S, et al. Early versus traditional post-operative feeding in patients undergoing resectional gastrointestinal surgery: a meta-analysis. JPEN J Parenter Enteral Nutr 2011;35:473–87.
[47] Lewis SJ, Andersen HK, Thomas S. Early enteral nutrition within 24 h of intestinal surgery versus later commencement of feeding: a systematic review and meta-analysis. J Gastrointest Surg 2009;13:569–75.
[48] Lee HS, Shim H, Jang JY. Early feeding is feasible after emergency gastrointestinal surgery. Yonsei Med J 2014;55(2):395–400.
[49] Klappenbach RF, Yazyi FJ, Alonso Quintas F. Early oral feeding versus traditional postoperative care after abdominal emergency surgery: a randomized controlled trial. World J Surg 2013;37(10):2293–9.
[50] Le Guen M, Fessler J, Fischler M. Early oral feeding after emergency abdominal operations: another paradigm to be broken? Curr Opin Clin Nutr Metab Care 2014;17(5):477–82.
[51] Mahan LK, Escott-Stump S. Krause's food, nutrition, and diet therapy. Philadelphia: WB Saunders Company; 2000.
[52] Yeung SE, Fenton TR. Colorectal surgery patients prefer simple solid foods to clear fluids as the first postoperative meal. Dis Colon Rectum 2009;52(9):1616–23.
[53] Binderow SR, Cohen SM, Wexner SD. Must early postoperative oral intake be limited to laparoscopy? Dis Colon Rectum 1994;37:584–9.
[54] Han-Geurts IJ, Hop WC, Kok NF. Randomized clinical trial of the impact of early enteral feeding on postoperative ileus and recovery. Br J Surg 2007;94:555–61.

[55] Hartsell PA, Frazee RC, Harrison JB. Early postoperative feeding after elective colorectal surgery. Arch Surg 1997;132:518–20.
[56] Lau C, Phillips E, Bresee C, et al. Early use of low residue diet is superior to clear liquid diet after elective colorectal surgery: a randomized controlled trial. Ann Surg 2014;260(4):641–7.
[57] Mizock BA. Immunonutrition and critical illness: an update. Nutrition 2010;26:701–7.
[58] Marik PE, Zaloga GP. Immunonutrition in high-risk surgical patients: a systemic review and analysis of the literature. JPEN J Parenter Enteral Nutr 2010;34:378–86.
[59] Cerantola Y, Hubner M, Grass F, et al. Immunonutrition in gastrointestinal surgery. Br J Surg 2011;98(1):37–48.
[60] Jiang ZM, Cao JD, Zhu XG. The impact of alanyl-glutamine on clinical safety, nitrogen balance, intestinal permeability, and clinical outcome in postoperative patients: a randomised, double-blind, controlled study of 120 patients. JPEN J Parenter Enteral Nutr 1999;23:S62–6.
[61] Morlion BJ, Stehle P, Wachtler P. Total parenteral nutrition with glutamine dipeptide after major abdominal surgery. Ann Surg 1998;227:302–8.
[62] Novak F, Heylandt DK, Avenell A. Glutamine supplementation in serious illness: a systemic review of the evidence. Crit Care Med 2002;30:2022–9.
[63] Loi C, Zazzo JF, Delpierre E. Increasing plasma glutamine in postoperative patients fed an arginine rich immune-enhancing diet—a pharmacokinetic randomized controlled study. Crit Care Med 2009;37:501–9.
[64] Morris SM Jr. Recent advances in arginine metabolism. Curr Opin Clin Nutr Metab Care 2004;7:45–51.
[65] Drover JW, Dhaliwal R, Weitzel L. Perioperative use of arginine supplemented diets: a systemic review of the evidence. J Am Coll Surg 2011;212(3):385–99.
[66] Sato N, Moore FA, Smith MA, et al. Immune-enhancing enteral nutrients differentially modulate the early proinflammatory transcription factors mediating gut ischemia/reperfusion. J Trauma 2005;58:455–61.
[67] Zaloga GP, Roberts PR, Marik P. Feeding the hemodynamically unstable patient: a critical evaluation of the evidence. Nutr Clin Pract 2003;18:285–93.

Advances in Surgery 49 (2015) 107–122

ADVANCES IN SURGERY

Principles in Management of Soft Tissue Sarcoma

Aimee M. Crago, MD, PhD*,
Murray F. Brennan, MFB, MD

Sarcoma Disease Management Team, Department of Surgery, Memorial Sloan Kettering Cancer Center, 1275 York Avenue, New York, NY 10065, USA

Keywords

- Soft tissue sarcoma • Multimodality therapy for sarcoma
- Retroperitoneal sarcoma

Key points

- Soft tissue sarcomas remain a divergent group of diseases with variable presentation by site and histology.
- Molecular diagnosis is increasingly used, defining tumors (eg, synovial sarcoma and solitary fibrous tumors) when presentation is atypical.
- Accurate diagnosis is essential because multimodality management protocols and surgical plan can differ significantly depending on histologic subtype.
- Surgical resection remains the primary modality of potentially curative treatment.
- Adjuvant radiation and chemotherapy can be used selectively, although with limited survival benefit.

SOFT TISSUE SARCOMA

Soft tissue sarcoma (STS) is diagnosed in approximately 15,000 patients yearly [1]. The rarity of STS has historically made it difficult to study. However, over the last 30 years, large clinical databases and tissue banks have led to a rapid increase in the understanding of STS [2]. What was once thought to be a single disease entity is now known to represent an umbrella diagnosis describing almost 100 individual pathologic abnormalities, each with a unique genomic underpinning (Table 1), progenitor cell, pattern of spread, prognosis (Fig. 1), and sensitivity to adjuvant therapies. An understanding of these unique subtypes has allowed the development of new diagnostic studies based on their

Disclosure: Dr. Brennan is on the Board of Ziopharm Oncology, Inc.

*Corresponding author. *E-mail address*: cragoa@mskcc.org

0065-3411/15/$ – see front matter
http://dx.doi.org/10.1016/j.yasu.2015.04.002

Table 1
Genomic alterations associated with common soft tissue sarcomas

Histologic subtype	Genomic alteration
Well-differentiated and dedifferentiated liposarcoma	12q13-15 amplification (CDK4/MDM2 overexpression) [57]
Myxoid/round cell liposarcoma	*FUS-CHOP* translocation [58]
Synovial sarcoma	*SYT-SSX* translocation [59]
Desmoid tumor	*CTNNB1* mutation (nuclear β-catenin expression) [60]
Solitary fibrous tumor	*NAB2-STAT6* translocation (nuclear STAT6 expression) [61,62]
Leiomyosarcoma	Complex copy number alterations [57]
Gastrointestinal stromal tumor	Activating *C-KIT* mutation [63]

associated genetic mutations (eg, fluorescence in situ hybridization for gene translocations or immunohistochemistry for aberrant protein expression, as in Table 1), improving diagnosis, and in some instances leading to targeted therapies currently in clinical trials (eg, imatinib for inhibition of activated c-Kit mutation in gastrointestinal stromal tumors). STS can occur in almost any region of the body, but is most common in the extremities (40%) and intra-abdominal and retroperitoneal regions (38%) [2]. Each of these locations is associated with a propensity to develop specific histologic subtypes (Fig. 2).

Risk factors associated with the development of STS are poorly understood. Trauma has been linked to the disease, but whether injury is the direct cause

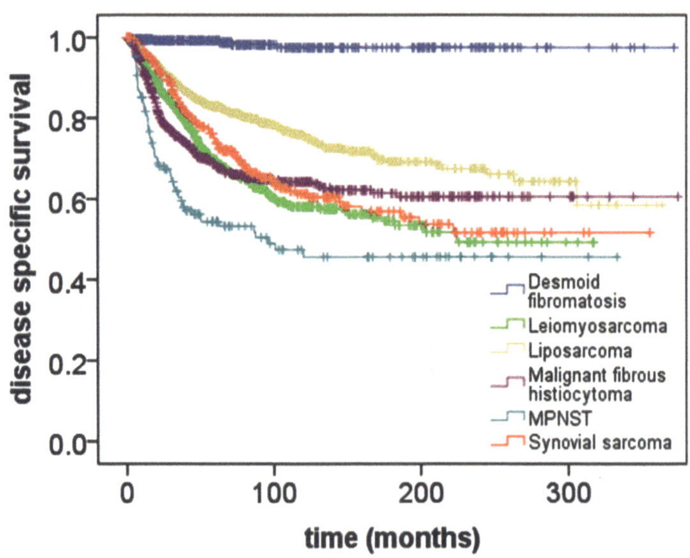

Fig. 1. Disease-specific survival following surgical resection of primary STS (n = 3840) between 1982 and 2014 at a single institution stratified by histologic subtype of primary STSs. MPNST, malignant peripheral nerve sheath tumor.

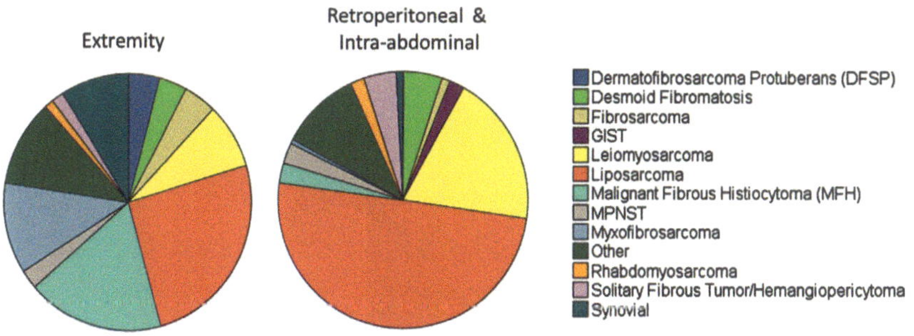

Fig. 2. Distribution of common histologic subtypes of primary STS resected from extremity (n = 3045) and retroperitoneal/intra-abdominal (n = 945) locations at a single institution between 1982 and 2014. MPNST, malignant peripheral nerve sheath tumor.

of tumor initiation is unclear. It is likely that in many cases trauma simply draws attention to a pre-existing lesion. Radiation exposure has clearly been associated with the development of aggressive STS with a poor prognosis [3]. Radiation exposure is closely linked with the development of tumors with complex chromosomal abnormalities and is a common cause of angiosarcoma of the breast when prescribed in the adjuvant setting following lumpectomy [4]. Angiosarcoma of the extremity has also been observed in the context of chronic lymphedema (Stewart-Treves syndrome) [5]. Hereditary syndromes predispose patients to developing STS, particularly Li-Fraumeni syndrome (*p53* mutation associated with malignant fibrous histiocytoma and myxofibrosarcoma), Gardner syndrome (*APC* mutation associated with polyposis and desmoid tumor), and neurofibromatosis (*NF1* mutation-associated malignant peripheral nerve sheath tumors [MPNST]) [6–8]. Less common causes of STS are environmental exposures linked to the development of specific histologic subtypes of STS (eg, hepatic angiosarcoma following vinyl chloride exposure) [9].

DIAGNOSIS AND MANAGEMENT OF EXTREMITY SARCOMAS

STS of the extremity generally presents as a painless mass. The lesion may appear rapidly or be associated with a prolonged history. Initial workup includes cross-sectional imaging in all but the smallest superficial lesions (<3 cm), which can be managed initially with both diagnostic and potentially therapeutic excision. MRI is somewhat more specific than computed tomography (CT) and can be used to delineate the anatomy associated with a tumor (eg, relation to neurovascular bundles) [10]. Carefully performed CT or MRI can be pathognomonic for well-differentiated and dedifferentiated liposarcoma and in many cases can be highly suggestive of histologic diagnosis (Fig. 3) [11].

When sarcoma histology cannot be clearly diagnosed by standard imaging as in the case of well-differentiated and dedifferentiated liposarcoma, core-needle biopsy is performed to obtain a histologic diagnosis, which will assist in both surgical planning and discussions regarding the utility of neoadjuvant chemotherapy.

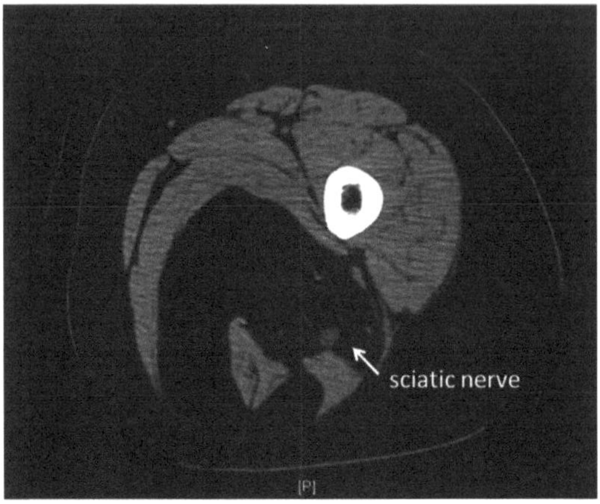

Fig. 3. Cross-sectional imaging (CT) demonstrating a well-differentiated liposarcoma in the posterior compartment of the thigh, encasing the sciatic nerve and hamstring muscles. On both CT and MRI, well-differentiated liposarcoma has imaging characteristics almost identical to normal fat. Enhancing septations may be present, and nodularity appears in the context of dedifferentiation.

Core-needle biopsy is more accurate than is fine-needle aspiration in its ability to define grade and histologic subtype and should be the default method for diagnosis; it will also allow the performance of specialized immunohistochemistry and cytogenetic analyses that define histology. In a study examining diagnosis based on 60 core-needle biopsies as compared with that made on evaluation of corresponding surgical specimens, correct histologic diagnosis was made in 75% of cases; grade was accurately determined in ~90% of patients [12]. Incisional biopsy is performed when core biopsy is not diagnostic and detailed information would change management recommendations.

Regardless of the method of biopsy, core, incisional, or excisional biopsy of small lesions, the surgeon should plan carefully so that the tract can be easily resected at the time of definitive surgery. This method generally requires that the biopsy incision be oriented along the length of the limb despite the fact that this may not result in the most cosmetically appealing scar as compared with a transversely designed incision. Re-excision following orientation of a biopsy scar transversely may preclude primary closure and necessitate placement of skin graft or soft tissue flap.

Once diagnosis is established, an extent of disease workup should be completed. In high-grade tumors, imaging of the chest is recommended, and a baseline CT scan is generally performed. Chest radiograph may be used for patients with tumors that carry relatively low risk of metastasis (eg, small, superficial sarcomas and low-grade lesions). There are rarely clinical indications to stage with PET scan because many malignant soft tissue lesions are not fluorodeoxyglucose avid, and other benign lesions (eg, schwannoma) can be PET avid.

SURGICAL RESECTION OF SOFT TISSUE TUMORS IN THE EXTREMITY

Amputation was historically considered the standard of care for patients with STS of the extremity. The role of amputation was questioned in a classic randomized trial, however, comparing outcomes in 16 patients undergoing amputation with 23 treated with wide excision and adjuvant radiation (designed 2:1 randomization). Amputation essentially eliminated risk of local recurrence, but no difference in overall survival or disease-specific survival was observed between the 2 groups. Despite what would be considered a seriously underpowered study by current criteria, the lack of difference in disease-specific survival has been maintained over 2 decades. This time span reflects the fact that patients experiencing isolated local recurrence (in the absence of metastatic disease) could be salvaged with amputation and indicates limb-sparing surgery is a preferred alternative to amputation for most patients with extremity sarcoma [13]. In modern series from specialty centers, amputation is rarely used for the management of primary STS.

Initially, limb-sparing procedures were planned to include the entire muscular body (origin to insertion) containing an STS. It is now recognized that a 1-cm margin circumferentially is adequate in most instances to achieve negative margins and minimize local recurrences. Specific consideration should be given to histologic subtypes with infiltrative borders, however. In the instance of myxofibrosarcoma, MRI demonstrates that infiltrative tails of microscopic tumor can grow far beyond the borders of the dominant tumor nodule (Fig. 4) [14].

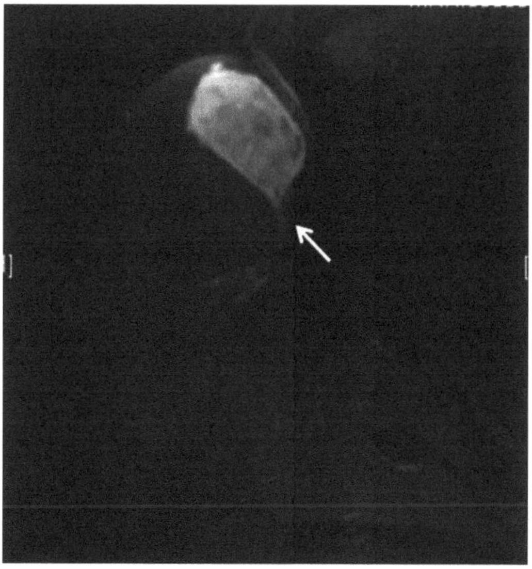

Fig. 4. T2-weighted images from cross-sectional MRI using gadolinium contrast and evaluating a primary myxofibrosarcoma of the right upper arm. An enhancing "tail sign" is demonstrated by the arrow.

Surgical resection should be planned to encompass these tails as well as a margin of normal tissue surrounding them to ensure complete resection. It is likely that early reports demonstrating high rates of local recurrence following resection of myxofibrosarcoma reflect the fact that the full extent of disease was not previously understood in many patients presenting with primary tumors [15].

As in the case of myxofibrosarcoma, dermatofibrosarcoma protuberans (DFSP) has historically been associated with high rates of local recurrence, and multiple resections may be required to remove all microscopic disease from the tumor bed. This finding is almost certainly a reflection that, in this disease, tendrils of microscopic tumor can extend radially from the dominant mass. Such information initially led many surgeons to plan resection with 4-cm margins to reduce rates of local recurrence. A recent review of surgical and pathologic specimens suggests that rates of reoperation are reasonable if 2-cm margins are planned at the time of surgical resection. Eighty-four percent of DFSP patients underwent complete microscopic resection at the time of the initial procedure when tumors were removed with 2-cm margins [16].

Even when a standard 1-cm margin is recommended, the extent of resection is generally limited by an adjacent neurovascular bundle, which often abuts deep tumors. In the instance that the tumor pushes on the bundle without encasing the structure, the tumor can be removed with the fibrous sheath encasing the bundle in an attempt to gain a negative margin. In almost all instances, the structures of the neurovascular bundle can be isolated above the tumor and protected as the tumor is retracted from the surgical bed. Rarely, the neurovascular bundle is encased by the tumor. If this is observed in the context of a low-grade tumor, the lesion can be bivalved to preserve major nerves and arteries, and sacrifice of the bundle can be reserved for the context of tumor recurrence. Of interest in all sarcomas is that a microscopic positive margin following complete gross resection does not uniformly result in subsequent local recurrence, so resection of an adjacent artery or nerve to obtain an R0 versus R1 resection is not indicated in the context of a primary lesion.

When a high-grade tumor surrounds or cannot be separated from major vascular structures to obtain a complete gross resection (eg, a leiomyosarcoma arising from a major vein), the vascular bundle is sacrificed (often with the associated nerve). Arterial resections may require vascular bypass. Attempts at venous bypass generally fail, and in the event of significant swelling, compression and elevation will temporize symptoms until collateral vessels develop. Resection of perineal or sciatic nerves can generally be managed with an ankle orthotic, although patients should be counseled regarding the sequelae of paresthesia on the dorsum of the foot resulting in unrecognized injuries if not examined on a regular basis [17]. Femoral nerve resection requires bracing of the knee to prevent long-term joint damage and falls related to buckling at the joint; such falls can contribute to an increased rate of fracture after limb-preserving procedures [18]. Resection of 1 of 3 of the major upper extremity nerves preserves opposition in the hand despite development of classically defined deficits.

ADJUVANT THERAPY FOR SARCOMA OF THE EXTREMITY

Adjuvant radiation and chemotherapy both play a role in the management of STS. When recommending multimodality therapy to a patient, the relative risk-to-benefit ratio of the treatment should be carefully considered in the context of results available from published clinical trials. Most trials have been performed on a heterogeneous subset of STS, but each specific histologic subtype carries unique propensity for local and distant recurrence, which can modulate a generalized algorithm for prescription of radiation and chemotherapy. Nomograms predicting histology-specific rates of local recurrence and disease-specific survival are widely available and can assist the clinician in counseling patients [19–22]. Tumors more likely to recur locally may benefit from more frequent prescription of adjuvant radiation, whereas tumors commonly associated with distal metastases may require more aggressive recommendations regarding systemic treatment. Sarcomas with low rates of local and distal recurrence may be best managed with surgery alone.

For example, a randomized trial examining the role of adjuvant radiation therapy after surgical resection has been performed in a cohort of 50 patients [23]. It is clear that radiation decreases the risk of local recurrence in STSs and could be considered standard therapy prescribed to patients following surgical resection; more than 30% of patients managed with surgery alone developed a local recurrence, whereas less than 5% of those receiving adjuvant radiation recurred locally ($P < 0.005$). Further analysis revealed, however, that no difference in overall survival was observed between patients treated with adjuvant radiation and those treated with surgery alone. Similar results were observed in a study examining the use of brachytherapy as an adjuvant to surgery in the management of STS. Patients with both high- and low-grade STS (n = 164) were randomized to receive surgery with or without brachytherapy. Again, local recurrence was reduced in patients treated with brachytherapy (89% 5-year actuarial local control rates as compared with 66% in those managed with surgery alone, $P = .04$), but no difference in distant recurrence (76% vs 83%, respectively; $P = .60$) or disease-specific survival (84% vs 81%; $P = .65$) were observed [24].

Based on these trials, adjuvant or neoadjuvant radiation is generally prescribed to patients with large, high-grade sarcomas with significant risk of local recurrence. Given, however, the long-term complications of radiation exposure (eg, secondary malignancies and joint fibrosis), the fact that radiation exposure does not improve disease-specific survival, and the low baseline risk of local recurrence in low-grade tumors and small, high-grade lesions (<5 cm), many physicians will generally recommend against adjuvant radiation in patients with these subtypes of sarcoma. Not using adjuvant radiation is based, in part, on subgroup analyses published as part of the randomized trial by Pisters and colleagues [24,25], which included 45 patients with low-grade STS among the cohort of patients randomized to receive adjuvant brachytherapy or surgery alone. At median follow-up of 67 months, local recurrence rates in patients with these tumors were similar (27% vs 22%) regardless of whether they received radiation; the benefit of adjuvant therapy was limited to patients with high-grade tumors. Again, although a small study, the result was independent of margin status and has been maintained even with follow-up of more than 20 years. Subsequently, a prospective trial examining outcomes in 74 patients with small extremity tumors (T1 tumors, ≤5 cm regardless of grade) was reported and suggests these low-risk tumors can be treated with surgery alone. Ten-year local recurrence rates of only 10.6% were observed when treatment of complete microscopic resection (R0 resection) was performed, and no radiation was administered [26]. When wide margins are obtained, radiation can be deferred in this patient population as well.

Radiation can be administered in the adjuvant or neoadjuvant setting. The risks and benefits of each option have been carefully delineated in a study, which randomized 94 patients to received 50 Gy preoperatively as compared with 66 Gy in the postoperative setting [27]. There was no difference in rates of local recurrence or long-term survival between the 2 cohorts of patients ($P = .71$); however, significant differences in complications were observed. In patients treated with preoperative therapy, wound complications necessitated secondary operations and prolonged drainage in 35% of patients (as compared with 18% of those receiving adjuvant radiation), particularly those with lower extremity tumors. Patients receiving radiation in the postoperative period had high rates of joint fibrosis (48% vs 32% grade 2 or greater in long-term follow-up) [28]. Given these findings, the authors' practice has been to consider radiation in the neoadjuvant setting when tumors are adjacent to a major joint and in cases where surgical resection will require soft tissue reconstruction for closure to avoid radiation of the flap. In general, to minimize surgical complications, most patients are prescribed adjuvant radiation therapy. In addition to joint fibrosis and wound infection, careful consideration should be paid to the long-term risk of bone fracture (~5%) [29]. This complication may be even more common in the context of tumors that are resected with the periosteum [30]. In this instance, patients with osteopenia or cortical thinning should be evaluated for prophylactic rodding if adjuvant radiation will be required.

Decisions regarding the ideal candidates for adjuvant or neoadjuvant chemotherapy are more difficult than are those regarding radiation. At many referral centers, adjuvant chemotherapy is not recommended to patients with soft tissue sarcomas outside of those with Ewing sarcoma and rhabdomyosarcoma, which have particularly poor outcomes [31]. This paradigm is based on data from a large number of randomized clinical trials examining patient outcomes that, in most cases, demonstrate no difference in outcome has been observed between patients receiving doxorubicin-based therapies and those receiving no systemic treatment [32]. The most recent of these trials has been performed under the auspices of the European Organisation for Research and Treatment of Cancer (EORTC) [33]. However, although no difference in overall survival was observed in the trial itself, a meta-analysis of clinical trials examining outcomes in 2145 patients receiving doxorubicin-based therapy and included in the group's report did show that the hazard ratio describing overall survival in patients receiving chemotherapy as compared with those who were observed was significant (0.86); patients may experience a small benefit if receiving adjuvant chemotherapy. In subgroup analysis of the trial participants, trends toward improved survival were observed in those patients with extremity tumors or high-grade tumors who received adjuvant therapy, leading most in the field to hypothesize that patients with these lesions are those who have the greatest potential to benefit from adjuvant chemotherapy and to selectively administer therapy to patients with these high-risk STSs.

In addition to these data, retrospective series have been used by some clinicians to justify administration of adjuvant or neoadjuvant chemotherapy in the context of select tumors associated with poor outcomes. For example, in a retrospective review of 356 patients with large, high-grade STSs, patients with greater than 10-cm, high-grade tumors who were treated with neoadjuvant doxorubicin and ifosfamide had improved disease-specific survival at 3 years as compared with those patients who did not receive therapy (83% vs 62%, respectively) [34]. Criticism regarding the utility of clinical trials has also been raised because most trials include a heterogeneous group of patients with a wide range of histologic subtypes of STS each with different chemosensitivity profiles, and retrospective analyses seeking to evaluate the role of chemotherapy in specific histologic subtypes of STS have also been reported to identify select patients who may benefit from adjuvant treatment. For example, in the context of synovial sarcoma and round cell liposarcoma, outcomes were better than predicted in patients receiving adjuvant treatment as compared with local therapy alone even in the context of smaller lesions (<7 cm) [22,35]. Patients with chemoresistant subtypes of sarcoma, such as dedifferentiated liposarcoma, have classically not been prescribed neoadjuvant chemotherapy by clinicians who believe in selected use of adjuvant therapy, although this pattern may alter as targeted therapies for these tumors are developed and clinical trials examining their activity become available.

Because of significant heterogeneity between histologic subtypes and individual tumors, as well as the unclear role of adjuvant therapy in improving survival, it has been the authors' practice, when considering prescription of neoadjuvant chemotherapy to patients with high-risk STS of the extremity, to administer the drug in the neoadjuvant setting. Administering the drug in the neoadjuvant setting allows the clinician to assess interval response to the drugs as opposed to committing to a full course of therapy in a cohort of patients who may have variable responses. Patients whose disease progresses through initial cycles of chemotherapy are not prescribed a prolonged course of systemic therapy but instead proceed to resection and radiation treatment.

PROGNOSIS AND MANAGEMENT OF RECURRENT DISEASE

Prognosis in patients presenting with STS of the extremity is highly variable and dependent on a range of clinicopathologic factors. Among these are tumor histology, size, grade, and site (upper vs lower extremity vs trunk). Unlike in most cancers, it is rare that a specialist would treat patients or predict outcome based on tumor stage, generally because the current American Joint Committee on Cancer staging systems do not incorporate data regarding histologic subtype, which can dictate both local and distal recurrence risk. For example, high-grade myxofibrosarcoma rarely recurs distantly, but instead is prone to local recurrence so that patients presenting with this disease have significantly better rates of disease-specific survival when presenting with large, high-grade tumors as compared with patients who present with similarly sized undifferentiated pleomorphic sarcomas. Perhaps a better method for predicting survival would be clinical nomograms, which incorporate multiple risk factors into a single model [20]. Many have been validated in multi-institutional studies and can be accessed online, and ranges have been developed to model outcomes in specific sarcoma subtypes [36–38].

In general, high-grade tumors tend to recur relatively quickly with more than half of the recurrences being observed in the first 2 years and almost all of the remaining recurrences happening in the first 5 years [34]. For this reason and because at least 40% of patients with tumors more than 5 cm in diameter will recur, the authors' routine has been to follow these patients every 4 months for the first 2 years after surgery, every 6 months until 5 years postoperatively, and then yearly after that point. Low-grade tumors may have smaller rates of recurrence; however, these recurrences may recur late after surgery. In fact, half recur more than 5 years postoperatively [39]. The authors would generally follow these patients every 6 months to a year for the first 5 years after surgery, but, as with high-grade lesions, they follow them indefinitely.

Patients routinely undergo physical examination to survey for recurrence, and imaging of the chest is obtained for all patients whose tumors carry metastatic potential. Abdominal and pelvic CT is completed for patients with a history of myxoid/round cell liposarcoma because metastases to the retroperitoneal fat pads can occur. The extremity itself is imaged if the tumor is deep, and recurrence would not be detected by examination. This imaging may be in the form of ultrasound or CT, but most commonly MRI, which can detect subtle differences between postoperative change and recurrence. Detecting subtle differences is particularly helpful in the context of tumors such as myxofibrosarcoma where infiltrative components may not be well visualized by modalities other than MRI.

Distant metastases are generally managed with systemic therapy, but solitary metastases or oligometastases (≤ 3) that occur after a long disease-free interval may be resected with curative intent [40]. The treatment paradigm for local recurrences is more complex. Tumors may be surgically resected using principles similar to those used in management of primary lesions. The entire surgical bed should be re-excised when possible. If limb-sparing surgery is not feasible or disease is widespread, amputation may be considered. If radiation were not used in management of the primary tumor, it is generally prescribed (except in the context of low-grade indolent lesions such as atypical lipomatous tumors/well-differentiated liposarcoma). In the context of rapidly recurring

(>5 cm lesions recurring <16 months after initial resection), high-grade tumors, outcomes are particularly poor (4-year disease-specific survival of 18%), and neoadjuvant chemotherapy should be considered before planning complex surgical resections or committing a patient to amputation [41].

MANAGEMENT OF ABDOMINAL AND RETROPERITONEAL TUMORS

Primary retroperitoneal sarcomas generally present as large lesions. The tumors can remain undetected for a prolonged period of time because patients may think they are simply gaining weight. Abdominal distention may lead to diagnosis or the lesions may be identified incidentally when patients undergo scans for an unrelated symptom. Imaging can show a bland or heterogeneous tumor in the retroperitoneum, mesentery, or adjacent to a loop of bowel and is often highly suggestive of histology. For this reason, unlike in the context of extremity tumors, retroperitoneal and intra-abdominal tumors evaluated at high-volume sarcoma treatment centers can often be treated without biopsy. Approximately 70% of retroperitoneal tumors are either well-differentiated and dedifferentiated liposarcomas or leiomyosarcomas. Liposarcomas are almost always associated with abnormal-appearing fat, which appears associated with an infiltrative process and in the context of dedifferentiated tumors have one or more solid, enhancing masses. Heterogeneous lesions in the retroperitoneum are often leiomyosarcoma; those located in the abdomen and associated with the small bowel may be leiomyosarcomas but often represent gastrointestinal stromal cell tumors (GIST). The differential diagnosis of retroperitoneal and intra-abdominal masses can be broad, and if there is any concern for other processes (eg, desmoid tumor, schwannoma, metastatic testicular cancer, and lymphoma), core-needle biopsy under image guidance or via endoscopic approach should be performed.

The treatment algorithm for primary retroperitoneal tumors is relatively straightforward. Surgical resection is the mainstay of therapy. The tumors are resected with a margin of normal bowel when arising from the visceral wall or with the entire retroperitoneal fat pad when localized to the retroperitoneum. A more extensive resection has been advocated by some investigators, who argue that routine removal of uninvolved but adjacent organs should minimize rates of local recurrence in patients with these diseases, and as local recurrence can often be life-limiting, due to associated bowel obstruction that will translate into improved patient survival [42,43]. Such a strategy is highly debated in the field [44]. There are no prospective data to support this position and many retroperitoneal tumors are adjacent to the major abdominal vessels. This plane becomes the closest margin of resection and cannot be addressed by resection of additional uninvolved organs. In addition, it is rare that adjacent organs are directly involved or invaded in the context of primary disease so that the authors' approach has been to remove the colon or kidney only when this is the case [45]. In most instances, the colon can be separated from the tumor, leaving a margin of the posterior mesenteric sheath with the tumor and the kidney preserved by resecting the renal capsule to provide an adequate margin.

Adjuvant chemotherapy has not been shown to provide any benefit in the context of abdominal and visceral tumors except for patients undergoing surgery for GIST. In that instance, adjuvant imatinib can be prescribed for high-risk lesions to prevent recurrence; these management algorithms have been extensively reviewed elsewhere [46]. Although neoadjuvant radiation is prescribed at many institutions in the context of retroperitoneal sarcomas, this is another point of contention with many in sarcoma oncology. Prospective trials suggest that neoadjuvant radiation in conjunction with surgery produces low rates of local recurrence; however, a direct comparison with surgery alone has not been performed [47]. Those who think surgery alone is sufficient to optimize outcomes argue that neoadjuvant radiation may make surgery more difficult to perform and may increase the rate of perioperative complications. Several randomized clinical trials sought to examine the role of radiation in retroperitoneal sarcomas, but to date most have failed to accrue sufficient numbers of patients to be powered to answer the question. A phase III trial has recently been opened by the EORTC and long-term rates of abdominal recurrence and disease-specific survival will be compared between groups undergoing surgical resection and surgical resection after administration of external beam radiation [48]. Results could have significant impact on treatment algorithms, although the studies are not stratified by histologic subtype, and many practitioners will argue that this compromises the ability to understand the role radiation will play in determining outcome.

Long-term outcomes after resection of retroperitoneal sarcomas and high-risk intra-abdominal lesions are generally poor. Imatinib may be able to control rates of local recurrence following resection of high-risk GIST, but more than 50% of patients with liposarcoma recur during the first 5 years following surgical resection of a primary tumor. Unlike after resection of extremity lesions, recurrence can be late with more than 80% of patients developing additional disease during long-term follow-up [49]. This finding is particularly true of patients with well-differentiated liposarcoma when many of the recurrences are detected more than 3 years after surgery. For these reasons, the authors have advocated for long-term imaging follow-up of patients to detect recurrence, which can potentially be managed surgically or with novel therapies. Patients diagnosed with high-grade disease undergo cross-sectional imaging every 4 months for 2 years after surgery, every 6 months between 2 and 5 years postoperatively, and yearly for an indefinite period of time. Patients with low-grade disease are followed every 6 months for 5 years and then yearly.

Treatment of recurrent retroperitoneal sarcomas can be difficult. Even after complete resection, the tumor almost always recurs and management must be thought of in terms of a chronic disease. The clinician constantly balances the risk of surgery, systemic therapy, and observation. Surgery is routinely used in the context of recurrence, but should be considered in the same context as metastasectomy for pulmonary metastases. The goal should be complete gross resection to ensure any chance of prolonged disease-free intervals. Unfortunately, even in selective series, complete gross resection rates decline with each succeeding operation. A simple algorithm is that complete resection rates of greater than 80% at initial operation decline to 60%, 40%, 20%, and 10% with each succeeding operation.

Incomplete gross resection may improve symptoms and prolong asymptomatic periods, but will not be curative. Prolonged disease-free intervals can be observed in patients with a limited number of sites of disease and late recurrences, but multifocality is associated with poor outcomes [50]. A recent review of patients presenting with recurrence after complete resection of a liposarcoma demonstrates that the rate of recurrence is also an important prognostic factor. Patients whose tumors recur at a rate of greater than 1 cm per month after complete gross resection do poorly. Even after complete removal of all visible disease, outcomes are comparable with those observed in patients who are managed with systemic therapy alone; disease-specific survival following surgical resection is just 13 months [51]. Ongoing research seeks to determine the genomic events that are associated with poor surgical outcomes in an effort to identify those patients best suited for surgery and to inform potential novel therapeutics. One such event, copy number loss on chromosome 19, is associated with rapid recurrence and death from disease [52].

When patients present with rapid recurrence or poor prognostic factors, systemic treatments should be considered. Liposarcoma may respond to gemcitabine-based chemotherapy or traditional doxorubicin-based regimens. Similar protocols have been shown to be efficacious in the context of recurrent or metastatic leiomyosarcoma [53]. More recently, target therapeutics have been examined to determine their role in management of retroperitoneal tumors. Leiomyosarcoma responds to trabectadin [54]. Well-differentiated and dedifferentiated liposarcoma specifically is characterized by amplification of the chromosome 12 genes *CDK4* and *MDM2*. Inhibitors of MDM2 have been examined in clinical trials and are associated with significant rates of grade 3 toxicities and few responses [55]. CDK4 inhibitors, however, may trigger response and prolong progression-free survival by more than 4 months [56].

SUMMARY AND CONCLUSIONS

STSs remain a divergent group of diseases with variable presentation by site and histology. Molecular diagnosis is increasingly used, defining tumors (eg, synovial sarcoma and solitary fibrous tumors) when presentation is atypical. Accurate diagnosis is essential as multimodality management protocols and surgical plan can differ significantly depending on histologic subtype. Surgical resection remains the primary modality of potentially curative treatment. Adjuvant radiation and chemotherapy can be used selectively, although with limited survival benefit. Molecular targets seem to be the most promising new approach to identify novel means to inhibit growth of these tumors and prevent death related to disease. A wide range of active research programs are rapidly advancing the understanding of a panel of diseases, which differ significantly in their clinical behavior, allowing continual improvement and optimizing therapy in individual patients.

References

[1] Jemal A, Siegel R, Ward E, et al. Cancer statistics. CA Cancer J Clin 2009;2009(59): 225–49.
[2] Brennan MF, Antonescu CR, Moraco N, et al. Lessons learned from the study of 10,000 patients with soft tissue sarcoma. Ann Surg 2014;260:416–21 [discussion: 421–2].
[3] Gladdy RA, Qin LX, Moraco N, et al. Do radiation-associated soft tissue sarcomas have the same prognosis as sporadic soft tissue sarcomas? J Clin Oncol 2010;28:2064–9.
[4] Billings SD, McKenney JK, Folpe AL, et al. Cutaneous angiosarcoma following breast-conserving surgery and radiation: an analysis of 27 cases. Am J Surg Pathol 2004;28: 781–8.
[5] Stewart FW, Treves N. Lymphangiosarcoma in postmastectomy lymphedema; a report of six cases in elephantiasis chirurgica. Cancer 1948;1:64–81.
[6] Li FP, Fraumeni JF Jr. Soft-tissue sarcomas, breast cancer, and other neoplasms. A familial syndrome? Ann Intern Med 1969;71:747–52.
[7] Gardner EJ, Richards RC. Multiple cutaneous and subcutaneous lesions occurring simultaneously with hereditary polyposis and osteomatosis. Am J Hum Genet 1953;5:139–47.
[8] LaFemina J, Qin LX, Moraco NH, et al. Oncologic outcomes of sporadic, neurofibromatosis-associated, and radiation-induced malignant peripheral nerve sheath tumors. Ann Surg Oncol 2013;20:66–72.
[9] Block JB. Angiosarcoma of the liver following vinyl chloride exposure. JAMA 1974;229: 53–4.
[10] Panicek DM, Gatsonis C, Rosenthal DI, et al. CT and MR imaging in the local staging of primary malignant musculoskeletal neoplasms: report of the Radiology Diagnostic Oncology Group. Radiology 1997;202:237–46.
[11] Peterson JJ, Kransdorf MJ, Bancroft LW, et al. Malignant fatty tumors: classification, clinical course, imaging appearance and treatment. Skeletal Radiol 2003;32:493–503.
[12] Heslin MJ, Lewis JJ, Woodruff JM, et al. Core needle biopsy for diagnosis of extremity soft tissue sarcoma. Ann Surg Oncol 1997;4:425–31.
[13] Rosenberg SA, Tepper J, Glatstein E, et al. The treatment of soft-tissue sarcomas of the extremities: prospective randomized evaluations of (1) limb-sparing surgery plus radiation therapy compared with amputation and (2) the role of adjuvant chemotherapy. Ann Surg 1982;196:305–15.
[14] Lefkowitz RA, Landa J, Hwang S, et al. Myxofibrosarcoma: prevalence and diagnostic value of the "tail sign" on magnetic resonance imaging. Skeletal Radiol 2013;42:809–18.
[15] Mentzel T, Calonje E, Wadden C, et al. Myxofibrosarcoma. Clinicopathologic analysis of 75 cases with emphasis on the low-grade variant. Am J Surg Pathol 1996;20:391–405.
[16] Farma JM, Ammori JB, Zager JS, et al. Dermatofibrosarcoma protuberans: how wide should we resect? Ann Surg Oncol 2010;17:2112–8.
[17] Brooks AD, Gold JS, Graham D, et al. Resection of the sciatic, peroneal, or tibial nerves: assessment of functional status. Ann Surg Oncol 2002;9:41–7.
[18] Jones KB, Ferguson PC, Deheshi B, et al. Complete femoral nerve resection with soft tissue sarcoma: functional outcomes. Ann Surg Oncol 2010;17:401–6.
[19] Dalal KM, Kattan MW, Antonescu CR, et al. Subtype specific prognostic nomogram for patients with primary liposarcoma of the retroperitoneum, extremity, or trunk. Ann Surg 2006;244:381–91.
[20] Kattan MW, Leung DH, Brennan MF. Postoperative nomogram for 12-year sarcoma-specific death. J Clin Oncol 2002;20:791–6.
[21] Cahlon O, Brennan MF, Jia X, et al. A postoperative nomogram for local recurrence risk in extremity soft tissue sarcomas after limb-sparing surgery without adjuvant radiation. Ann Surg 2012;255:343–7.

[22] Eilber FC, Brennan MF, Eilber FR, et al. Chemotherapy is associated with improved survival in adult patients with primary extremity synovial sarcoma. Ann Surg 2007;246:105–13.
[23] Yang JC, Chang AE, Baker AR, et al. Randomized prospective study of the benefit of adjuvant radiation therapy in the treatment of soft tissue sarcomas of the extremity. J Clin Oncol 1998;16:197–203.
[24] Pisters PW, Harrison LB, Leung DH, et al. Long-term results of a prospective randomized trial of adjuvant brachytherapy in soft tissue sarcoma. J Clin Oncol 1996;14:859–68.
[25] Pisters PW, Harrison LB, Woodruff JM, et al. A prospective randomized trial of adjuvant brachytherapy in the management of low-grade soft tissue sarcomas of the extremity and superficial trunk. J Clin Oncol 1994;12:1150–5.
[26] Pisters PW, Pollock RE, Lewis VO, et al. Long-term results of prospective trial of surgery alone with selective use of radiation for patients with T1 extremity and trunk soft tissue sarcomas. Ann Surg 2007;246:675–81 [discussion: 681–2].
[27] O'Sullivan B, Davis AM, Turcotte R, et al. Preoperative versus postoperative radiotherapy in soft-tissue sarcoma of the limbs: a randomised trial. Lancet 2002;359:2235–41.
[28] Davis AM, O'Sullivan B, Turcotte R, et al. Late radiation morbidity following randomization to preoperative versus postoperative radiotherapy in extremity soft tissue sarcoma. Radiother Oncol 2005;75:48–53.
[29] Alektiar KM, Brennan MF, Singer S. Influence of site on the therapeutic ratio of adjuvant radiotherapy in soft-tissue sarcoma of the extremity. Int J Radiat Oncol Biol Phys 2005;63:202–8.
[30] Lin PP, Schupak KD, Boland PJ, et al. Pathologic femoral fracture after periosteal excision and radiation for the treatment of soft tissue sarcoma. Cancer 1998;82:2356–65.
[31] Esnaola NF, Rubin BP, Baldini EH, et al. Response to chemotherapy and predictors of survival in adult rhabdomyosarcoma. Ann Surg 2001;234:215–23.
[32] Adjuvant chemotherapy for localised resectable soft-tissue sarcoma of adults: meta-analysis of individual data. Sarcoma Meta-analysis Collaboration. Lancet 1997;350:1647–54.
[33] Woll PJ, Reichardt P, Le Cesne A, et al. Adjuvant chemotherapy with doxorubicin, ifosfamide, and lenograstim for resected soft-tissue sarcoma (EORTC 62931): a multicentre randomised controlled trial. Lancet Oncol 2012;13:1045–54.
[34] Grobmyer SR, Maki RG, Demetri GD, et al. Neo-adjuvant chemotherapy for primary high-grade extremity soft tissue sarcoma. Ann Oncol 2004;15:1667–72.
[35] Eilber FC, Eilber FR, Eckardt J, et al. The impact of chemotherapy on the survival of patients with high-grade primary extremity liposarcoma. Ann Surg 2004;240:686–95 [discussion: 695–7].
[36] Eilber FC, Brennan MF, Eilber FR, et al. Validation of the postoperative nomogram for 12-year sarcoma-specific mortality. Cancer 2004;101:2270–5.
[37] Crago AM, Denton B, Salas S, et al. A prognostic nomogram for prediction of recurrence in desmoid fibromatosis. Ann Surg 2013;258:347–53.
[38] Canter RJ, Qin LX, Maki RG, et al. A synovial sarcoma-specific preoperative nomogram supports a survival benefit to ifosfamide-based chemotherapy and improves risk stratification for patients. Clin Cancer Res 2008;14:8191–7.
[39] Canter RJ, Qin LX, Ferrone CR, et al. Why do patients with low-grade soft tissue sarcoma die? Ann Surg Oncol 2008;15:3550–60.
[40] Temple LK, Brennan MF. The role of pulmonary metastasectomy in soft tissue sarcoma. Semin Thorac Cardiovasc Surg 2002;14:35–44.
[41] Eilber FC, Brennan MF, Riedel E, et al. Prognostic factors for survival in patients with locally recurrent extremity soft tissue sarcomas. Ann Surg Oncol 2005;12:228–36.
[42] Gronchi A, Lo Vullo S, Fiore M, et al. Aggressive surgical policies in a retrospectively reviewed single-institution case series of retroperitoneal soft tissue sarcoma patients. J Clin Oncol 2009;27:24–30.
[43] Bonvalot S, Miceli R, Berselli M, et al. Aggressive surgery in retroperitoneal soft tissue sarcoma carried out at high-volume centers is safe and is associated with improved local control. Ann Surg Oncol 2010;17:1507–14.

[44] Pisters PW. Resection of some–but not all–clinically uninvolved adjacent viscera as part of surgery for retroperitoneal soft tissue sarcomas. J Clin Oncol 2009;27:6–8.
[45] Russo P, Kim Y, Ravindran S, et al. Nephrectomy during operative management of retroperitoneal sarcoma. Ann Surg Oncol 1997;4:421–4.
[46] Joensuu H, DeMatteo RP. The management of gastrointestinal stromal tumors: a model for targeted and multidisciplinary therapy of malignancy. Annu Rev Med 2012;63:247–58.
[47] Pawlik TM, Pisters PW, Mikula L, et al. Long-term results of two prospective trials of preoperative external beam radiotherapy for localized intermediate- or high-grade retroperitoneal soft tissue sarcoma. Ann Surg Oncol 2006;13:508–17.
[48] A phase III randomized study of preoperative radiotherapy plus surgery versus surgery alone for patients with Retroperitoneal sarcomas (RPS) - STRASS. Available at: http://www.cancer.gov/clinicaltrials/search/view?cdrid=699225&version=HealthProfessional. Accessed April 30, 2015.
[49] Singer S, Antonescu CR, Riedel E, et al. Histologic subtype and margin of resection predict pattern of recurrence and survival for retroperitoneal liposarcoma. Ann Surg 2003;238: 358–70 [discussion: 370–1].
[50] Anaya DA, Lahat G, Liu J, et al. Multifocality in retroperitoneal sarcoma: a prognostic factor critical to surgical decision-making. Ann Surg 2009;249:137–42.
[51] Park JO, Qin LX, Prete FP, et al. Predicting outcome by growth rate of locally recurrent retroperitoneal liposarcoma: the one centimeter per month rule. Ann Surg 2009;250:977–82.
[52] Crago AM, Socci ND, Decarolis P, et al. Copy number losses define subgroups of dedifferentiated liposarcoma with poor prognosis and genomic instability. Clin Cancer Res 2012;18:1334–40.
[53] Maki RG, Wathen JK, Patel SR, et al. Randomized phase II study of gemcitabine and docetaxel compared with gemcitabine alone in patients with metastatic soft tissue sarcomas: results of sarcoma alliance for research through collaboration study 002 [corrected]. J Clin Oncol 2007;25:2755–63.
[54] Samuels BL, Chawla S, Patel S, et al. Clinical outcomes and safety with trabectedin therapy in patients with advanced soft tissue sarcomas following failure of prior chemotherapy: results of a worldwide expanded access program study. Ann Oncol 2013;24:1703–9.
[55] Ray-Coquard I, Blay JY, Italiano A, et al. Effect of the MDM2 antagonist RG7112 on the P53 pathway in patients with MDM2-amplified, well-differentiated or dedifferentiated liposarcoma: an exploratory proof-of-mechanism study. Lancet Oncol 2012;13:1133–40.
[56] Dickson MA, Tap WD, Keohan ML, et al. Phase II trial of the CDK4 inhibitor PD0332991 in patients with advanced CDK4-amplified well-differentiated or dedifferentiated liposarcoma. J Clin Oncol 2013;31:2024–8.
[57] Barretina J, Taylor BS, Banerji S, et al. Subtype-specific genomic alterations define new targets for soft-tissue sarcoma therapy. Nat Genet 2010;42:715–21.
[58] Crozat A, Aman P, Mandahl N, et al. Fusion of CHOP to a novel RNA-binding protein in human myxoid liposarcoma. Nature 1993;363:640–4.
[59] Clark J, Rocques PJ, Crew AJ, et al. Identification of novel genes, SYT and SSX, involved in the t(X;18)(p11.2;q11.2) translocation found in human synovial sarcoma. Nat Genet 1994;7:502–8.
[60] Alman BA, Li C, Pajerski ME, et al. Increased beta-catenin protein and somatic APC mutations in sporadic aggressive fibromatoses (desmoid tumors). Am J Pathol 1997;151: 329–34.
[61] Chmielecki J, Crago AM, Rosenberg M, et al. Whole-exome sequencing identifies a recurrent NAB2-STAT6 fusion in solitary fibrous tumors. Nat Genet 2013;45:131–2.
[62] Robinson DR, Wu YM, Kalyana-Sundaram S, et al. Identification of recurrent NAB2-STAT6 gene fusions in solitary fibrous tumor by integrative sequencing. Nat Genet 2013;45: 180–5.
[63] Hirota S, Isozaki K, Moriyama Y, et al. Gain-of-function mutations of c-kit in human gastrointestinal stromal tumors. Science 1998;279:577–80.

Advances in Surgery 49 (2015) 123–129

ADVANCES IN SURGERY

Hospital Accreditation and Bariatric Surgery: Is It Important?

Juan J. Blondet, MD[a], John M. Morton, MD, MPH[b], Ninh T. Nguyen, MD[a,*]

[a]University of California Irvine Medical Center, 333 City Boulevard West, Suite 1600, Orange, CA 92868, USA; [b]Bariatric and Minimally Invasive Surgery, Stanford School of Medicine, 300 Pasteur Drive, H3680, Stanford, CA 94305, USA

Keywords

• Bariatric surgery accreditation • Center of excellence • ASMBS • CMS • MBSAQIP • Surgical outcomes

Key points

- National facility accreditation in bariatric surgery was first implemented in 2004 by the American Society for Metabolic and Bariatric Surgery and by the American College of Surgeons in 2005.
- Accreditation in bariatric surgery signifies that the center has the infrastructure and equipment to care for the morbidly obese, has experienced and qualified staff and surgeons, and participates in 100% data reporting and quality improvement initiatives.
- Substantial data have shown that the presence of bariatric facility accreditation is associated with improved outcomes.

INTRODUCTION

Bariatric surgery is the most effective therapy for the treatment of individuals with severe obesity. The implementation of laparoscopy in the late 1990s revolutionized bariatric surgery. Between 1998 and 2003, there was exponential growth in the number of bariatric operations being performed in the United States [1]. With reduction in the invasiveness of the operation, more patients were willing to undergo bariatric surgery. Bariatric surgery is now one of the most common gastrointestinal surgical procedures. During the early 2000s, there were questions regarding the safety of bariatric surgery [2]. Individual

The authors have nothing to disclose.

*Corresponding author. *E-mail address:* ninhn@uci.edu

0065-3411/15/$ – see front matter
http://dx.doi.org/10.1016/j.yasu.2015.03.012

third-party payers then initiated their own centers of excellence (COE) to improve the quality of care for patients undergoing bariatric surgery. A major consideration in the COE concept is the relationship between hospital case volume and outcomes. Multiple studies have reported lower morbidity and mortality associated with bariatric surgery when performed at high-volume centers. Using the volume and outcome relationship in bariatric surgery as the basis, the concept of bariatric surgery accreditation was first developed by the American Society for Metabolic and Bariatric Surgery (ASMBS) and the American College of Surgeons (ACS). This article reviews the relationship between volume and outcomes in bariatric surgery, the history of bariatric surgery accreditation, components of facility accreditation, and data regarding the value of accreditation.

Relationship between volume and outcomes in bariatric surgery

Bariatric surgery, particularly Roux-en-Y gastric bypass, is a complex operation performed in a high-risk patient population with many comorbid conditions. The complexity of the procedure and patient population lead investigators to evaluate for modifiable and nonmodifiable factors predictive of morbidity and mortality. One of these factors is the hospital or surgeon annual case volume. The volume and outcome relationship is well known in several high-risk, complex operations, such as esophagectomy, pancreatectomy, abdominal aortic aneurysm repair, and coronary bypass grafting. The premise behind the volume and outcome relationship is that patients treated at high-volume centers or by high-volume surgeons tend to have better outcomes than patients treated at low-volume hospitals [3].

Several studies have been published showing a relationship between hospital volume and outcomes in bariatric surgery [4–7]. In 2004, Nguyen and colleagues [5] reported that Roux-en-Y gastric bypass performed at hospitals with more than 100 cases annually is associated with a shorter length of stay, lower morbidity and mortality, and decreased costs. In a comprehensive systematic review of the literature published in 2012, Zevin and colleagues [7] analyzed 24 studies with a total of 458,032 bariatric patients and found a strong positive association between annual hospital volume and patient outcomes in 14 of 17 studies. More recently, using the Nationwide Inpatient Sample (NIS) database, Jafari and colleagues [4] analyzed 277,760 laparoscopic stapling bariatric procedures (laparoscopic Roux-en-Y gastric bypass and laparoscopic sleeve gastrectomy) performed between 2006 and 2010 and compared the outcomes between low-volume centers (centers performing <50 stapling bariatric cases per year) and high-volume centers (centers performing 50 or more stapling bariatric cases per year). They found that in the laparoscopic era, the in-hospital mortality rate was higher at low-volume centers (0.17%) than at high-volume centers (0.07%). Multivariate analysis showed that low-volume centers had higher rates of mortality (odds ratio [OR], 2.5; 95% confidence interval, 1.3–4.8; $P<.01$) and serious morbidity (OR, 1.2; 95% confidence interval, 1.1–1.4; $P<.01$).

In contrast to hospital annual volume, other studies have shown a linear relationship between an annual surgeon's volume and outcomes in bariatric surgery. In the Zevin and colleagues [7] systematic review, they found a strong positive association between annual surgeon volume and patient outcomes in 11 of 13 studies. In a study from the Longitudinal Assessment of Bariatric Surgery, Smith and colleagues [8] found that for every 10 cases per year increase in surgeon volume, the adjusted risk ratio for an adverse composite event (defined as venous thromboembolism, pulmonary embolism, reoperation, nondischarge at 30 days, rehospitalization within 30 days, or death) decreased by 10%.

HISTORY OF ACCREDITATION

In 2004, the ASMBS initiated the COE concept to improve safety and quality in bariatric surgery in response to the increasing number of bariatric surgeries being performed in the United States. This initiative was followed by the creation of the ACS Bariatric Surgery Center Network (BSCN) in 2005 [9]. Both of these initiatives developed structure and processes that focused on establishing an infrastructure to care for the morbidly obese that included a multidisciplinary team, streamline standards of practice, a threshold of 125 bariatric cases per year, experienced staff and surgeons, and establishing a prospective database for collection of patient-level data. In 2006, national bariatric accreditation was adopted by the Centers for Medicare and Medicaid Services (CMS) within the National Coverage Determination (NCD) in bariatric surgery. The CMS bariatric surgery decision mandated Medicare patients to undergo bariatric surgery only at accredited centers, but this decision was later overturned in 2013. Bariatric facility accreditation also became widely accepted and supported by insurance companies as the baseline for participation in their networks including Blue Cross Blue Shield, Optum, Aetna, and Cigna, to name a few. In 2012, the two national bariatric accreditation programs (ASMBS-COE and ACS-BSCN) unified into a single program: the Metabolic and Bariatric Surgery Accreditation and Quality Improvement Program (MBSAQIP). MBSAQIP focuses on providing standards that allow for wider participation by new programs, provides well-defined data definitions and standardized collection methods consistent with the ACS National Surgical Quality Improvement Program standards, instituted 100% case reporting, and created a framework for local and regional collaboration to improve outcomes through the local institutional Metabolic and Bariatric Surgery Committees [10].

In September of 2013, CMS decided to drop the requirement for bariatric surgery accreditation largely because of concerns of limiting access to bariatric surgery [11]. Even before this decision was implemented, multiple publications in the literature have been trying to address the fundamental questions regarding the value of accreditation: does accreditation improve quality, and lower morbidity, mortality, and costs? And does accreditation establish a culture of safety and quality improvement? In contrast, a major argument against accreditation is the issue that requirement for bariatric surgery to only be performed at accredited centers may lead to an unintended consequence of impeding access to care.

Components of accreditation

The original ASMBS COE had a single level of accreditation with 10 criteria that included institutional commitment to in-service education, facility volume of at least 125 cases per year, a designated bariatric medical director, full consultative staff and critical care services, full line of bariatric equipment and instruments, qualified bariatric surgeons, standardized perioperative care pathways, designated nurse or physician extenders, availability of support groups, and a system for long-term follow-up and outcome reporting. The original ACS BSCN had two levels of accreditation. A level 1 bariatric surgery center performed at least 125 weight loss operations annually, with at least two experienced and credentialed bariatric surgeons capable of managing complex bariatric patients. A level 2 bariatric surgery center provided high-quality care with a lower volume of annual cases (a minimum of 25 per year) limited to lower-risk patients (ie, patients with lower body mass index) and no elective revisional cases. In the current MBSAQIP accreditation there are four designations: (1) comprehensive, (2) low acuity, (3) band center, and (4) adolescent center. Comprehensive center designation is the most common designation. This designation requires a facility to have a minimum of 50 stapling cases per year, a commitment to quality care, appropriate equipment and instruments, presence of critical care support, continuum of care and commitment to long-term follow-up, data collection of 100% of cases, and a continuous quality improvement process. Currently there are more than 700 accredited bariatric surgery centers in the United States and Canada [12].

Data regarding accreditation

The advantages of participation in an accreditation program are the establishment of a uniform structure, processes of care, and collection of prospective data. Outcomes of individual centers can be compared with the national average and centers with outliers in morbidity or mortality can be identified, and feedback may result in interventions to improve outcomes. Many studies have been published on the outcomes of bariatric surgery performed at accredited versus nonaccredited centers and also on the outcomes of bariatric surgery performed before versus after initiation of the Medicare NCD in 2006. Discussed next are relevant data supporting accreditation and data against accreditation.

Data supporting accreditation

Using the University Health Consortium database, Nguyen and colleagues [13] analyzed 35,284 bariatric operations and found that bariatric surgery performed at accredited centers was associated with shorter length of stay (mean difference, 0.3 days), lower mortality (0.06% accredited vs 0.21% nonaccredited), and lower cost (mean difference of $3758). Similarly, Kwon and colleagues [14] used the national MarketScan Commercial Claims and Encounter

Database to show that accredited centers had significant reduction in inpatient mortality, 90-day reoperations, complications, and readmissions. Using the NIS database Jafari and colleagues [4] analyzed 277,760 laparoscopic stapling bariatric procedures and showed that high-volume centers (centers performing 50 or more stapling cases per year) that were also accredited COE had significantly lower in-hospital mortality but higher rate of serious morbidity compared with nonaccredited centers. This combination of lower complications but higher mortality at nonaccredited centers may suggest that patients experiencing complications at nonaccredited centers are more likely to die from their complications. This may represent a concept previously described as "failure to rescue."

Recently, three more studies were published supporting the role of bariatric center accreditation. Morton and colleagues [15] used the 2010 NIS database and found that compared with accredited centers, nonaccredited centers had a higher mean length of stay (2.25 vs 1.99 days), higher total charges ($51,189 vs $42,212), higher incidence of complications (12.3% vs 11.3%), higher mortality (0.13% vs 0.07%), and higher rate of "failure to rescue" (0.97% vs 0.55%). Using a multivariate logistic regression analysis they identified that nonaccredited status was a positive predictor for higher incidence of complications and mortality. Another study from Young and colleagues [16] evaluated outcomes of 775,040 bariatric surgical patients performed over a 10-year period (2001–2010) using the NIS database. Compared with Medicare patients who underwent bariatric surgery before the 2006 Medicare NCD, Medicare patients who underwent bariatric surgery after the NCD had a 59% (statistically significant) reduction of in-hospital mortality. They also found that since the 2006 NCD, access to bariatric surgery does not seem to be an issue because the number of bariatric procedures performed in Medicare beneficiaries increased by 71%. They similarly found improvements in in-hospital mortality and serious morbidity when bariatric surgery was performed at accredited compared with nonaccredited centers. Lastly, Gebhart and colleagues [17] reported that resources established for bariatric surgery accreditation may have the secondary benefit of improving outcomes for morbidly obese patients undergoing other general laparoscopic operations. Using the NIS database between 2008 and 2011, they analyzed 277,068 bariatric operations. Multivariate analysis showed that morbidly obese patients who underwent laparoscopic cholecystectomy (OR, 2.4; $P<.05$) and antireflux surgery (OR, 2.03; $P<.01$) at nonaccredited bariatric surgery centers had higher rates of serious complications compared with patients who underwent these operations at accredited centers.

Data against accreditation

Three studies have been cited against bariatric surgery accreditation. The first study by Livingston [18] examined the 2005 NIS database and found no difference in morbidity and mortality between the 24 COE versus the 229 non-COE. A major limitation of this study is the premature analysis of the effect of accreditation on outcomes because accreditation only started in 2004. By

2005, only a small number of centers had achieved accreditation (only 6% of the centers were COE in the study). The second study by Birkmeyer and colleagues [19] compared 17 accredited with 8 nonaccredited centers in the Michigan Bariatric Surgery Collaborative (MBSC) and found no significant difference in the rate of serious complications (2.7% accredited vs 2.0% nonaccredited). The main limitation of this study is that all hospitals in Michigan participating within the MBSC require an annual volume of 25 cases and participate in data submission and quality improvement efforts. Therefore, the nonaccredited centers within the MBSC have structure and processes that are similar to that of accredited centers. Finally, Dimick and colleagues [20] compared the outcomes of Medicare beneficiaries before versus after the NCD and used the non-Medicare population as a control. They found a significant reduction of serious complication rates after the NCD for both Medicare and non-Medicare patients. When taking the trends in improvement of outcomes from the non-Medicare population into account, they concluded that there was no significant difference in the rate of complications before versus after the NCD. The non-Medicare population is a poor control group, however, because the non-Medicare patient population was similarly exposed to the accreditation process at around the same time period and improvement in outcomes in this population might be related to the initiation of accreditation by the ASMBS and ACS. Another limitation of this study was that mortality was not analyzed, even though mortality has been shown to be the most accurate end point within administrative data.

SUMMARY

National facility accreditation in bariatric surgery was first implemented in 2004 by the ASMBS and by the ACS in 2005. The two programs unified to a single program in 2012: the MBSAQIP. Accreditation in bariatric surgery signifies that the center has the infrastructure and equipment to care for the morbidly obese, has experienced and qualified staff and surgeons, has standardized clinical pathways, and participates in 100% data reporting and quality improvement initiatives. Substantial data have shown that the presence of bariatric facility accreditation is associated with improved outcomes. Now that there are more than 700 accredited centers in the United States and Canada, accreditation of metabolic and bariatric surgery is here to stay.

References

[1] Nguyen NT, Masoomi H, Magno CP, et al. Trends in use of bariatric surgery, 2003–2008. J Am Coll Surg 2011;213(2):261–6.

[2] Flum DR, Salem L, Elrod JA, et al. Early mortality among Medicare beneficiaries undergoing bariatric surgical procedures. JAMA 2005;294(15):1903–8.

[3] Nguyen NT, Higa K, Wilson SE. Improving the quality of care in bariatric surgery: the volume and outcome relationship. Adv Surg 2005;39:181–91.

[4] Jafari MD, Jafari F, Young MT, et al. Volume and outcome relationship in bariatric surgery in the laparoscopic era. Surg Endosc 2013;27:4539–46.

[5] Nguyen NT, Paya M, Stevens CM, et al. The relationship between hospital volume and outcome in bariatric surgery at academic medical centers. Ann Surg 2004;240(4): 586–93 [discussion: 593–4].
[6] Ballantyne GH, Belsley S, Stephens D, et al. Bariatric surgery: low mortality at high-volume center. Obes Surg 2008;18:660–7.
[7] Zevin B, Aggarwal R, Grantcharov TP. Volume-outcome association in bariatric surgery: a systematic review. Ann Surg 2012;256:60–71.
[8] Smith MD, Patterson E, Wahed AS, et al. Relationship between surgeon volume and adverse outcomes after RYGB in Longitudinal Assessment of Bariatric Surgery (LABS) study. Surg Obes Relat Dis 2010;6(2):118–25.
[9] Champion JK, Pories WJ. Centers of excellence for bariatric surgery. Surg Obes Relat Dis 2005;1(2):148–51.
[10] Blackstone R, Dimick JB, Nguyen NT. Accreditation in metabolic and bariatric surgery: pro versus con. Surg Obes Relat Dis 2014;10(2):198–202.
[11] Proceedings of the National Coverage Analysis (NCA) for Bariatric Surgery for the Treatment of Morbid Obesity – Facility Certification Requirement (CAG-00250 R3). 2013.
[12] Metabolic and Bariatric Surgery Accreditation and Quality Improvement Program. American College of Surgeons and American Society for Metabolic and Bariatric Surgery. Available at: http://www.facs.org/quality-programs/mbsaqip. Accessed November 12, 2014.
[13] Nguyen NT, Nguyen B, Nguyen VQ, et al. Outcomes of bariatric surgery performed at accredited vs nonaccredited centers. J Am Coll Surg 2012;215:467–74.
[14] Kwon S, Wang B, Wong E, et al. The impact of accreditation on safety and cost of bariatric surgery. Surg Obes Relat Dis 2013;9:617–22.
[15] Morton JM, Garg T, Nguyen N. Does hospital accreditation impact bariatric surgery safety? Ann Surg 2014;260(3):504–8 [discussion: 508–9].
[16] Young MT, Jafari MD, Gebhart A, et al. A decade analysis of trends and outcomes of bariatric surgery in Medicare beneficiaries. J Am Coll Surg 2014;219(3):480–8.
[17] Gebhart A, Young M, Phelan M, et al. Impact of accreditation in bariatric surgery. Surg Obes Relat Dis 2014;10(5):767–73.
[18] Livingston EH. Bariatric surgery outcomes at designated centers of excellence vs nondesignated programs. Arch Surg 2009;144(4):319–25.
[19] Birkmeyer NJ, Dimick JB, Share D, et al. Hospital complication rates with bariatric surgery in Michigan. JAMA 2010;304(4):435–42.
[20] Dimick JB, Nicholas LH, Ryan AM, et al. Bariatric surgery complications before vs after implementation of a national policy restricting coverage to centers of excellence. JAMA 2013;309(8):792–9.

Advances in Surgery 49 (2015) 131–141

ADVANCES IN SURGERY

Trainee Participation in Emergency Surgery

What Are the Consequences?

George Kasotakis, MD, MPH[a,*], Gerard Doherty, MD[b]

[a]Section of Trauma, Acute Care Surgery & Surgical Critical Care, Department of Surgery, Boston Medical Center, Boston University School of Medicine, 840 Harrison Avenue, Dowling 2 South, Suite #2414, Boston, MA 02118, USA; [b]Department of Surgery, Boston Medical Center, Boston University School of Medicine, 88 East Newton Street, Suite C500, Boston, MA 02118, USA

Keywords

• Emergency surgery • Residents • Trainees • Outcomes
• Graduate medical education • Operative time • Supervision

Key points

- Research on the effect of surgical trainee involvement in emergency surgery is mostly retrospective, and focuses on mostly safe, common procedures (appendectomy, cholecystectomy).
- Resident participation in emergency general surgery is associated with longer operative times, and possibly a small increase in postoperative complications.
- Resident involvement does not appear to affect mortality after emergency surgery, although its effect on hospital length of stay is unclear; when length of stay is prolonged, it appears that costs also increase.

INTRODUCTION

The enactment of the Patient Protection and Affordable Care Act of 2010 has significantly expanded medical coverage [1], whereas an aging population with a greater number of chronic conditions, coupled with only a modest projected expansion in the physician workforce, has led to a widening gap in the clinician supply-and-demand equation [2,3]. At the epicenter of this conundrum is graduate medical education, which is tasked to balance two important needs: provide affordable, efficient, and quality health care to those who need it, and at the same time safely train junior physicians in their specialty of choice. Extensive research has demonstrated both beneficial and adverse effects associated with resident participation in many fields of medicine, including, but not

*Corresponding author. *E-mail address*: gkasot@bu.edu

0065-3411/15/$ – see front matter
http://dx.doi.org/10.1016/j.yasu.2015.04.001

limited to, radiology [4], cardiology [5], gastrointestinal medicine [6], and elective surgery [7–10]. Polanczyk and colleagues [11] demonstrated lower mortality after acute coronary events at teaching institutions, and Buchner and colleagues [6] demonstrated higher colonic malignancy-detection rates in endoscopies performed with resident involvement. Contrary to these reports, however, a substantial body of evidence suggests that trainee participation may be associated with adverse outcomes. In a study investigating the diagnostic competency of radiology residents, most junior trainees misidentified prominent trauma abnormalities on imaging [4], and in primary care, adverse outcomes have been linked to more prescribing errors made by junior trainees compared with their senior counterparts [12].

Among the most commonly cited factors for adverse outcomes when trainees are involved are lack of experience and inadequate supervision. These aspects may be even more pronounced in surgical training programs, in which trainees' lack of sophisticated technical skills, experience, and familiarity with complex procedures and evolving surgical technologies may play important roles [7,13]. A growing body of evidence suggests that surgical procedures tend to require longer operative times when trainees are involved, with a small, yet appreciable effect on clinical outcomes related to the longer operating room (OR) stay [14–16]. On the other hand, it appears that resident participation may improve outcomes when complications arise postoperatively, as more health care professionals assess patients with increased frequency, allowing early recognition of potential clinical deterioration [17,18].

The question remains, however, what the trainee effect is in patients undergoing *emergency* surgery. The unique characteristic of this type of surgical intervention is that time is of the essence: total time from presentation to definitive source control may affect outcomes to a greater extent than seen in elective surgery, as an appreciably deranged host physiology and prolongation of the inflammatory phase may exert their deleterious effects [19]. With this article, we aim to review currently available literature on the "resident effect" on outcomes in patients undergoing *emergency* surgery.

SUMMARY OF THE "RESIDENT EFFECT" ON SPECIFIC OUTCOMES AND DISCUSSION

Effect of resident participation on operative time and postoperative morbidity

We recently demonstrated, through an extensive retrospective review and analysis of the American College of Surgeons National Surgical Quality Improvement Program (ACS-NSQIP), that residents required longer time in the OR to perform common emergency operations (75.1 ± 54.8 minutes vs 59.2 ± 44.8 minutes, $P<.001$), after matching our resident (RES) and no-resident (NO-RES) cohorts on patient demographic and clinical characteristics, as well as procedure-related factors [19]. A small increase in intraoperative and postoperative morbidity, such as unplanned returns to the OR, need for intraoperative transfusions, surgical site infections and sepsis, and pulmonary and thromboembolic complications, was also noted (Table 1). We also demonstrated that operative time was another important factor associated with intraoperative and postoperative transfusions; unplanned reoperations; and wound, pulmonary, infectious, and thromboembolic complications, adjusting for baseline comorbidities, case complexity, and resident participation. It appears that when trainees are involved, prolongation of the inflammatory state, OR time, immobility on the surgical table, and time on mechanical ventilation required for general anesthesia, may affect outcomes unfavorably. A limitation of our study, however, was lack of a 1-to-1 procedure matching in the RES and NO-RES

Table 1
Clinically relevant 30-day postoperative outcomes

	Matched cohort, n = 83,790		
Outcome	NO-RES, n = 41,895	RES, n = 41,895	*P* value
Mortality	2.96	3.25	.082
Length of stay	4.59 ± 7.98	4.97 ± 9.63	.019
Operative technique			
Operative time	59.17 ± 44.78	75.10 ± 54.77	<.001
Anesthesia time	99.92 ± 55.45	122.42 ± 66.22	<.001
Intraoperative transfusion	2.55	3.43	<.001
Postoperative bleed requiring transfusion	1.28	1.12	.031
Unplanned return to operating room	3.80	4.22	.002
Wound complications			
Superficial wound infection	2.78	3.50	<.001
Deep wound infection	0.89	0.73	.011
Organ space infection	1.77	2.27	<.001
Wound dehiscence	0.69	0.63	.266
Pulmonary complications			
Postoperative pneumonia	1.67	1.85	.043
Unplanned reintubation	1.15	1.64	<.001
Prolonged ventilation (>48 h)	2.06	2.87	<.001
Cardiovascular complications			
Myocardial infarction	0.26	0.27	.637
Cardiopulmonary arrest	0.32	0.39	.071
Cerebrovascular accident	0.13	0.16	.205
Deep venous thrombosis	0.62	0.80	.002
Pulmonary embolism	0.28	0.43	<.001
Renal complications			
Acute renal failure	0.31	0.34	.427
Renal failure requiring dialysis	0.43	0.37	.209
Urinary tract infection	1.14	1.45	<.001
Life-threatening infectious complications			
Sepsis	2.13	2.42	.005
Septic shock	1.41	1.51	.205

Abbreviations: NO-RES, no-resident cohort; RES, resident cohort.

Adapted from Kasotakis G, Lakha A, Sarkar B, et al. Trainee participation is associated with adverse outcomes in emergency general surgery: an analysis of the National Surgical Quality Improvement Program database. Ann Surg 2014;260:486; with permission.

groups. Scarborough and colleagues [20] similarly showed an increased incidence of serious and overall postoperative complications when appendectomies were performed with resident participation, adjusting for baseline comorbidities and total operative time. However, they demonstrated that operative times and risk for postoperative morbidity increased with postgraduate year of training, and attributed this effect to the increased level of autonomy senior residents enjoy in the operating theater. However, they did not risk-adjust these 2 outcomes in their analysis for such a conclusion to be definitively drawn. Contrasting this finding is the study by Papandria and colleagues [16], which also reviewed a subset of the ACS-NSQIP dataset. Papandria and colleagues [16] assessed the effect of resident participation on the 3 most commonly performed general surgery procedures, namely laparoscopic appendectomy and cholecystectomy, and open inguinal herniorrhaphy. Even though they did not investigate the trainee effect specifically on emergency procedures, most appendectomies were classified as emergent (>72%), and so were a significant number of cholecystectomies (>4000 cases) and inguinal herniorrhaphies (300). The investigators demonstrated longer operative times in all cases performed with resident involvement, even after controlling for potential confounders ($P<.001$). Interestingly, they did not find a difference in operative times between cases performed by junior versus senior residents, a result they ascribed to senior residents enjoying greater autonomy in the OR. In our own study, we found that operative times may indeed be prolonged when senior trainees are involved, but this seems to be a result of resident self-selection to more complex cases (Figs. 1 and 2). Similar results were echoed in other ACS-NSQIP analyses also, yet with more modest operative time and morbidity increases [21].

The group at the University of Texas at Austin established their surgical residency training program in 2009 and retrospectively studied the trainee effect on certain procedures, including laparoscopic and open cholecystectomies and appendectomies [22]. Although the investigators did not divide their cases into elective versus urgent ones, they demonstrated that, of the 4 procedures, only laparoscopic cholecystectomies took longer to perform when trainees were involved (71 ± 32 minutes RES vs 66 ± 28 minutes NO-RES, $P = .02$). However, the investigators did not adjust for case complexity, which may have been an important factor as evidenced by the wide SDs, or for attending seniority. The latter can be an important confounder also, as the increased efficiency in the OR that is expected of attending surgeons with growing experience, may counteract the lack of advanced laparoscopic skills of junior residents. A more consistent increase in operative times when trainees were involved was identified in a study by Castillo and colleagues [23] in a new surgical residency program in Florida. Even though the investigators did not divide laparoscopic cholecystectomies into elective versus urgent ones, they demonstrated a significant increase in operative time in both laparoscopic cholecystectomies and appendectomies whenever residents were involved (53.4 ± 19.9 minutes RES vs 37.2 ± 18.4 minutes NO-RES, $P<.001$, and 45.4 ± 14.6 minutes RES vs 30.6 ± 14.6 minutes NO-RES, $P<.001$, respectively).

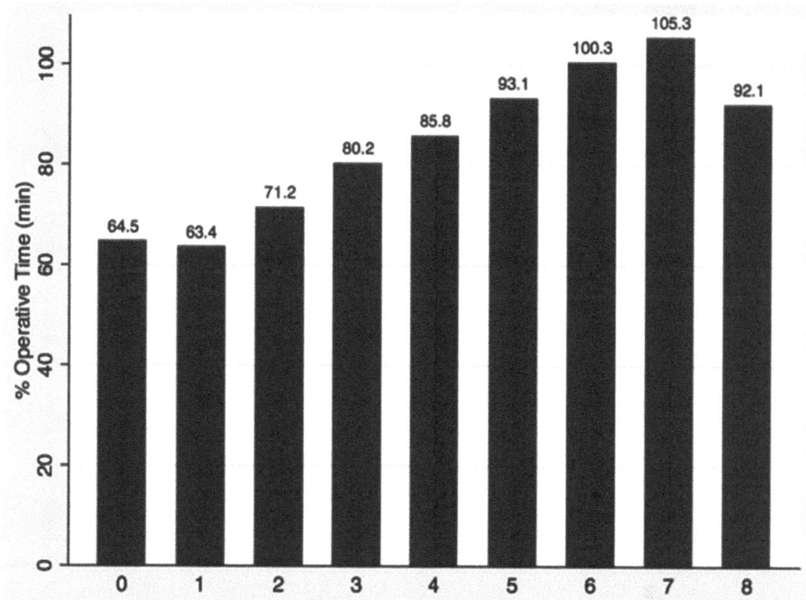

Fig. 1. Operative time (minutes) versus postgraduate year (year 0 corresponds to cases performed by attending surgeons alone). (*Adapted from* Kasotakis G, Lakha A, Sarkar B, et al. Trainee participation is associated with adverse outcomes in emergency general surgery: an analysis of the National Surgical Quality Improvement Program database. Ann Surg 2014;260:488; with permission.)

Looking specifically at appendectomies, Hwang and associates [24,25] also demonstrated that both laparoscopic and open appendectomies that were performed with resident involvement required longer time (58.9 minutes RES vs 44.4 minutes NO-RES, $P<.05$, and 63.3 minutes RES vs 48.0 minutes NO-RES, $P<.05$, respectively). This study, although also retrospective, occurred at a unique setting, where 2 groups of staff surgeons, 1 with resident coverage and 1 without, alternate call at the same institution and manage surgical emergencies as they present. This study also identified a higher complication rate in laparoscopic appendectomies when trainees were involved (5.9% vs 4.4%, $P<.05$) [25]. Although this setting may be ideal in helping eliminate patient and disease severity–related differences between the RES and NO-RES groups, a skill differential across the 2 attending groups may still exist. Graat and colleagues [26] also found residents required longer operative times if appendectomies were performed by unsupervised trainees compared with staff surgeons alone at a teaching institution in the Netherlands (50.0 ± 18.3 minutes RES vs 46.7 ± 17.1 minutes NO-RES, $P = .019$). The same study also found no difference in major complications, even though staff surgeons and supervised residents were more likely to operate on patients with higher American Society of Anesthesiology (ASA) class and with perforated appendicitis.

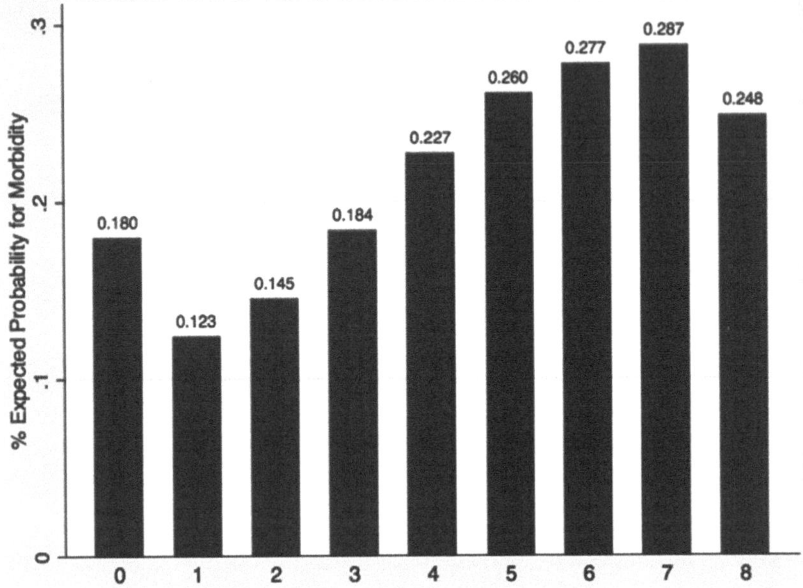

Fig. 2. Expected probability of morbidity versus postgraduate year (year 0 corresponds to cases performed by attending surgeons alone). (*Adapted from* Kasotakis G, Lakha A, Sarkar B, et al. Trainee participation is associated with adverse outcomes in emergency general surgery: an analysis of the National Surgical Quality Improvement Program database. Ann Surg 2014;260:488; with permission.)

When Naiditch and colleagues [27] and Mizrahi and colleagues [28] assessed the effect of trainee participation on pediatric laparoscopic appendectomies, they too found that longer operative times were needed in cases performed by junior residents. However, although the study by Naiditch and colleagues [27] demonstrated a greater incidence of organ space infection requiring intervention (odds ratio 2.31 compared with supervised junior residents, $P = .02$) when fellows were involved, Mizrahi and colleagues [28] did not identify a difference in overall complications (5% RES vs 7% NO-RES, $P = .29$) or readmission rates (2% RES vs 5% NO-RES, $P = .52$). Advani and colleagues [29] demonstrated both longer operative times for laparoscopic appendectomies when trainees participated (49 [interquartile range 38–64] minutes RES vs 35 [27–46] minutes NO-RES, $P < .001$), and greater incidence of overall and specific complications (Table 2).

Singh and colleagues [30], retrospectively analyzing a multicenter, prospectively collected dataset of appendectomies mostly from the United Kingdom, published one of the few studies that demonstrated higher morbidity (pelvic abscess) in cases performed by attending surgeons; however, it appears that these cases involved older subjects with higher ASA scores.

Table 2
Complication profile of laparoscopic appendectomies performed with and without resident involvement

Laparoscopic appendectomy	Resident involvement, n = 11,451, %	No resident involvement, n = 5398, %	*P* value
Serious morbidity	1.8	1.3	.01
Overall morbidity	3.7	2.8	.004
Return to the operating room	0.7	1	.03
Infectious complications	3	2	.01
Wound complications	3	2	.02
Cardiac complications	0.4	0.2	.02
Vascular complications	0.1	0.1	.96
Neurologic and renal complications	0.3	0.3	.48
Septic complications	0.7	0.5	.07

Adapted from Advani V, Ahad S, Gonczy C, et al. Does resident involvement effect surgical times and complication rates during laparoscopic appendectomy for uncomplicated appendicitis? An analysis of 16,849 cases from the ACS-NSQIP. Am J Surg 2012;203(3):349; with permission.

Regarding laparoscopic cholecystectomy, another commonly performed, occasionally urgent procedure, Kauvar and colleagues [31] demonstrated that junior residents took longer to complete the case compared with their senior counterparts and regardless of surgeon seniority. Similarly, Bencini and colleagues [14] showed that in their institution, laparoscopic cholecystectomies took longer when residents were involved (67 minutes RES vs 50 minutes NO-RES, $P<.001$), even though fewer additional procedures were required (3% RES vs 7% NO-RES, $P = .009$) and patients were less complicated in the trainee group (ASA group 3 or 4, 2% RES vs 8% NO-RES, $P = .04$). Thankfully, the incidence of iatrogenic bile duct injury was not found to be greater when residents were involved [32,33], even though, with such a rare complication, very large sample sizes would be needed, which both the aforementioned studies lack. Finally, Kauvar and associates [31] demonstrated that at the Brooke Army Medical Center in San Antonio, TX, resident seniority influenced operative time, and cases with junior resident assistance had a higher complication rate (5.6% RES vs 0.78% NO-RES, $P<.05$), most commonly cystic duct leak.

Effect of trainee involvement on mortality

Most literature on emergency surgery is concentrated on procedures with low mortality (typically appendectomies and cholecystectomies), and currently available data do not suggest an association between trainee participation and higher mortality after emergency surgery. Uecker and colleagues [22] showed no difference in mortality (0.17% RES vs 0.35% NO-RES, $P = .45$) in their studied appendectomized or cholecystectomized subjects, a finding that was also echoed in the article by Hwang and colleagues [24] (0% mortality for both cholecystectomies and appendectomies). In our review of a larger list of emergency operations, including procedures with non-negligible mortality (such as exploratory laparotomy, bowel resection, repair of perforated viscus, and abdominal wall hernia repairs), we noted a trend toward slightly higher mortality (3.25% RES vs 2.96% NO-RES, $P = .082$); however, this did not reach statistical significance [19]. One additional caveat of most currently available research is that essentially all studies assess in-hospital or 30-day deaths, not mortality that may have occurred outside this short window, and may still be associated with the index surgical disease or procedure.

Effect of resident participation on hospital length of stay and associated costs

The "resident effect" on hospital length of stay is somewhat more controversial, and conflicting reports suggesting an increase or shortening of the length of stay, or no effect whatsoever, all exist. Uecker and associates [22] demonstrated that shorter hospital stays were achieved after the establishment of the residency program (2.6 days RES vs 3.7 days NO-RES, $P < .001$), a finding they attributed to a greater number of health care providers rounding on patients more frequently and helping their care move along. However, improvements in the quality of care and hospital/OR workflow efficiency that typically occur with time in mature institutions were not looked into. Mizrahi and colleagues [28] reported a similar finding in pediatric patients after appendectomy when trainees were involved (4.0 ± 0.2 days RES vs 4.5 ± 0.2 days NO-RES, $P = .03$).

On the other hand, Hwang and colleagues [24,25] demonstrated that resident involvement was associated with longer hospital stays in 5 index procedures, which included cholecystectomy and appendectomy, and higher costs, when procedures were performed by staff surgeons who had resident coverage. They attributed the increased costs to the longer hospital stays, as resource utilization was otherwise largely similar in the 2 groups. However, attending seniority and efficiency metrics were not assessed, and emergency procedures were lumped with elective ones.

In contrast, Kazaure and colleagues [21] demonstrated that, after adjusting for patient baseline characteristics and operative factors, there was no resident effect on hospital length of stay. Similarly, even though we identified a minimal increase in length of stay of questionable clinical significance (4.97 ± 9.63 days RES vs 4.59 ± 7.98 days NO-RES, $P = .019$), in our multivariate analysis, trainee involvement was not identified as an independent risk factor for longer hospital stays (odds ratio 0.07, 95% confidence interval −0.04–0.17, $P = .242$), when patient characteristics and procedure-related factors were controlled for [19]. Reconciling these findings, it is unlikely that resident participation significantly affects length of stay in a meaningful way, but when it does, higher costs are likely incurred.

Issues with current research and summary

Even though the main associations with various clinical outcomes when surgical residents are involved in emergency procedures were stated earlier, it has to be remembered that the quality of currently available evidence, from which these conclusions were drawn, is mediocre. Essentially all research is based on retrospective, observational reviews or secondary analyses of prospectively collected databases that were not specifically designed to assess the "resident effect." In the era of the 80-hour work week and the resulting restricted operative time for surgical trainees, conducting a prospective trial in which subjects are randomized to resident or no-resident involvement would be unethical and likely to be met with upheaval from the trainee bodies. In addition, a large body of evidence is derived from analysis of data from the ACS-NSQIP database, which although well validated and highly reliable, are skewed toward larger, tertiary medical centers that perform more complex procedures, whereas smaller hospitals may be underrepresented. The residents' autonomy and how it is recorded is subject to significant observation bias, and in addition may fluctuate significantly depending on case complexity (trainees may enjoy much greater autonomy in the OR in abscess-drainage procedures and appendectomies, for example, as opposed to colon resections for malignancy or laparotomies for hollow viscus perforations). Finally, a large number of studies either lump urgent and emergency procedures with elective ones, or assess the effect of trainee participation on relatively safe procedures (appendectomies, cholecystectomies).

Keeping these limitations in mind, currently available data suggest that resident involvement is associated with longer operative times, and possibly a small increase in postoperative complications (pulmonary, wound-related, and thromboembolic) as a direct consequence of the prolonged time under general anesthesia, immobility, and wound exposure. This effect is likely more pronounced in emergency surgery, as patients are already typically in an inflammatory state and frequently underresuscitated and underfed, compared with their elective counterparts. While still in this inflammatory phase, they receive an additional inflammatory insult (that of surgery) that appears to account for the outcome differential between emergency and elective procedures. Unnecessary prolongation of this secondary insult may be the link to the slightly worse outcomes when trainees are involved. Surgery resident involvement does not appear to adversely affect mortality, whereas the effect on hospital length of stay is still a topic of debate.

References

[1] Blumenthal D, Collins SR. Health care coverage under the affordable care act–a progress report. N Engl J Med 2014;371:275–81.
[2] Grover A, Niecko-Najjum LM. Physician workforce planning in an era of health care reform. Acad Med 2013;88:1822–6.
[3] Dall TM, Gallo PD, Chakrabarti R, et al. An aging population and growing disease burden will require a large and specialized health care workforce by 2025. Health Aff 2013;32:2013–20.
[4] McLauchlan CA, Jones K, Guly HR. Interpretation of trauma radiographs by junior doctors in accident and emergency departments: a cause for concern? J Accid Emerg Med 1997;14:295–8.

[5] Sandhu A, Moscucci M, Dixon S, et al. Differences in the outcome of patients undergoing percutaneous coronary interventions at teaching versus non-teaching hospitals. Am Heart J 2013;166:401–8.
[6] Buchner AM, Shahid MW, Heckman MG, et al. Trainee participation is associated with increased small adenoma detection. Gastrointest Endosc 2011;73:1223–31.
[7] Davis SS Jr, Husain FA, Lin E, et al. Resident participation in index laparoscopic general surgical cases: impact of the learning environment on surgical outcomes. J Am Coll Surg 2013;216:96–104.
[8] Iannuzzi JC, Chandra A, Rickles AS, et al. Resident involvement is associated with worse outcomes after major lower extremity amputation. J Vasc Surg 2013;58: 827–31.e1.
[9] Iannuzzi JC, Rickles AS, Deeb AP, et al. Outcomes associated with resident involvement in partial colectomy. Dis Colon Rectum 2013;56:212–8.
[10] Kern SQ, Lustik MB, McMann LP, et al. Comparison of outcomes after minimally invasive versus open partial nephrectomy with respect to trainee involvement utilizing the American College of Surgeons National Surgical Quality Improvement Program. J Endourol 2014;28: 40–7.
[11] Polanczyk CA, Lane A, Coburn M, et al. Hospital outcomes in major teaching, minor teaching, and nonteaching hospitals in New York State. Am J Med 2002;112:255–61.
[12] Ryan C, Ross S, Davey P, et al. Prevalence and causes of prescribing errors: the PRescribing Outcomes for Trainee Doctors Engaged in Clinical Training (PROTECT) study. PLoS One 2014;9:e79802.
[13] Tseng WH, Jin L, Canter RJ, et al. Surgical resident involvement is safe for common elective general surgery procedures. J Am Coll Surg 2011;213:19–26 [discussion: 26–8].
[14] Bencini L, Bernini M, Martini F, et al. Safety of laparoscopic cholecystectomy performed by surgical residents. Chir Ital 2008;60:819–24.
[15] Kiran RP, Ahmed Ali U, Coffey JC, et al. Impact of resident participation in surgical operations on postoperative outcomes: National Surgical Quality Improvement Program. Ann Surg 2012;256:469–75.
[16] Papandria D, Rhee D, Ortega G, et al. Assessing trainee impact on operative time for common general surgical procedures in ACS-NSQIP. J Surg Educ 2012;69:149–55.
[17] Ferraris VA, Bolanos M, Martin JT, et al. Identification of patients with postoperative complications who are at risk for failure to rescue. JAMA Surg 2014;149(11):1103–8.
[18] Bukur M, Singer MB, Chung R, et al. Influence of resident involvement on trauma care outcomes. Arch Surg 2012;147:856–62.
[19] Kasotakis G, Lakha A, Sarkar B, et al. Trainee participation is associated with adverse outcomes in emergency general surgery: an analysis of the National Surgical Quality Improvement Program database. Ann Surg 2014;260:483–90 [discussion: 90–3].
[20] Scarborough JE, Bennett KM, Pappas TN. Defining the impact of resident participation on outcomes after appendectomy. Ann Surg 2012;255:577–82.
[21] Kazaure HS, Roman SA, Sosa JA. The resident as surgeon: an analysis of ACS-NSQIP. J Surg Res 2012;178:126–32.
[22] Uecker J, Luftman K, Ali S, et al. Comparable operative times with and without surgery resident participation. J Surg Educ 2013;70:696–9.
[23] Castillo A, Zarak A, Kozol RA. Does a new surgical residency program increase operating room times? J Surg Educ 2013;70:700–2.
[24] Hwang CS, Pagano CR, Wichterman KA, et al. Resident versus no resident: a single institutional study on operative complications, mortality, and cost. Surgery 2008;144:339–44.
[25] Hwang CS, Wichterman KA, Alfrey EJ. The cost of resident education. J Surg Res 2010;163:18–23.
[26] Graat LJ, Bosma E, Roukema JA, et al. Appendectomy by residents is safe and not associated with a higher incidence of complications: a retrospective cohort study. Ann Surg 2012;255: 715–9.

[27] Naiditch JA, Lautz TB, Raval MV, et al. Effect of resident postgraduate year on outcomes after laparoscopic appendectomy for appendicitis in children. J Laparoendosc Adv Surg Tech A 2012;22:715–9.
[28] Mizrahi I, Mazeh H, Levy Y, et al. Comparison of pediatric appendectomy outcomes between pediatric surgeons and general surgery residents. J Surg Res 2013;180:185–90.
[29] Advani V, Ahad S, Gonczy C, et al. Does resident involvement effect surgical times and complication rates during laparoscopic appendectomy for uncomplicated appendicitis? An analysis of 16,849 cases from the ACS-NSQIP. Am J Surg 2012;203:347–51 [discussion 51–2].
[30] Singh P, Turner EJ, Cornish J, et al, National Surgical Research Collaborative. Safety assessment of resident grade and supervision level during emergency appendectomy: analysis of a multicenter, prospective study. Surgery 2014;156:28–38.
[31] Kauvar DS, Braswell A, Brown BD, et al. Influence of resident and attending surgeon seniority on operative performance in laparoscopic cholecystectomy. J Surg Res 2006;132:159–63.
[32] Schwartz SI, Yaghoubian AT, Andacheh ID, et al. Senior residents as teaching assistants during laparoscopic cholecystectomy in the 80-hour workweek era: effect on biliary injury and overall complication rates. J Surg Educ 2013;70:796–9.
[33] Harrison VL, Dolan JP, Pham TH, et al. Bile duct injury after laparoscopic cholecystectomy in hospitals with and without surgical residency programs: is there a difference? Surg Endosc 2011;25:1969–74.

Advances in Surgery 49 (2015) 143–156

ADVANCES IN SURGERY

ELSEVIER
MOSBY

Laparoscopic Pancreaticoduodenectomy

Is It an Effective Procedure for Pancreatic Ductal Adenocarcinoma?

May C. Tee, MD, MPH, Michael L. Kendrick, MD, Michael B. Farnell, MD*

Section of Hepato-Pancreatic-Biliary Surgery, Division of Subspecialty General Surgery, Department of Surgery, Mayo Clinic, 200 First Street Southwest, Rochester, MN 55905, USA

Keywords

- Laparoscopic pancreaticoduodenectomy/Whipple procedure
- Oncologic outcomes • Technical safety

Key points

- Laparoscopic pancreaticoduodenectomy is a safe procedure with comparable perioperative morbidity and mortality to open pancreaticoduodenectomy.
- Evidence consistently shows decreased length of hospital stay and less blood loss with laparoscopic compared with open pancreaticoduodenectomy.
- Short-term oncologic outcomes following laparoscopic pancreaticoduodenectomy are equivalent and possibly superior to open pancreaticoduodenectomy.
- Long-term oncologic outcomes following laparoscopic pancreaticoduodenectomy are equivalent with no difference in overall survival and possibly improved disease-free survival with laparoscopic compared with open pancreaticoduodenectomy.

INTRODUCTION

Evolution of laparoscopic pancreaticoduodenectomy

Since the first reported pancreaticoduodenectomy (PD) by Whipple in 1935 [1], several advances have been observed with standard open PD [2,3] and minimally invasive approaches to pancreatic surgery [4]. Although laparoscopy has been performed on nearly every abdominal organ, the first minimally

The authors have nothing to disclose.

*Corresponding author. *E-mail address:* mfarnell@mayo.edu

0065-3411/15/$ – see front matter
http://dx.doi.org/10.1016/j.yasu.2015.03.003

invasive PD was not reported until 1994 by Gagner and Pomp [5]. The first laparoscopic PD was performed electively in Canada on a patient with pancreatic divisum and chronic pancreatitis [5]. Operative time was more than 10 hours and length of stay was 30 days because of a postoperative course that was complicated by jejunal ulceration and delayed gastric emptying [5]. This laparoscopic PD was subsequently followed by a case series (n = 23 of laparoscopic pancreatectomies, 10 of which were laparoscopic PD) that reported a 40% conversion rate, average operative time of 8.5 hours, and length of stay of 22 days [6]. No clear benefit of laparoscopic PD was demonstrated, leading the authors to conclude that there was minimal value added of laparoscopic compared with open PD [6].

Subsequent groups have since supported the safety and efficacy of totally laparoscopic PD (TLPD) [7–9]. Palanivelu and colleagues [9] reported a retrospective case series of 42 patients undergoing elective TLPD and demonstrated a mean operative time of 370 minutes, 10.2-day length of stay, 30% perioperative morbidity, 2% perioperative mortality, and a 5-year overall survival of 30% in patients with pancreatic malignancy. This engendered enthusiasm and larger case series were subsequently reported [7–9]. Kendrick and Cusati [8] reviewed 62 patients undergoing laparoscopic PD for all indications and reported a mean operative time of 368 minutes, 10-day median length of stay, 18% pancreatic fistula rate, and 1.6% mortality. In a comparative review of 53 patients undergoing laparoscopic PD, Asbun and Stauffer [7] reported a mean operative time of 541 minutes, 8-day mean length of stay, 24.5% major perioperative morbidity, and 5.7% perioperative mortality. Significant differences identified were a shorter length of stay (8 days laparoscopic vs 12 days open, $P<.001$) and greater operative time (541 minutes laparoscopic vs 401 minutes open, $P<.001$) for laparoscopic PD compared with open PD [7].

Currently, the definition of minimally invasive pancreatectomy is heterogeneous and encompasses TLPD, laparoscopic-assisted, robotic-assisted, and robotic pancreatectomy [10,11]. Meta-analyses have combined the experiences of TLPD and robotic PD, pooling 6 studies (n = 542 total subjects) in an overall evaluation of minimally invasive PD [11]. Minimally invasive PD was associated with decreased intraoperative blood loss (weighted mean difference of 1460 mL, $P<.001$), but longer operating times (weighted mean difference of 131 minutes, $P = .003$). There was also an associated decrease in length of hospital stay with minimally invasive compared with open PD (weighted mean difference of 3.7 days, $P = .02$). Thus, the safety of minimally invasive approaches to PD has been demonstrated by several groups, although potential oncologic benefits to this approach have only been recently described.

Technique of laparoscopic pancreaticoduodenectomy

The techniques of TLPD with and without vein resection have been previously described [8,12]. These steps are summarized in Box 1. Suggested trocar placement for TLPD is illustrated in Fig. 1.

Box 1: Technique of laparoscopic pancreaticoduodenectomy

Port placement and positioning

- Supine position
- Six working ports placed semi-circumferentially
- Camera initially in the periumbilical region
- Diagnostic laparoscopy to confirm absence of peritoneal or hepatic metastatic deposits
- Laparoscopic ultrasound used as needed to localize the lesion and inform operative planning

Mobilization and resection

- Lesser sac is entered by dividing the gastrocolic omentum with an energy device
- Posterior attachments of the stomach are released and fan retractor placed to elevate stomach and expose pancreas
- Common hepatic artery is identified and hepatic artery lymph node is removed to improve exposure
- Common hepatic artery neurolysis is performed, and the gastroduodenal and right gastric arteries are ligated, clipped, and divided
- Portal vein is identified superiorly and the superior mesenteric vein inferiorly
- Tunnel is created under the pancreatic neck using suction and blunt dissector to the portal confluence
- Umbilical tape is introduced to wrap around the pancreatic neck for retraction
- D1 is divided with endoscopic stapler distal to the pylorus (for pylorus-preserving PD)
- Ligament of Treitz is identified and dissected using an energy device to the other side of the inferior vena cava in an essentially reverse-style Kocher maneuver
- Proximal jejunum is divided with an endoscopic stapler and passed into the supramesocolic compartment
- The Kocher maneuver is completed in the standard fashion with a fan retractor on the duodenum for countertraction
- Once the duodenal-jejunal flexures are mobilized, the first jejunal vein is taken along with fibro-fatty tissue around the pancreas
- Cholecystectomy is performed
- Hilar lymphadenectomy is performed sharply to skeletonize hilar structures
- Bile duct is divided on confirmation of complete portal dissection up to the hilar plate
- Pancreatic parenchyma is transected using an energy device (endoscopic scissors are used to divide the pancreatic duct)

	• Pancreatic duct is dilated with a blunt dissector • Uncinate process is dissected free using an energy device with pancreaticoduodenal tributaries taken between metal clips • Infraumbilical incision is extended and the specimen is removed using an endoscopic retrieval bag • Specimen margins are marked at the portomesenteric groove and superior mesenteric artery (SMA) using different colored ink
Vein resection	• Involved portion of the portomesenteric vein is isolated by a combined anterior approach to the SMA and uncinate process • The portal vein, superior mesenteric vein, and splenic vein are exposed for vascular control before resection • The above pancreaticoduodenectomy dissection is completed with the venous transection performed as the final step to minimize mesoportal clamp time • Intravenous heparin (70 units/Kg) is administered before mesoportal clamping • Atraumatic endoscopic vessel clamps are placed before division • Vein resection is then performed en bloc with the specimen after obtaining vascular control
Reconstruction	• Extraction site fascia is closed and pneumoperitoneum is re-established • Negative resection margin status on frozen section of the specimen is confirmed before intracorporeal reconstruction • End-to-side, duct-to-mucosa, pancreaticojejunostomy anastomosis is performed in 2 layers using the Blumgart technique (Vicryl is used for the inner layer and PDS is used for the outer layer) • End-to-side hepaticojejunostomy is performed in a single layer (Vicryl is used) • Jejunum is secured and closure of the mesenteric defect at the ligament of Treitz is performed • End-to-side antecolic duodenojejunostomy is performed in 2 layers (inner running layer and outer interrupted layer using Vicryl) • Vein reconstruction (if resected) is performed either by primary end-to-end anastomosis, by patch repair (autologous or allogenic), or via an interposition graft using the left renal vein. The specimen is removed from the abdomen at the completion of vein reconstruction
Closure	• Trocar sites are closed and drains placed as needed

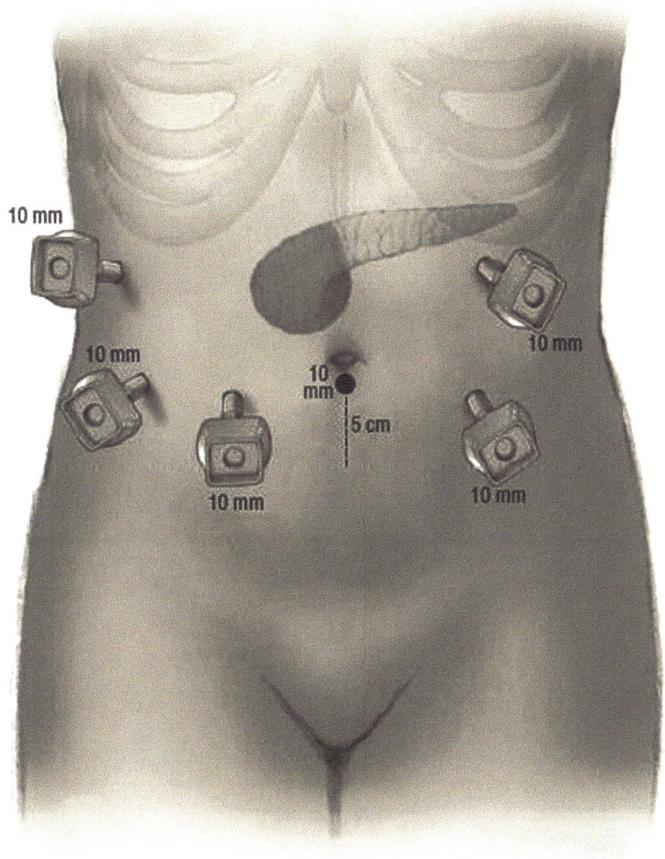

Fig. 1. Suggested trocar placement. (*From* Kendrick ML, Cusati D. Total laparoscopic pancreaticoduodenectomy: feasibility and outcome in an early experience. Arch Surg 2010;145(1):20; with permission.)

DISCUSSION

Safety of laparoscopic pancreaticoduodenectomy

A summary of the literature to include prospective, retrospective, and case series on surgical outcomes following minimally invasive PD is listed in Tables 1 and 2. A total of 12 studies beyond small case series and case reports were identified from centers that offered such a procedure with a combined experience of 377 minimally invasive PD cases [10,11]. Of these 12 summarized studies, 3 examined laparoscopic-assisted PD, 2 examined robotic-assisted PD, 2 examined robotic PD, 4 examined TLPD, and 1 examined TLPD with vein resection and reconstruction in the context of borderline resectable pancreatic cancer.

A case series of 65 patients by Kendrick and Cusati [8] undergoing TLPD for benign and malignant indications demonstrated comparable outcomes in

Table 1
Summary of outcomes following minimally invasive pancreatectomy

Study, year	Design	Surgery	Total N	OR time (min)	EBL (mL)	Lymph nodes	R1/R2 resection (%)	Morbidity (%)	Mortality (%)	Pancreatic fistula	Delayed gastric emptying	Length of stay (d)
Dulucq et al [13], 2006	Prospective case series	LAPD	25	287 ± 39	107 ± 48	18 ± 4	0	31.8	4.5	4.5	9.1	16.2 ± 2.7
Palinevu et al [9], 2007	Case series	TLPD	42	357 (range 270–650)	74 (range 35–410)	14 (range 8–22)	2.6	26.7	1.33	6.67	NR	8.2 (range 6–42)
Kendrick et al [8], 2010	Case series	TLPD	62	368 (range 258–608)	240 (30–1200)	15 (range 6–31)	11	41.9	1.6	17.7	14.5	7 (range 4–69)
Kendrick et al [12], 2011	Case series	TLPD with vein resection	11	413 (range: 301–666)	500 (range 75–2800)	19 (9–45)	10	54	0	27.3	9.1	7 (range 4–45)

Data are represented as mean ± standard deviation unless otherwise specified.

Abbreviations: EBL, estimated blood loss; LAPD, laparoscopy-assisted pancreaticoduodenectomy; OR, operating room; R1, presence of microscopic residual disease; R2, presence of macroscopic residual disease.

Table 2
Comparative studies between minimally invasive and open pancreaticoduodenectomy

Study, year	Design	Surgery	Total N	OR time (min)	EBL (mL)	Lymph nodes	R1/R2 resection (%)	Morbidity (%)	Mortality (%)
Cho et al [14], 2009	Prospective	LAPD	15	338 ± 48	445 ± 384	18.5 ± 5.9	0	27	0
		Open	15	287 ± 117	552 ± 336	20 ± 8.9	0	27	0
Buchs et al [32], 2011	Retrospective	RTPD	44	444 ± 93.5	387 ± 334	16.8 ± 10	9.1	36.4	4.5
		Open	39	559 ± 135	827 ± 439	11 ± 6.3	18.5	48.7	2.6
Zhou et al [33], 2011	Prospective	RTPD	8	718 ± 186	153 ± 43	NR	0	25	0
		Open	8	420 ± 127	210 ± 53	NR	16.7	75	12.5
Zureikat et al [15], 2011	Retrospective	TLPD	14	456 ± 110	300 ± 225	18.5	0	20	7
		Open	14	372 ± 117	400 ± 750	19.1	0	7.1	0
Asbun et al [7], 2012	Prospective	TLPD	53	541 ± 88	195 ± 136	23.4 ± 10.1	5.1	17	5.7
		Open	215	401 ± 108	1032 ± 1151	16.8 ± 10.6	17	29.3	8.8
Chalikonda et al [34], 2012	Prospective	RAPD	30	476	485	13.2	0	30	4
		Open	30	366.5	775	11.7	13	43	0
Kuroki et al [35], 2012	Retrospective	LAPD	20	657 ± 191	377 ± 291	NR	NR	20	0
		Open	31	555 ± 119	1510 ± 1000	NR	NR	19	0
Lai et al [36], 2012	Retrospective	RAPD	20	491.5	247	10 ± 6	26.7	50	0
		Open	67	264.9	775	10 ± 8	35.9	49.3	3

Data are represented as mean ± standard deviation unless otherwise specified.

Abbreviations: EBL, estimated blood loss; LAPD, laparoscopy-assisted pancreaticoduodenectomy; OR, operating room; R1, presence of microscopic residual disease; R2, presence of macroscopic residual disease; RAPD, robotic (assisted) pancreaticoduodenectomy; RTPD, robotic (total) pancreaticoduodenectomy.

postoperative blood loss, operative time, postoperative morbidity, length of stay, and 30-day in-hospital mortality to reports of open PD. Other case series of TLPD were also reported with similar findings [7,9,13]. Although these series suggested feasibility and safety of minimally invasive PD, a formal evaluation in the setting of malignancy was lacking. As technical abilities advanced, evaluation of the feasibility and safety of major vascular resection at the time of PD was also reported [12]. A series of 11 patients with pancreatic cancer undergoing TLPD with vein resection and reconstruction was evaluated [12]. Outcomes such as operative time, blood loss, mesoportal clamp time, margin negative resection, and 30-day mortality and morbidity were reported and appeared comparable to those reported with the open approach [12].

Several comparative studies have also confirmed the safety of laparoscopic PD [7,14,15]. Asbun and Stauffer [7] compared perioperative outcomes of TLPD to open PD and reported TLPD was associated with decreased intraoperative blood loss (195 mL vs 1032 mL, $P<.001$), transfusions (0.64 units vs 4.7 units, $P<.001$), length of hospital stay (8.0 days vs 12.4 days, $P<.001$), and length of intensive care unit (ICU) stay (1.1. days vs 3.0 days, $P<.001$). Risk of postoperative pancreatic fistula, delayed gastric emptying, and operative mortality were found to be equivalent between the 2 groups, although TLPD was associated with longer operative time compared with the open approach (541 minutes vs 401 minutes, $P<.001$) [7]. Although these studies did not evaluate long-term oncologic outcomes, short-term markers, such as rate of histologically negative resection margins and lymph node harvest, were found to be equivalent or slightly better with the laparoscopic group compared with the open group [7,14,15].

Oncologic benefits of laparoscopic pancreaticoduodenectomy

Short-term markers of oncologic outcomes have been examined in terms of the rate of negative resection margins and lymph node harvest in subgroup analyses of patients undergoing TLPD for malignant indications [7,14,15]. Cho and colleagues [14] prospectively compared TLPD to open PD (n = 15 subjects in each arm) and did not detect any differences in status of surgical margins or number of lymph nodes harvested, although the analysis may have been underpowered and did not adjust for confounding factors such as tumor size and grade. Zureikat and colleagues [15] performed a matched case-control study comparing TLPD with open PD (n = 14 subjects in each arm) and similarly did not detect any differences in status of surgical margins or number of lymph nodes harvested, although this study may have also been underpowered. Notably, when examining cancer stage, there was no significant difference between laparoscopic compared with open PD; however, tumor size was significantly smaller in the laparoscopic compared with the open PD group (2.2 cm vs 3.6 cm, $P=.02$), suggesting potential selection bias that may have accounted for such results [15].

A larger study comparing TLPD (n = 53) to open PD (n = 215) by Asbun and Shaeffer [7] demonstrated improved lymph node harvest with TLPD compared with open PD (23 vs 16 lymph nodes, $P<.001$). The adequacy of lymph node retrieval was further characterized by the lymph node ratio (defined as the ratio of the number of lymph nodes harboring metastatic cancer to the total number of lymph nodes examined), an important prognostic factor following pancreatectomy [16]. Lymph node ratio among N1 patients was significantly decreased in the TLPD compared with the open PD group (0.159 vs 0.241, $P<.001$) [7]. In contrast with previously reported studies, there was no difference in tumor size and stage between the TLPD and open PD groups [7]. There was also no significant difference in negative resection margin status or number of positive lymph nodes harvested between the 2 groups [7]. This study seemed adequately powered to detect differences in short-term oncologic outcomes with similar prognostic factors of tumor size and stage between the TLPD and the open PD groups that were unlikely to confound results.

A meta-analysis of laparoscopic and robotic PD included 6 studies comparing minimally invasive PD (n = 169 cases) with open PD (n = 373 cases) [11]. Minimally invasive PD demonstrated significantly lower operative blood loss (weighted mean difference 1460 mL, $P<.001$), greater lymph node retrieval (weighted mean difference of 3.2, $P = .03$), and lower risk of R1/R2 resection (odds ratio 0.4, $P = .007$), compared with open PD. Notably, tumor size was also significantly smaller in the minimally invasive versus open PD group (weighted mean difference 0.6 cm, $P = .02$). As most of these studies were retrospective case series, the noted difference could have reflected bias that selected earlier stage cancers in the minimally invasive compared with open PD group [11].

Each of the above studies did not demonstrate any significant difference in residual disease following resection, which is most strongly associated with long-term disease-free survival [17,18]. With respect to minimally invasive lymphadenectomy, the technical aspects of TLPD may be suitable to better visualization by providing the operating surgeon magnified views and angles that may not otherwise be appreciated via the open approach. This finding is particularly evident when performing lymphadenectomy around major vascular structures, such as the SMA, superior mesenteric vein, and portal vein [7].

Decreased intraoperative blood loss and need for blood transfusion have also been attributed to the improved visualization offered by a laparoscopic approach [7]. Visualization of major and minor vascular structures during dissection is enhanced, which may facilitate more accurate and precise dissection. Blood loss requiring transfusion may have long-term oncologic sequelae, because allogenic blood transfusion may impair host immune responses responsible for preventing recurrence and metastases of primary tumors [19]. In a retrospective, risk-adjusted analysis of subjects with ampullary cancer undergoing open PD (n = 67), 5-year survival was significantly decreased in patients who received 3 or more units of transfused blood than patients who did not receive any transfused blood (30.2% vs 70.8%, $P = .005$) [19].

A similar negative biological effect of blood transfusion on cancer recurrence following resection has been demonstrated for other gastrointestinal malignancies, including the colon/rectum, stomach, and liver [20–22]. A study from the National Cancer Institute demonstrated that each additional unit of blood transfused in the perioperative period increased the risk of disease recurrence by 5% and death by 7% in patients undergoing partial hepatectomy for colorectal liver metastases [22]. Blood transfusions in primary liver tumors, such as hepatocellular carcinoma, also showed similar results: patients who received any blood transfusions in the perioperative period had a significantly worse disease-free survival and overall survival compared with patients who did not receive any blood transfusions [23]. Exposure to leukocytes in allogenic blood products is thought to contribute to immunosuppressive effects that may be responsible for increased risk of cancer recurrence and surgical site infections in postoperative patients [24].

Improved surgical morbidities following pancreatectomy have also been shown to increase overall survival and disease-free recurrence [17]. Postoperative morbidity with respect to pancreatic fistula, delayed gastric emptying, after-pancreatectomy hemorrhage, bile leakage, reoperation, and mortality is equivalent between TLPD and open PD [8,10,11]. Recent meta-analyses and systematic reviews have further demonstrated improved wound infection rate, blood loss, and length of hospital stay when comparing laparoscopic with open PD [10,11]. Postoperative complications contribute to the need for additional interventions and increased hospital stay, all of which may delay the initiation of systemic chemotherapy to promote disease-free survival.

Pancreatic cancer has uniformly poor survival because of the risk of recurrent disease [25]. Recent advances in systemic therapy, however, have shown reasonable results with respect to mitigating disease progression [26,27]. Lengthy hospital stays, unplanned ICU admissions, and severe postoperative complications delay postoperative recovery and potentially interfere with timely administration of systemic therapy. The combination of complete oncologic resection with adequate lymphadenectomy in addition to systemic adjuvant therapy is the treatment regimen that maximizes the chance of long-term cure.

Data from the Mayo Clinic represent one of the largest experiences with TLPD worldwide. Long-term survival and oncologic data have been analyzed for patients undergoing TLPD and compared with a risk-adjusted cohort of similar patients undergoing open PD for ductal adenocarcinoma of the pancreas [28]. Croome and colleagues [28] examined 322 patients undergoing elective PD, of which 108 underwent TLPD and 214 underwent open PD over the same time period. The 2 groups did not differ with respect to tumor size, neoadjuvant therapy, node positivity, and positive resection margin status. Primary end points of the study included overall and disease-free survival. Secondary end points examined perioperative outcomes, length of hospital stay, and time to receive adjuvant chemotherapy.

The results of this analysis by Croome and colleagues [28] demonstrated similar perioperative outcomes as reported by other investigators. TLPD was associated with significantly decreased blood loss (TLPD 492 mL vs open PD 867 mL, $P<.001$) and blood transfusion requirements (TLPD 19% vs open PD 33%, $P = .01$) compared with open PD. Notably, there was no significant difference in operative time (TLPD 379 minutes vs open PD 388 minutes, $P = .45$) [28]. The minimal difference in operative time between the 2 procedures may reflect the expertise of a single institution that has mastered the learning curve for this procedure by accruing a large volume of cases. Length of hospital stay was also significantly lower in the TLPD group versus the open group (TLPD 6 days vs open PD 9 days, $P < .001$), a finding that has been corroborated by several other studies evaluating TLPD [7,10,11]. Readmission rates were not directly reported in this study, but analysis based on the authors' institutional data does not reveal any difference in 30-day hospital readmission rates between the TLPD and open PD groups (TLPD 23.1% vs open PD 18.4%, $P = .16$).

Long-term outcomes following TLPD were also examined, which demonstrate improved disease-free survival following TLPD compared with open PD [28]. Overall survival between the 2 groups did not differ significantly, but there seemed to be an increased risk of local recurrence with open PD (27%) compared with TLPD (15%). A multivariate survival model was constructed to evaluate predictors of poor survival, which included age, body mass index, tumor size, positive margins, positive nodes, and a delay of receiving chemotherapy beyond 3 months following surgery or none at all because of postoperative complications. There was only one modifiable risk factor for survival following pancreatectomy: time to receive chemotherapy was significantly longer in patients undergoing open PD versus TLPD (open PD 59 vs TLPD 48 days, $P = .001$). A greater delay beyond 8 weeks to receive adjuvant therapy was also observed in the open versus laparoscopic group (open PD 41% vs TLPD 27%, $P = .01$). More importantly, a delay in receiving chemotherapy because of postoperative complications beyond 3 months or none at all was significantly greater in the open compared with the laparoscopic group (open PD 12% vs TLPD 5%, $P = .04$) [28].

Several limitations should be mentioned regarding this study [28]. The retrospective nature of the study design makes selection bias between the cohorts a real possibility, although the only difference identified between the TLPD and open PD groups were with respect to patient gender ($P = .02$). Sensitivity analyses by gender were performed and no significant difference was subsequently identified for overall survival ($P = .86$) or disease-free survival ($P = .15$). The length of follow-up for survival curves was also limited to a very small number of patients at risk and thus the long-term survival data would require interpretation with caution. Given the single institution nature of these results, it would also be important for such results to be reproduced at several other institutions before shifts in practice and management may be safely recommended.

With this said, other gastrointestinal malignancies have not shown inferiority with respect to laparoscopic approaches compared with conventional approaches. A multi-institution randomized trial comparing laparoscopic-assisted versus open colectomy for colorectal cancer did not demonstrate any differences between the 2 groups with respect to overall survival and cancer recurrence [29]. The lack of difference in overall survival between the 2 groups may reflect a tumor biology that is far less aggressive than that of pancreatic cancer. In terms of other hepatobiliary tumors, however, data suggest that laparoscopic hepatectomy may confer survival advantage over open hepatectomy for malignant lesions with additional benefits of decreased length of stay, lower operative blood loss, and decreased risk of postoperative complications [30]. These findings from laparoscopic hepatectomy, which parallel the findings for laparoscopic pancreatectomy for cancer, suggest that prognosis for hepatobiliary tumors very much depends on operative technique and minimization of surgical morbidity.

Implications and future directions

The learning curve for laparoscopic pancreatectomy and technical demands of the operation may not make it as accessible to most hepatobiliary surgeons. Current training programs in hepatobiliary surgery are incorporating advanced laparoscopy skills into their curricula, and major shifts in practice may not be seen for several years. Robotic technologies may offer a bridge to the technical limitations of laparoscopic surgery by increasing the range of motion and dexterity of operating instruments [31]. Technical advantages of the robot must be balanced by the increased cost, which may make widespread implementation of this technology prohibitive for most centers. Other variations of TLPD include laparoscopic-assisted or robotic-assisted resections wherein reconstructions are done either in the conventional open manner or via the robot.

These other minimally invasive modalities offer short-term advantages similar to TLPD [10]. The evidence with respect to oncologic outcomes is likely transferrable from studies evaluating TLPD, but no formal studies have yet addressed such a question. Although a randomized controlled trial would provide the highest level of evidence to evaluate the efficacy and effectiveness of TLPD as well as other minimally invasive techniques, this may not be practical because of patient-driven demands that newer technologies be offered in their care. In summary, the evidence regarding TLPD suggests it is associated with decreased length of hospital stay, decreased postoperative morbidity, decreased need for blood transfusion, and decreased time to receipt of adjuvant systemic therapy, factors of which may contribute to improved disease-free survival following resection for pancreatic cancer.

References

[1] Whipple AO, Parsons WB, Mullins CR. Treatment of carcinoma of the ampulla of vater. Ann Surg 1935;102(4):763–79.
[2] Crist DW, Sitzmann JV, Cameron JL. Improved hospital morbidity, mortality, and survival after the Whipple procedure. Ann Surg 1987;206(3):358–65.
[3] Winter JM, Cameron JL, Campbell KA, et al. 1423 pancreaticoduodenectomies for pancreatic cancer: a single-institution experience. J Gastrointest Surg 2006;10(9):1199–210 [discussion: 1210–1].
[4] Nakeeb A. The role of minimally invasive surgery for pancreatic pathology. Adv Surg 2005;39:455–69.
[5] Gagner M, Pomp A. Laparoscopic pylorus-preserving pancreatoduodenectomy. Surg Endosc 1994;8(5):408–10.

[6] Gagner M, Pomp A. Laparoscopic pancreatic resection: is it worthwhile? J Gastrointest Surg 1997;1(1):20–5 [discussion: 25–6].
[7] Asbun HJ, Stauffer JA. Laparoscopic vs open pancreaticoduodenectomy: overall outcomes and severity of complications using the Accordion Severity Grading System. J Am Coll Surg 2012;215(6):810–9.
[8] Kendrick ML, Cusati D. Total laparoscopic pancreaticoduodenectomy: feasibility and outcome in an early experience. Arch Surg 2010;145(1):19–23.
[9] Palanivelu C, Jani K, Senthilnathan P, et al. Laparoscopic pancreaticoduodenectomy: technique and outcomes. J Am Coll Surg 2007;205(2):222–30.
[10] Lei P, Wei B, Guo W, et al. Minimally invasive surgical approach compared with open pancreaticoduodenectomy: a systematic review and meta analysis on the feasibility and safety. Surg Laparosc Endosc Percutan Tech 2014;24:296–305.
[11] Correa-Gallego C, Dinkelspiel HE, Sulimanoff I, et al. Minimally-invasive vs open pancreaticoduodenectomy: systematic review and meta-analysis. J Am Coll Surg 2014;218(1): 129–39.
[12] Kendrick ML, Sclabas GM. Major venous resection during total laparoscopic pancreaticoduodenectomy. HPB (Oxford) 2011;13(7):454–8.
[13] Dulucq JL, Wintringer P, Mahajna A. Laparoscopic pancreaticoduodenectomy for benign and malignant diseases. Surg Endosc 2006;20(7):1045–50.
[14] Cho A, Yamamoto H, Nagata M, et al. Comparison of laparoscopy-assisted and open pylorus-preserving pancreaticoduodenectomy for periampullary disease. Am J Surg 2009;198(3):445–9.
[15] Zureikat AH, Breaux JA, Steel JL, et al. Can laparoscopic pancreaticoduodenectomy be safely implemented? J Gastrointest Surg 2011;15(7):1151–7.
[16] Pawlik TM, Gleisner AL, Cameron JL, et al. Prognostic relevance of lymph node ratio following pancreaticoduodenectomy for pancreatic cancer. Surgery 2007;141(5):610–8.
[17] Howard TJ, Krug JE, Yu J, et al. A margin-negative R0 resection accomplished with minimal postoperative complications is the surgeon's contribution to long-term survival in pancreatic cancer. J Gastrointest Surg 2006;10(10):1338–45 [discussion: 1345–6].
[18] Corsini MM, Miller RC, Haddock MG, et al. Adjuvant radiotherapy and chemotherapy for pancreatic carcinoma: the Mayo Clinic experience (1975-2005). J Clin Oncol 2008;26(21):3511–6.
[19] Yao HS, Wang Q, Wang WJ, et al. Intraoperative allogeneic red blood cell transfusion in ampullary cancer outcome after curative pancreatoduodenectomy: a clinical study and meta-analysis. World J Surg 2008;32(9):2038–46.
[20] Burrows L, Tartter P. Effect of blood transfusions on colonic malignancy recurrent rate. Lancet 1982;2(8299):662.
[21] Hyung WJ, Noh SH, Shin DW, et al. Adverse effects of perioperative transfusion on patients with stage III and IV gastric cancer. Ann Surg Oncol 2002;9(1):5–12.
[22] Stephenson KR, Steinberg SM, Hughes KS, et al. Perioperative blood transfusions are associated with decreased time to recurrence and decreased survival after resection of colorectal liver metastases. Ann Surg 1988;208(6):679–87.
[23] Shiba H, Ishida Y, Wakiyama S, et al. Negative impact of blood transfusion on recurrence and prognosis of hepatocellular carcinoma after hepatic resection. J Gastrointest Surg 2009;13(9):1636–42.
[24] Goodnough LT, Brecher ME, Kanter MH, et al. Transfusion medicine. First of two parts–blood transfusion. N Engl J Med 1999;340(6):438–47.
[25] Hidalgo M. Pancreatic cancer. N Engl J Med 2010;362(17):1605–17.
[26] Oettle H, Neuhaus P, Hochhaus A, et al. Adjuvant chemotherapy with gemcitabine and long-term outcomes among patients with resected pancreatic cancer: the CONKO-001 randomized trial. JAMA 2013;310(14):1473–81.
[27] Conroy T, Desseigne F, Ychou M, et al. FOLFIRINOX versus gemcitabine for metastatic pancreatic cancer. N Engl J Med 2011;364(19):1817–25.

[28] Croome KP, Farnell MB, Que FG, et al. Total laparoscopic pancreaticoduodenectomy for pancreatic ductal adenocarcinoma: oncologic advantages over open approaches? Ann Surg 2014;260(4):633–40.
[29] Clinical Outcomes of Surgical Therapy Study Group. A comparison of laparoscopically assisted and open colectomy for colon cancer. N Engl J Med 2004;350(20):2050–9.
[30] Croome KP, Yamashita MH. Laparoscopic vs open hepatic resection for benign and malignant tumors: an updated meta-analysis. Arch Surg 2010;145(11):1109–18.
[31] Zeh HJ 3rd, Bartlett DL, Moser AJ. Robotic-assisted major pancreatic resection. Adv Surg 2011;45:323–40.
[32] Buchs NC, Addeo P, Bianco FM, et al. Robotic versus open pancreaticoduodenectomy: a comparative study at a single institution. World J Surg 2011;35(12):2739–46.
[33] Zhou NX, Chen JZ, Liu Q, et al. Outcomes of pancreatoduodenectomy with robotic surgery versus open surgery. Int J Med Robot 2011;7(2):131–7.
[34] Chalikonda S, Aguilar-Saavedra JR, Walsh RM. Laparoscopic robotic-assisted pancreaticoduodenectomy: a case-matched comparison with open resection. Surg Endosc 2012;26(9):2397–402.
[35] Kuroki T, Adachi T, Okamoto T, et al. A non-randomized comparative study of laparoscopy-assisted pancreaticoduodenectomy and open pancreaticoduodenectomy. Hepatogastroenterology 2012;59(114):570–3.
[36] Lai EC, Yang GP, Tang CN. Robot-assisted laparoscopic pancreaticoduodenectomy versus open pancreaticoduodenectomy–a comparative study. Int J Surg 2012;10(9):475–9.

Advances in Surgery 49 (2015) 157–171

ADVANCES IN SURGERY

Bariatric Surgery versus Intensive Medical Weight Management for Type 2 Diabetes

Monica Sethi, MD[a,b], Manish Parikh, MD[a,b,*]

[a]Department of Surgery, New York University Medical Center, 550 First Avenue NBV 15 South 7, New York, NY 10016, USA; [b]Department of Surgery, Bellevue Hospital Center, 550 First Avenue NBV 15 South 7, New York, NY 10016, USA

Keywords

• Diabetes • Obesity • Bariatric surgery • Metabolic surgery
• Medical weight management

Key points

- Medical weight management (MWM) trials in obese patients with type 2 diabetes mellitus (T2DM) show that weight loss is modest, is infrequently sustained beyond 1 year, and leads to limited improvement in glycemic control, with hemoglobin A_{1c} (HbA_{1c}) rarely dropping below 7%.
- Surgery leads to significant weight loss and better glycemic control and T2DM remission rates compared with MWM.
- Bariatric surgery can improve insulin resistance by mechanisms independent of weight loss, including altering the gastrointestinal hormonal milieu (enhanced glucagon-like peptide-1 [GLP-1] and decreased ghrelin levels).
- For patients with T2DM who are eligible for bariatric surgery, surgery is the ideal treatment.

INTRODUCTION

T2DM is a chronic and debilitating metabolic disorder associated with significant long-term morbidity including heart disease, stroke, blindness, renal failure, and lower extremity amputation. According to the 2014 National Diabetes Statistics Report, 29.1 million people, or 9.3% of the US population,

The authors have nothing to disclose.

*Corresponding author: Department of Surgery, Bellevue Hospital Center, 550 First Avenue NBV 15 South 7, New York, NY 10016. *E-mail address*: Manish.parikh@nyumc.org

0065-3411/15/$ – see front matter
http://dx.doi.org/10.1016/j.yasu.2015.04.004

have diabetes [1]. The vast majority of these patients have T2DM. Hispanic Americans and non-Hispanic African Americans are disproportionately affected by diabetes and diabetes-related complications [1].

Nearly 2 million new cases of diabetes are diagnosed in US adults each year. The incidence is likely to increase, because nearly 86 million Americans aged 20 years or older met criteria for prediabetes in 2012 [1]. This increase has closely paralleled the obesity epidemic. Obesity is associated with multiple medical comorbidities, including T2DM, heart disease, sleep apnea, stroke, gallbladder disease, liver disease, cancer, musculoskeletal disease, and infertility. Between 1988 and 2008, the prevalence of obesity increased in adults at all income and education levels [2]. At present, more than one-third of adults and 17% of youth in the United States are obese [3].

The connection between obesity and diabetes has been well established. Among all patients with T2DM, 46% have a body mass index (BMI; calculated as the weight in kilograms divided by the height in meters square) of at least 30 [4]. Obesity is a central feature in the pathophysiologic development of diabetes, because visceral adiposity induces insulin resistance, hyperinsulinemia, and glucose intolerance, leading to significant metabolic complications. The risk of developing diabetes increases dramatically as the degree of obesity increases [4].

Intensive weight management, including diet, behavioral therapies, exercise, and pharmacologic agents, has been the cornerstone of T2DM treatment; however, management has been evolving, especially in obese patients, as multiple studies have demonstrated that surgical treatment of obesity may result in remission of T2DM. Evidence exists that bariatric procedures can improve insulin resistance independent of weight loss, by altering the gastrointestinal hormonal milieu. This article reviews the current literature regarding medical and surgical treatment of T2DM.

DIAGNOSIS AND TREATMENT OF TYPE 2 DIABETES MELLITUS

Diagnosis is based on either of the following [5]:

1. Plasma glucose levels
   a. Fasting plasma glucose (FPG) level of 126 mg/dL or more
   b. Two-hour plasma glucose value of 200 mg/dL or more after a 75-g oral glucose tolerance test
2. HbA_{1c} value of 6.5% or more

Treatment has traditionally consisted of diet and exercise, as well as tight glycemic control. The pharmacologic agents used to achieve glycemic control are usually oral and/or injectable medications, including

- Metformin and thiazolidinediones: these target insulin resistance
- Sulfonylureas and thiazolidinediones: these target β-cell function
- GLP-1 agonists: incretin hormones
- Insulin

As T2DM progresses, insulin therapy is eventually needed for many patients (Box 1) [5].

To achieve weight loss, the American Diabetes Association (ADA) recommends intensive lifestyle interventions, including dietary changes, physical activity, and supportive measures for behavior change [5].

As evidence of this treatment strategy, the Look AHEAD Research Group [8] performed a landmark multicenter randomized controlled trial (RCT) comparing the long-term effects of intensive lifestyle intervention with standard supportive therapy. The details may be summarized as follows:

- Study group: 5145 overweight (mean BMI 36) individuals with T2DM
- Outcomes: changes in weight, diabetes, and other cardiovascular risk factors
- Duration: 4 years
- Interventions
  - Study group (intensive lifestyle intervention)
    - Diet modification consisting of a low-calorie diet (1200–1800 kcal based on initial weight)
    - Free liquid meal replacements
    - Physical activity goal of at least 175 minutes per week
    - Weekly follow-up for the initial 6 months, and at least once a month for the next 2–4 years
  - Control group (standard supportive therapy)
    - Voluntary informational session held 3 times per year
- Results
  - Averaged across 4 years
    - Weight loss (study vs control): 6.15% versus 0.88%, $P<.0001$
    - HbA_{1c} (study vs control): −0.36% versus −0.09%, $P<.0001$
  - At 4 years: HbA_{1c} trended toward baseline levels
  - At 4 years, a small but statistically significant proportion of the intensive weight loss group achieved complete or partial remission of diabetes (3.5% vs 0.5%) [9]

Overall, the Look AHEAD trial showed that weight loss and HbA_{1c} reductions were initially greater among the intensive lifestyle intervention group than controls but that these changes were not sustained at the end of the 4-year follow-up.

Box 1: Diet and intensive MWM

According to the 2014 ADA recommendations, diet and exercise are recommended for all patients with diabetes, because:

- Even modest weight loss may provide clinical benefits, especially to those early in the disease process [5]
- Weight loss can improve glycemic control without the risk of pharmacotherapy-induced hypoglycemia, a common problem with sulfonylureas and insulin [6]
- Weight loss can lead to a significant reduction in the risk of cardiovascular disease and diabetes-related mortality [7]

A Cochrane Database review of nonpharmacologic medical weight loss interventions for overweight adults (mean BMI 33.2) with T2DM was performed in 2005. The details are as follows:

- Interventions: various diets, behavioral therapies, and exercise regimens
- Duration: between 10 weeks and 5 years
- Follow-up: between 1 and 5 years
- Findings
  - Average of 1.7 kg (3.1% baseline body weight) loss after any intervention with 1- to 2-year follow-up
  - Reduction in HbA_{1c} corresponded to weight loss; however, these changes were not significant
  - Sustained intensive interventions and very-low-calorie diets (VLCD) had the greatest effect on weight loss [10]

Nutritional interventions alone

Trials that focus on nutritional advice alone have shown that the most effective nutritional interventions are low-calorie diets and VLCD [11]. VLCD are associated with HbA_{1c} reduction ranging from 0.9% to 2.0% after 3 to 6 months, with larger reductions seen in patients with newly diagnosed T2DM [12]. Lim and colleagues [13] have shown that more extreme caloric restriction (600 kcal/d) for 8 weeks can normalize β-cell function and result in reversal of type 2 diabetes.

Weight loss medications

In addition to diet, exercise, and behavioral therapy, weight loss medications can be effective and lead to improvements in glycemic control [6]. In an RCT, orlistat was shown to reduce body weight (5.4 kg vs 2.4 kg, $P<.0001$) and HbA_{1c} (1% vs 0.6%, $P = .0008$) in patients with T2DM over a 24-week period [14]. Fluoxetine and sibutramine produce similar weight loss effects [15]. Nonetheless, weight loss medications have limited weight loss effects, may be unsuccessful in the long term, and may have long-term side effects. The exact role of these medications in the treatment of T2DM is still uncertain, and they are best used as adjuncts to a multifaceted weight loss program (Box 2) [6].

At the population level, these changes may have significant health benefits, but a small decrease in weight is unlikely to induce diabetes remission, especially in obese patients. In fact, the UK Prospective Diabetes Study showed that in patients

Box 2: Summary of MMW studies

Several meta-analyses, RCTs, and observational studies have demonstrated the benefits of medical weight loss in the management of type 2 diabetes; however:

- Weight loss is modest, ranging from 3 to 5 kg or 2 to 3 BMI units
- Weight loss is infrequently sustained beyond 1 year
- Improvement in glycemic control can be achieved, but is limited
- HbA_{1c} rarely drops below 7%

Box 3: Meta-analysis of bariatric surgery studies in patients with T2DM

- A total of 4070 patients with T2DM (mean BMI 47.9) underwent bariatric surgery.
- Combined analysis showed that 78% of patients had complete remission of diabetes (defined as normalization of blood glucose levels in the absence of medications) after any bariatric surgery, and remission was generally sustained for over 2 years.
- Weight loss and diabetes remission were greatest for patients undergoing biliopancreatic diversion/duodenal switch, followed by Roux-en-Y gastric bypass, followed by gastric banding procedures [17].

with elevated FPG levels 28% weight loss was necessary to achieve glycemic control [16]. This degree of weight loss is very difficult to achieve with medical interventions alone and unlikely to be sustained in the long term [10].

BARIATRIC SURGERY

Surgery has the potential to offer substantial and durable weight loss that can significantly improve glycemic control and even lead to diabetes remission. Bariatric surgery is an important treatment strategy for obese patients (BMI > 35) with T2DM. The ADA has recognized the importance of bariatric surgery to treat T2DM in adults with BMI greater than 35 [5].

There have been numerous studies evaluating the effect of bariatric surgery in patients with T2DM. Buchwald and colleagues [17] performed a meta-analysis of all bariatric surgery studies in patients with T2DM (Box 3, Table 1).

The patients who are more likely to experience diabetes remission typically

- Have shorter duration of diabetes (<5 years)
- Have less-severe T2DM (not requiring insulin)
- Have the greatest weight loss after bariatric surgery [18]

Secondary and long-term outcomes after bariatric surgery

Many studies have shown additional metabolic benefits for patients with T2DM undergoing bariatric surgery. Ikramuddin and colleagues [19] showed

Table 1
Overview of weight loss, surgical procedure, and diabetes resolution

	Total	Gastric banding	Gastroplasty	Gastric bypass	BPD/DS
% EBWL	55.9	46.2	55.5	59.7	63.6
% Resolved overall	78.1	56.7	79.7	80.3	95.1
% Resolved <2 y	80.3	55	81.4	81.6	94
% Resolved ≥2 y	74.6	58.3	77.5	70.9	95.9

Abbreviations: %EBWL, percentage excess body weight loss; BPD/DS, biliopancreatic diversion/duodenal switch.

(*Data from* Buchwald H, Estok R, Fahrbach K, et al. Weight and type 2 diabetes after bariatric surgery: systematic review and meta-analysis. Am J Med 2009;122:248–56.e5.)

Table 2
Summary of comparative trials of MWM versus bariatric surgery in patients with T2DM

Study	Study type Follow-up	T2DM (severity/duration)	Intervention	Pre-TX BMI	Post-TX weight loss measure	% T2DM remission (R)	Additional outcomes
Ribaric [22]	Meta-analysis 17.3 mo	T2DM	Conventional therapy control group (n = 3055)	39.4	11.3% EWL	$R^1 = 15.6$	The odds of patients undergoing bariatric surgery achieving T2DM remission ranged from 9.8 to 15.8 times the odds of patients treated with conventional therapy
			Bariatric surgery (n = 3076)	40.9	75.3% EWL	$R^1 = 63.5$	
Mean BMI >35							
Sjostrom [21]	Prospective matched cohort 15 y	T2DM	Nonstandardized obesity & DM care ranging from lifestyle intervention to behavior modification (n = 260)	40.0	3.6% BWL	$R^2 = 6.5$	Microvascular complications occurred at a frequency of 41.8/1000 person-years for controls vs 20.6/1000 person-years in surgical patients
			Gastric banding (n = 61), VBG (n = 227), RYGB (n = 55)	42.1	18% BWL	$R^2 = 30.4$	
Dixon [23]	RCT 2 y	T2DM (<2 y)	Intensive weight loss program with focus on lifestyle change (n = 30)	37.2	4.3% EWL	$R^3 = 13$	Remission of T2DM was related to weight loss and lower baseline HbA_{1c} levels
			Intensive weight loss program + LAGB (n = 30)	37.0	62.5% EWL	$R^3 = 73$	

Mingrone [24]	RCT 2 y	T2DM (≥ 5 y)	Conventional medical therapy and lifestyle modification program with visits q 3 mo (n = 20)	45.6	9.3% EWL	$R^4 = 0$	Blood pressure decreased in all groups. Lipid profiles decreased in the BPD group only
			BPD (n = 20)	45.1	69.4% EWL	$R^4 = 95$	
			RYGB (n = 20)	44.9	68.1% EWL	$R^4 = 75$	
Halperin [25]	RCT 1 y	T2DM (>1 y)	12-wk multidisciplinary lifestyle, medical, and education sessions (n = 19)	36.5	N/A	$R^5 = 16$	At 1 y, the surgical group had improved weight, waist circumference, blood pressure, triglyceride levels, cardiovascular risk scores, and quality of life scores when compared with controls
			RYGB (n = 19)	36.0	N/A	$R^5 = 58$	
Kashyap [26]	RCT 2 y	T2DM uncontrolled (mean $HbA_{1c} \geq 9.7$)	Intensive medical therapy (n = 17)	35.8	−0.5 kg	$R^6 = 5.9$	Body fat reduction was similar for RYGB and SG groups, but truncal fat was reduced in the RYGB group relative to the SG group. Insulin sensitivity and pancreatic β-cell function increased in the RYGB group, but not in the SG group or in controls
			Intensive medical therapy + RYGB (n = 18)	36.1	−25.4 kg	$R^6 = 33.3$	
			Intensive medical therapy + SG (n = 19)	36.4	−22.5 kg	$R^6 = 10.5$	

(*continued on next page*)

Table 2
(*continued*)

Study	Study type Follow-up	T2DM (severity/ duration)	Intervention	Pre-TX BMI	Post-TX weight loss measure	% T2DM remission (R)	Additional outcomes
Schauer [27]	RCT 3 y	T2DM uncontrolled (mean HbA_{1c} 9.3%)	Intensive medical therapy with lifestyle counseling and visits q 3 mo (n = 40)	36.4	4.2% BWL	$R^6 = 5$	The use of glucose-lowering medications including insulin, lipid-lowering and antihypertensive medications, body weight loss, and quality of life were significantly improved in the surgical group compared with the medical therapy group
			Intensive medical therapy + RYGB (n = 48)	37.1	24.5% BWL	$R^6 = 38$	
			Intensive medical therapy + SG (n = 49)	36.1	21.1% BWL	$R^6 = 24$	
Courcoulas [28]	RCT 1 y	T2DM (mean HbA_{1c} 7.9%)	Intensive lifestyle weight loss intervention with weekly to biweekly personal sessions (n = 20)	35.7	10.2% BWL	$R^7 = 0$	Significant reduction in use of antidiabetic medications occurred in both surgical groups
			RYGB (n = 20)	35.5	27.0% BWL	$R^7 = 50$	
			LAGB (n = 21)	35.5	17.3% BWL	$R^7 = 27$	

Mean BMI <35							
Ikramuddin [19]	RCT 1 y	T2DM (≥6 mo)	Intensive lifestyle and MWM (n = 60)	34.3	7.9% BWL	$R^6 = 9$	At 12 mo, 19% of controls and 49% of surgical patients met the composite outcome (HbA_{1c}<7%, LDL levels<100 mg/dL, SBP<130 mm Hg)
			Intensive lifestyle and medical management + RYGB (n = 60)	34.9	26.9% BWL	$R^6 = 44$	
Parikh [29]	RCT 6 mo	T2DM (mean HbA1c = 7.8)	MWM (n = 28)	32.4	−1.0 BMI	$R^5 = 0$	Surgery is effective in the short-term treatment of T2DM in patients with BMI 30–35. Higher baseline sRAGE was associated with better weight loss outcomes
			Surgery: RYGB, LSG, LAGB (n = 29)	32.8	−7.0 BMI	$R^5 = 65$	

Note: There are varying definitions of T2DM remission (R) in the bariatric surgery literature; for each article, the remission definition is stated below: R^1 defined independently by each article in the meta-analysis; R^2 defined as blood glucose levels less than 110 mg/dL without the use of antidiabetic medications; R^3 defined as FPG less than 126 mg/dL and HbA_{1c} less than 6.2% without the use of antidiabetic medications; R^4 defined as FPG less than 100 mg/dL and HbA_{1c} less than 6.5% for at least 1 year; R^5 defined as FPG less than 126 mg/dL and HbA_{1c} less than 6.5%; R^6 defined as HbA_{1c} less than 6%; R^7 (partial remission) defined as HbA_{1c} levels less than 6.5% and FPG levels less than 125 mg/dL without the use of antidiabetic medications.

Abbreviations: BPD, biliopancreatic diversion; BWL, body weight loss; DM, Diabetes Mellitus; EWL, excess weight loss; LAGB, laparoscopic adjustable gastric band; LDL, low-density lipoprotein; LSG, laparoscopic sleeve gastrectomy; N/A, not available; SBP, systolic blood pressure; SG, sleeve gastrectomy; sRAGE, soluble receptor for advanced end-glycation end products; Tx, treatment; VBG, vertical banded gastroplasty.

that adding Roux-en-Y gastric bypass (RYGB) to MWM was associated with a greater likelihood of achieving the composite outcome of HbA_{1c} less than 7%, low-density lipoprotein levels less than 100 mg/dL, and systolic blood pressure less than 130 mm Hg (49% vs 19%; odds ratio [OR], 4.8; 95% confidence interval [CI], 1.9–11.7).

A study by Brethauer and colleagues [20] assessed the long-term effects (median 6 years) of RYGB, laparoscopic sleeve gastrectomy (LSG), and gastric banding in patients with T2DM and found the following:

- Mean excess weight loss of 55%
- Reduction in HbA_{1c} from 7.5% to 6.5%
- Reduction in fasting blood glucose levels from 155.9 to 114.8 mg/dL
- Diabetes remission in 50%, improvement in 34%, unchanged in 16%
- Recurrence of T2DM after initial remission in 19% (associated with longer duration of T2DM and poor weight loss)

This study also found that gastric bypass had the highest rate of long-term diabetes remission and the lowest recurrence.

The Swedish Obesity Study demonstrated that bariatric surgery was associated with more-frequent T2DM remission and fewer complications than usual care. At 15 years, the T2DM remission rate was 6.5% for control patients versus 30.4% for patients who underwent bariatric surgery (OR 6.3; 95% CI 2.1–18.9; $P<.001$) [21].

SUMMARY OF COMPARATIVE TRIALS OF MEDICAL WEIGHT MANAGEMENT VERSUS BARIATRIC SURGERY IN PATIENTS WITH TYPE 2 DIABETES MELLITUS

Several comparative studies have been performed comparing bariatric surgery to MWM for the treatment of T2DM. Table 2 is a summary of comparative studies.

In a recent meta-analysis, Ribaric and colleagues [22] reviewed 16 RCTs and observational studies that directly compared bariatric surgery and conventional medical therapy (Box 4).

Box 4: Controlled trials and observational studies comparing bariatric surgery and conventional medical therapy

- Study population: 3055 MWM versus 3076 surgery
- Follow-up: 17.3 months (median)
- Results: T2DM remission rate (surgery vs medical) 63.5% versus 15.6% ($P<.001$). The odds of patients undergoing bariatric surgery having remission of T2DM ranged from 9.8 to 15.8 times the odds of patients treated with MWM.

Data from Ribaric G, Buchwald JN, McGlennon TW. Diabetes and weight in comparative studies of bariatric surgery vs conventional medical therapy: a systematic review and meta-analysis. Obes Surg 2014;24:437–55.

DISCUSSION

Pathophysiology of bariatric surgery in the treatment of type 2 diabetes mellitus

Bariatric surgery leads to significant weight loss, increased insulin sensitivity, decreased insulin resistance, and improved β-cell function. Although the diabetes improvement is considered to be primarily weight loss driven, there are patients who have been noted to be off diabetes medications before hospital discharge, preceding substantial weight loss [30].

There are several potential mechanisms for this. The reduced caloric intake immediately after surgery leads to a negative caloric balance and the rapid resolution of diabetes before significant weight loss occurs [31]. This negative energy balance is similar to that induced by VLCD, which have been shown to normalize β-cell function and result in reversal of type 2 diabetes [13]. Second, the exclusion of food from the hormonally active antrum, duodenum, and proximal jejunum may alter the gastrointestinal hormonal milieu [32,33]. The presentation of undigested food to the midjejunum may also play a role (Box 5).

Hindgut hypothesis

The hindgut hypothesis is explained by the increased rate of nutrient delivery to the hindgut after RYGB, stimulating the ileal break and the release of GLP-1 and peptide YY. These hindgut hormones decrease food intake, increase insulin secretion, and are increased after RYGB and biliopancreatic diversion. In addition to RYGB, LSG may also impact glucose homeostasis by similar incretin effects. It is hypothesized that an increased rate of gastric emptying or lack of gastric signaling to intestinal L-cells after LSG can lead to enhanced GLP-1 secretion [33–35].

Foregut hypothesis

Studies have shown that bypassing the hormonally active gastric fundus, duodenum, and jejunum leads to a decrease in ghrelin secretion. Ghrelin has anti-incretin effects, suppresses insulin levels and impairs glucose tolerance [36]. Ghrelin levels are decreased in patients undergoing RYGB and may be an integral factor in the enhanced glycemic control after bariatric surgery [32,37].

Additional hypotheses

Other possible mechanisms include alterations in gut microbiota, alterations in bile acids, and changes in neural signaling [32]. Research on these and the hormonal implications of bariatric surgery is critical, because there are likely

Box 5: Theories regarding the potential metabolic effects of bypassing the stomach

1. The hindgut hypothesis: shortcut of nutrients to the distal intestine.
2. The foregut hypothesis: exclusion of the hormonally active proximal gastrointestinal tract [32,33].

Box 6: Results of systematic review and meta-analysis performed for bariatric surgery in patients with T2DM and BMI < 35

- A total of 39 studies, 1389 patients with T2DM (mean BMI 30.5)
- Almost 55% estimated T2DM remission at 1 year (Fig. 1)

Data from Parikh M, Issa R, Vieira D, et al. Role of bariatric surgery as treatment for type 2 diabetes in patients who do not meet current NIH criteria: a systematic review and meta-analysis. J Am Coll Surg 2013;217:527–32.

numerous other gastrointestinal hormones and signaling molecules that have yet to be examined.

EARLY INTERVENTION AND LOW BODY MASS INDEX

At present, only patients with T2DM and BMI greater than 35 are eligible for bariatric surgery, based on the 1991 National Institutes of Health guidelines. Although the Food and Drug Administration recently lowered the BMI criteria for gastric banding to BMI of 30 with comorbidities, most US insurance companies do not approve bariatric surgery in patients with BMI less than 35. Nevertheless, there is emerging evidence supporting the use of bariatric surgery to treat T2DM in less-obese (BMI < 35) patients (see Table 2). The Agency for Healthcare Research and Quality has identified this area as a research priority for comparative effectiveness research (Box 6).

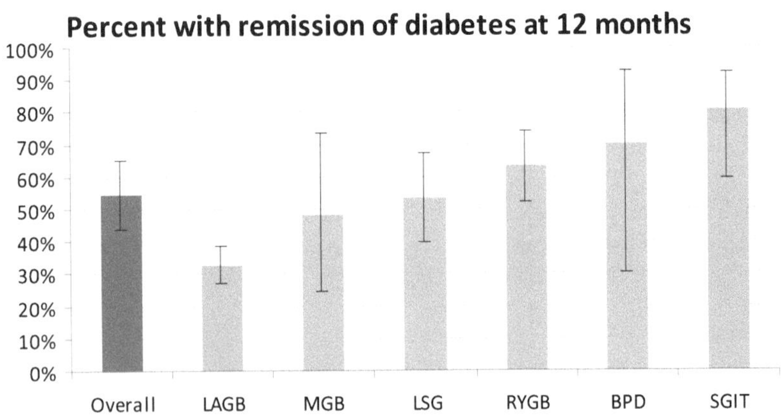

	Overall	LAGB	MGB	LSG	RYGB	BPD	SGIT
# studies	39	8	5	6	10	6	6
# patients	1389	163	265	98	322	64	176

Fig. 1. Estimated T2DM remission rates for BMI greater than 35. BPD, biliopancreatic diversion (with or without duodenal switch); LAGB, laparoscopic adjustable gastric banding; MGB, mini–gastric bypass; SGIT, sleeve gastrectomy with ileal transposition. (*From* Parikh M, Issa R, Vieira D, et al. Role of bariatric surgery as treatment for type diabetes in patients who do not meet current NIH criteria: a systematic review and meta-analysis. J Am Coll Surg 2013;217:530; with permission.)

A similar meta-analysis demonstrated that the magnitude of change in HbA_{1c} among patients with low BMI with T2DM is similar to that of patients with BMI greater than 35, despite less postoperative weight loss [38]. Although there are clear benefits of bariatric surgery in patients with type 2 diabetes with BMI less than 35, larger RCTs with longer-term follow-up are still needed.

SUMMARY

Based on current evidence, bariatric surgery is superior to MWM for treating patients with T2DM with mild to severe obesity. More randomized trials are needed in the BMI 30 to 35 cohort.

References

[1] Centers for Disease Control and Prevention. National diabetes statistics report: estimates of diabetes and its Burden in the United States, 2014. Atlanta (GA): U.S. Department of Health and Human Services; 2014.
[2] Ogden CL, Lamb MM, Carroll MD, et al. Obesity and socioeconomic status in adults: United States, 1988-1994 and 2005-2008. NCHS data brief No. 50 2010. Hyattsville (MD): National Center for Health Statistics; 2010.
[3] Ogden CL, Carroll MD, Flegal KM, et al. Prevalence of obesity in the United States. JAMA 2014;312:189–90.
[4] National Task Force on the Prevention and Treatment of Obesity. Overweight, obesity, and health risk. Arch Intern Med 2000;160:898–904.
[5] American Diabetes Association. Standards of medical care in diabetes - 2014. Diabetes Care 2014;37:S14–80.
[6] Wilding JP. The importance of weight management in type 2 diabetes mellitus. Int J Clin Pract 2014;68:682–91.
[7] Williamson DF, Thompson TJ, Thun M, et al. Intentional weight loss and mortality among overweight individuals with diabetes. Diabetes Care 2000;23:1499–504.
[8] The Look AHEAD Research Group, Wing RR. Long-term effects of a lifestyle intervention on weight and cardiovascular risk factors in individuals with type 2 diabetes mellitus: four-year results of the Look AHEAD trial. Arch Intern Med 2010;170:1566–75.
[9] Gregg EW, Chen H, Wagenknecht LE, et al. Association of an intensive lifestyle intervention with remission of type 2 diabetes. JAMA 2012;308:2489–96.
[10] Norris SL, Zhang X, Avenell A, et al. Long-term non-pharmacologic weight loss interventions for adults with type 2 diabetes. Cochrane Database Syst Rev 2005;(2):CD004095.
[11] Metz JA, Stern JS, Kris-Etherton P, et al. A randomized trial of improved weight loss with a prepared meal plan in overweight and obese patients: impact on cardiovascular risk reduction. Arch Intern Med 2000;160:2150–8.
[12] Pastors JG, Warshaw H, Daly A, et al. The evidence for the effectiveness of medical nutrition therapy in diabetes management. Diabetes Care 2002;25:608–13.
[13] Lim EL, Hollingsworth KG, Aribisala BS, et al. Reversal of type 2 diabetes: normalisation of beta cell function in association with decreased pancreas and liver triacylglycerol. Diabetologia 2011;54:2506–14.
[14] Shi YF, Pan CY, Hill J, et al. Orlistat in the treatment of overweight or obese Chinese patients with newly diagnosed Type 2 diabetes. Diabet Med 2005;22:1737–43.
[15] Norris SL, Zhang X, Avenell A, et al. Pharmacotherapy for weight loss in adults with type 2 diabetes mellitus. Cochrane Database Syst Rev 2005;(1):CD004096.
[16] UKPDS Group. UK Prospective Diabetes Study 7: response of fasting plasma glucose to diet therapy in newly presenting type II diabetic patients. Metabolism 1990;39:905–12.
[17] Buchwald H, Estok R, Fahrbach K, et al. Weight and type 2 diabetes after bariatric surgery: systematic review and meta-analysis. Am J Med 2009;122:248–56.e5.

[18] Schauer PR, Burguera B, Ikramuddin S, et al. Effect of laparoscopic Roux-en Y gastric bypass on type 2 diabetes mellitus. Ann Surg 2003;238:467–84.
[19] Ikramuddin S, Korner J, Lee WJ, et al. Roux-en-Y gastric bypass vs intensive medical management for the control of type 2 diabetes, hypertension, and hyperlipidemia: the Diabetes Surgery Study randomized clinical trial. JAMA 2013;309:2240–9.
[20] Brethauer SA, Aminian A, Romero-Talamas H, et al. Can diabetes be surgically cured? Long-term metabolic effects of bariatric surgery in obese patients with type 2 diabetes mellitus. Ann Surg 2013;258:628–36.
[21] Sjostrom L, Peltonen M, Jacobson P, et al. Association of bariatric surgery with long-term remission of type 2 diabetes and with microvascular and macrovascular complications. JAMA 2014;311:2297–304.
[22] Ribaric G, Buchwald JN, McGlennon TW. Diabetes and weight in comparative studies of bariatric surgery vs conventional medical therapy: a systematic review and meta-analysis. Obes Surg 2014;24:437–55.
[23] Dixon JB, O'Brien PE, Playfair J, et al. Adjustable gastric banding and conventional therapy for type 2 diabetes: a randomized controlled trial. JAMA 2008;299:316–23.
[24] Mingrone G, Panunzi S, De Gaetano A, et al. Bariatric surgery versus conventional medical therapy for type 2 diabetes. N Engl J Med 2012;366:1577–85.
[25] Halperin F, Ding SA, Simonson DC, et al. Roux-en-Y Gastric bypass surgery or lifestyle with intensive medical management in patients with type 2 diabetes: feasibility and 1-year results of a randomized clinical trial. JAMA Surg 2014;149:716–26.
[26] Kashyap SR, Bhatt DL, Wolski K, et al. Metabolic effects of bariatric surgery in patients with moderate obesity and type 2 diabetes: analysis of a randomized control trial comparing surgery with intensive medical treatment. Diabetes Care 2013;36: 2175–82.
[27] Schauer PR, Bhatt DL, Kirwan JP, et al. Bariatric surgery versus intensive medical therapy for diabetes–3-year outcomes. N Engl J Med 2014;370:2002–13.
[28] Courcoulas AP, Goodpaster BH, Eagleton JK, et al. Surgical vs medical treatments for type 2 diabetes mellitus: a randomized clinical trial. JAMA Surg 2014;149:707–15.
[29] Parikh M, Chung M, Sheth S, et al. Randomized pilot trial of bariatric surgery versus intensive medical weight management on diabetes remission in type 2 diabetic patients who do not meet NIH criteria for surgery and the role of soluble rage as a novel biomarker of success. Ann Surg 2014;260:617–24.
[30] Pories W, Swanson M, MacDonald K, et al. Who would have though it? An operation proves to be the most effective therapy for adult onset diabetes mellitus. Ann Surg 1995;222:339–52.
[31] Rubino F, Forgione A, Cummings DE, et al. The mechanism of diabetes control after gastrointestinal bypass surgery reveals a role of the proximal small intestine in the pathophysiology of type 2 diabetes. Ann Surg 2006;244:741–9.
[32] Patel RT, Shukla AP, Ahn SM, et al. Surgical control of obesity and diabetes: the role of intestinal vs. gastric mechanisms in the regulation of body weight and glucose homeostasis. Obesity 2014;22:59–69.
[33] Lee WJ, Chong K, Ling YH, et al. Laparoscopic sleeve gastrectomy versus single anastomosis (mini-) gastric bypass for the treatment of type 2 diabetes mellitus: 5-year results of a randomized trial and study of incretin effect. Obes Surg 2014;24:1552–62.
[34] Mallipedhi A, Prior SL, Barry DJ, et al. Temporal changes in glucose homeostasis and incretin hormone response at 1 and 6 months after laparoscopic sleeve gastrectomy. Surg Obes Relat Dis 2014;10:860–9.
[35] Al-Sabah S, Alasfar F, Al-Khaledi G, et al. Incretin response to a standard test meal in a rat model of sleeve gastrectomy with diet-induced obesity. Obes Surg 2014;24: 95–101.
[36] Murata M, Okimura Y, Lida K, et al. Ghrelin modulates the downstream molecules of insulin signaling in hepatoma cells. J Biol Chem 2002;277:5667–74.

[37] Yenumula P, Goncalves CG, Brethauer SA, et al. Diabetes in the bariatric surgery patient, in minimally invasive bariatric surgery. In: Schauer PR, Schrimer BD, Brethauer SA, editors. Minimally Invasive Bariatric Surgery. New York: Springer; 2007. p. 449–59. Available at: http://link.springer.com/chapter/10.1007/978-0-387-68062-0_54. Accessed May 18, 2015.
[38] Ngiam KY, Lee WJ, Lee YC, et al. Efficacy of metabolic surgery on HbA1c decrease in type 2 diabetes mellitus patients with BMI <35 kg/m2–a review. Obes Surg 2014;24:148–58.

Advances in Surgery 49 (2015) 173–184

ADVANCES IN SURGERY

Should Steroids Be Used During Endovascular Aortic Repair?

Louise de la Motte, MD, PhD[a,*],
Torben V. Schroeder, MD, DMSc[b], Henrik Kehlet, MD, PhD[c]

[a]Department of Vascular Surgery 3111, Rigshospitalet, University of Copenhagen, Blegdamsvej 9, Copenhagen DK-2100, Denmark; [b]Center for Clinical Education 5404, Rigshospitalet, University of Copenhagen, Capital Region of Denmark, Blegdamsvej 9, Copenhagen DK-2100, Denmark; [c]Section for Surgical Pathophysiology 4074, Rigshospitalet, University of Copenhagen, Blegdamsvej 9, Copenhagen DK-2100, Denmark

Keywords

• Abdominal aortic aneurysm • EVAR • Glucocorticoids • Length of stay
• Postimplantation syndrome • Systemic inflammatory response syndrome
• Surgical stress response • Recovery

Key points

- Endovascular aortic repair (EVAR) is a minimally invasive procedure for abdominal aortic aneurysm (AAA).
- The postimplantation syndrome is an obstacle to uncomplicated recovery.
- Preoperative methylprednisolone during EVAR could potentially enhance recovery.
- Further randomized trials are indicated before general recommendations on steroids during EVAR can be applied.

INTRODUCTION

Treatment options for abdominal aortic aneurysms

Open repair of abdominal aortic aneurysm (AAA) is a well-established durable treatment. However, there is a continuing trend toward less invasive techniques via small incisions (mini laparotomy), retroperitoneal access, or laparoscopic repair [1–4] and by optimization of perioperative care [5,6]. Endovascular aneurysm repair, first introduced about 30 years ago [7,8], has contributed

The authors have nothing to disclose.

*Corresponding author. *E-mail address:* Louisedelamotte@dadlnet.dk

0065-3411/15/$ – see front matter
http://dx.doi.org/10.1016/j.yasu.2015.03.001

substantially to making aneurysm repair minimally invasive. Endovascular aortic repair (EVAR) consists of endoluminal deployment of a stent graft (a metal mesh lined by a synthetic graft) in the aorta by access via the femoral arteries (Fig. 1). By deployment of a stent graft inside the aorta via the femoral arteries, minimal skin incisions, no manipulation of the intestine, and minimal blood loss are achieved. Owing to the minimally invasive character of the procedure, EVAR was soon adapted and is now the most frequent choice of preventive treatment in the United States and Europe [9,10].

The systemic inflammatory response related to endovascular aortic repair

Improved stent graft devices and technical experience have resulted in better outcomes, as well as EVAR has been suggested to attenuate the inflammatory response compared with open surgery [11–19]. However, a postimplantation syndrome (PIS), characterized by fever, flulike symptoms, neutrophil leukocytosis, and coagulation disturbances, has been observed in terms of the systemic inflammatory response syndrome (SIRS) in 13% to 60% of patients within the first 5 days after EVAR [20–23].

SIRS defines a physiologic state consisting of at least 2 of 4 criteria defined by the American College of Chest Physicians and Society of Critical Care Medicine Consensus Conference Committee (Box 1) [24].

Although the surgical trauma in EVAR is much less than the injury inflicted by open surgery, efforts have been made to determine the cause of the PIS. Factors such as stent graft material, contrast media, endothelial injury, acute formation of thrombus in the AAA sac, and manipulation of the intraluminal thrombus (ILT) have been suggested [25–30]. As yet, there is no satisfactory explanation to this marked response.

Previous studies have shown a high level of the cytokine interleukin (IL)-6 in the ILT lining the aneurysm and in the systemic circulation after EVAR

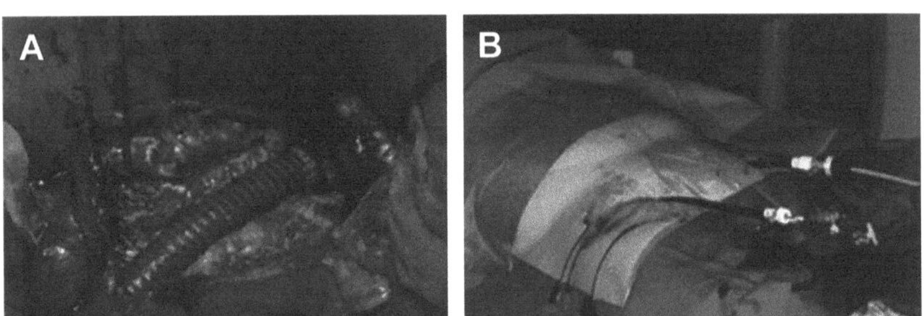

Fig. 1. (*A*) Open operative procedure. (*B*) Endovascular procedure. (*From* de la Motte L, Jensen LP. Endovascular and open aortic repair of abdominal aortic aneurysm are still both warranted - a systematic review. Ugeskr Laeger 2012;174(20):1376 [in Danish]; with permission.)

Box 1: Definition of systemic inflammatory response syndrome (SIRS)

Presence of 2 or more of the following criteria

- A temperature of greater than 38°C or less than 36°C
- A heart rate of greater than 90 beats per minute
- A respiratory rate of greater than 20 breaths per minute, or $Paco_2$ of less than 4.3 kPa
- A white blood cell count of greater than $12.0 \times 10^9/L$, or less than $4.0 \times 10^9/L$, or greater than 10% immature (band) forms

[18,25,26,28,29,31,32]. Other biomarkers demonstrated to be present at elevated levels after EVAR are C-reactive protein, D-dimer, the proinflammatory mediators IL-1β, tumor necrosis factor-α, IL-8, and the antiinflammatory mediator IL-10 [18,25,33,34].

Although this inflammatory response often remains at subclinical levels, it can also lead to major organ dysfunction [35]. Primarily the elderly and patients with more comorbidities are prone to the adverse effects of a transient systemic inflammatory response. Consequently, SIRS may prolong recovery and increase the risk of morbidity [25,36,37]. A technically successful EVAR should lead to a length of stay (LOS) of about 1 to 2 days, even in high-risk patients, if the increased organ demands owing to SIRS could be eliminated. In this context, the literature is inconclusive; some centers have reported a short LOS and even an outpatient procedure in selected EVAR patients [38,39] in contrast with other reports of LOS of more than 4 days [14,15,22,36,40,41].

Late implications of the postimplantation syndrome

Apart from the immediate discomfort to the patient a concern, at least theoretically, could be that the PIS may increase the risk of late complications such as endoleak (Fig. 2), stent graft migration, or aneurysm rupture. Continued inflammatory activity after EVAR compared with open aneurysm resection has been suggested by a sustained elevated plasma level of IL-6 [31]. In addition, analysis of the ILT, which is left in situ after EVAR, has shown a high content of IL-6 [29,32]. The ILT has also been identified as a source of proteases (one of which is matrix metalloproteinase [MMP]-9), active in the growth of the aneurysms [42] and speculated to be involved in development of the late complications related to EVAR [43–45].

The importance of a transient SIRS to the sustained biological activity after EVAR is unclear, but it seems relevant to speculate that an increase in plasma neutrophils and IL-6 in relation to the procedure, could have an effect on the high levels of IL-6 and MMP-9 reported to be present long after the procedure [31,43,44].

Preoperative glucocorticoids

Several trials have demonstrated a reduction in the inflammatory response, postoperative nausea and vomiting and pain by administration of preoperative

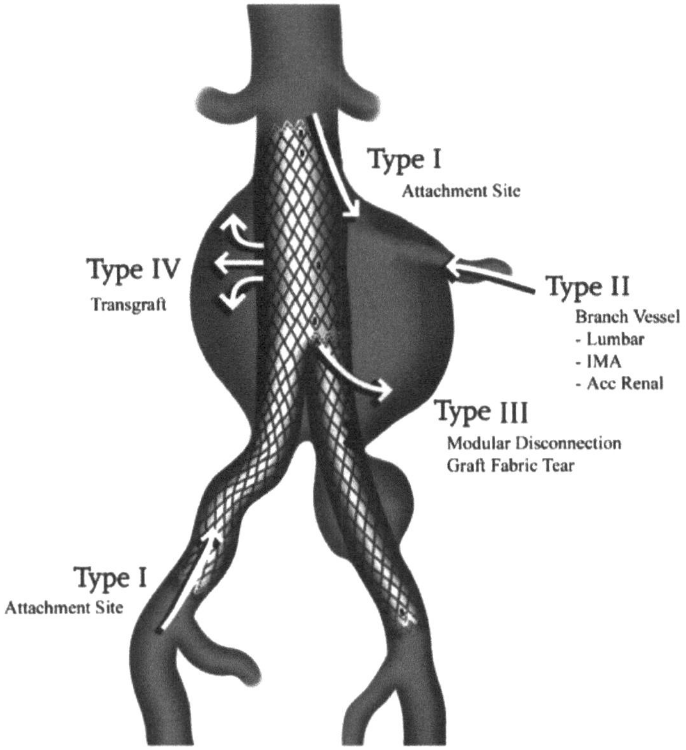

Fig. 2. Endoleak is a complication unique to endovascular aortic repair (EVAR). Detection is essential because an endoleak may lead to aneurysm expansion and rupture. Therefore, EVAR patients are offered surveillance with ultrasonography, CT, and/or x-ray for the detection of endoleak and stent graft migration. There are different types of endoleaks. Type I are leaks at the proximal (type 1a) or distal (type 1b) attachment sites. Type II endoleaks are caused by retrograde flow through side branches into the aneurysm sac. Type III endoleaks are defects in the fabric or separation of the stent graft modules. Type IV endoleaks are owing to porosity of the graft fabric and are not seen in newer generation stent grafts. (*Courtesy of* Medtronic; with permission.)

glucocorticoids (GC; Box 2)[46–51]. The well-documented antiinflammatory effects [52] of GC include inhibition of proinflammatory biomarkers and an increase in the antiinflammatory response [51]. Of particular interest in vascular surgery is the previously demonstrated injury-induced disruption of endothelial glycocalyx [53], where GC have been shown to preserve the endothelial glycocalyx and the vascular barrier, and to reduce interstitial edema [54]. These positive effects have been shown during ischemic injury [54], as well as during tumor necrosis factor-α–induced glycocalyx disruption [55]. The administration of GC is also known to increase leukocyte count and blood glucose level. However, the transitory hyperglycemic response after a single high-dose GC has not been related to increased postoperative complications [56]

Box 2: Effects of a single preoperative dose of glucocorticoid

- Decreases proinflammatory mediators
- Reduces postoperative hyperthermia
- Decreases postoperative nausea and vomiting
- Decreases local edema, resulting in reduced pain
- Increases leukocyte count and glucose concentration in peripheral blood

supported by the findings in a recent randomized, controlled trial (RCT) of methylprednisolone (MP) in EVAR, taking into account the limited number of patients in the subgroup of diabetics [51]. The increase in blood leukocyte count is mainly a neutrocytosis, but the neutrocyte activity is altered, in part by a transient impairment of the neutrophil oxidative burst by MP [57], which is supported by the finding of an unaltered myeloperoxidase level despite a higher concentration of neutrocytes after administration of MP [51].

A wide variety of operative procedures have been submitted to "fast-track" protocols resulting in lower morbidity and a reduction in postoperative LOS [58]. Schulze and colleagues [59] found a significant reduction of postoperative pain, fever, and fatigue by the administration of 30 mg/kg MP before colon resection and cholecystectomy [60]. They also found that preoperative administration of MP reduced the increase in plasma IL-6 and C-reactive protein seen after colectomy [61]. Another, more recent study confirmed the same effect of MP independent of the extent of surgical trauma [62]. In addition, preoperative administration of MP is shown to exert cardioprotective effects [63]. Patients with AAA have a high rate of cardiac comorbidity [64,65] and IL-6, which is increased in plasma from AAA patients [66], has been identified as an independent risk factor for cardiovascular death [67]. Furthermore, Dawson and colleagues [31] have shown that open repair but not EVAR decreases the plasma level of IL-6.

Timing of steroid administration in relation to surgery

The timing of GC administration is essential to attenuate the surgical stress response. Cytokines are produced within hours as response to tissue trauma and activation of the earliest mediators occurs immediately after the surgical incision. They act as signal molecules that recruit inflammatory cells to the tissue and activate the cells [68]. Steroids generally exert their effect via regulation of protein synthesis, the optimal timing of administration would therefore be 1 to 2 hours before surgery to obtain full biological effect of the steroid at the time of incision [46,69]. However, there is a lack of definitive clinical studies on the specific role of timing of GC treatment versus effect size.

Steroids during endovascular aortic repair

An attenuation of the systemic inflammatory response after EVAR by preoperative administration of GC seems feasible and complimentary effects on cardiac morbidity might be achieved. Although GC have been used in EVAR

[28,36,38], this approach has only been tested once in a recent RCT [51] that studied the effect of high-dose MP (30 mg/kg) before EVAR, resulting in a pronounced reduction of the postoperative components of the SIRS response from 92% to 27%. In addition, the decrease in the inflammatory responses and proinflammatory biomarkers (Fig. 3) was associated with an increase in the antiinflammatory response in IL-10, and the unaltered myeloperoxidase level despite a higher concentration of neutrocytes in the MP group may support previous findings of a transient impairment of the neutrophil oxidative burst by MP [57]. Importantly, these physiologic effects of MP resulted in a reduction in time to meet discharge criteria without any apparent safety issues.

The other nonrandomized reports on steroids during EVAR come from the outpatient report by Lachat and colleagues [38] in which they described the administration of prolonged (5 days) low-dose prednisone therapy starting some hours after the EVAR procedure to reduce PIS. Gerasimidis and colleagues [28] reported the use of 500 mg of hydrocortisone during the EVAR procedure and finally Nano and colleagues [36] described the administration of 1 g of hydrocortisone intravenously on the third postoperative day in case of PIS. In all 3 reports, the timing of GC is suboptimal considering the physiologic functions of steroids [46,69].

DISCUSSION

EVAR is a durable and minimally invasive treatment option for AAA [9,12,14,15,41]. Long-term mortality rates are similar and fewer complications are seen after EVAR, as compared with open repair, considering both aneurysm-related and procedure-related complications [14]. However, there is room for improvement regarding LOS, wound complications, and endoleaks.

The undesirable inflammatory response to EVAR may lead to major organ dysfunction [35], especially in the elderly and patients with severe comorbidities [25]. Moreover, SIRS may be interpreted as an infectious complication mandating prolonged antibiotic management. Interestingly, postoperative IL-6 levels may decrease earlier after open AAA operation compared with EVAR [31], supporting the notion of a continuous inflammatory response after EVAR. In this context, the high rate of SIRS seen after EVAR affects the potential for a fast track protocol [58], supporting the potential for future routine administration of preoperative GC to attenuate the inflammatory response.

In recent years, there has been an increased interest in the use of preoperative pharmacologic doses of GC, not only for postoperative nausea and vomiting prophylaxis, but also owing to the reduction in pain and opioid requirements [47,48,50]. GC have several well-documented antiinflammatory effects [52], such as inhibition of the proinflammatory response and increase of antiinflammatory mediators [51]. The ability of GC to preserve the endothelial glycocalyx [54,55] and thereby the vascular barrier is of particular interest in vascular surgery, where injury-induced disruption of the endothelial glycocalyx results in impairment of the vascular barrier and promotion of interstitial edema [53]. Although, procedure-specific dose–response studies are still needed, the positive

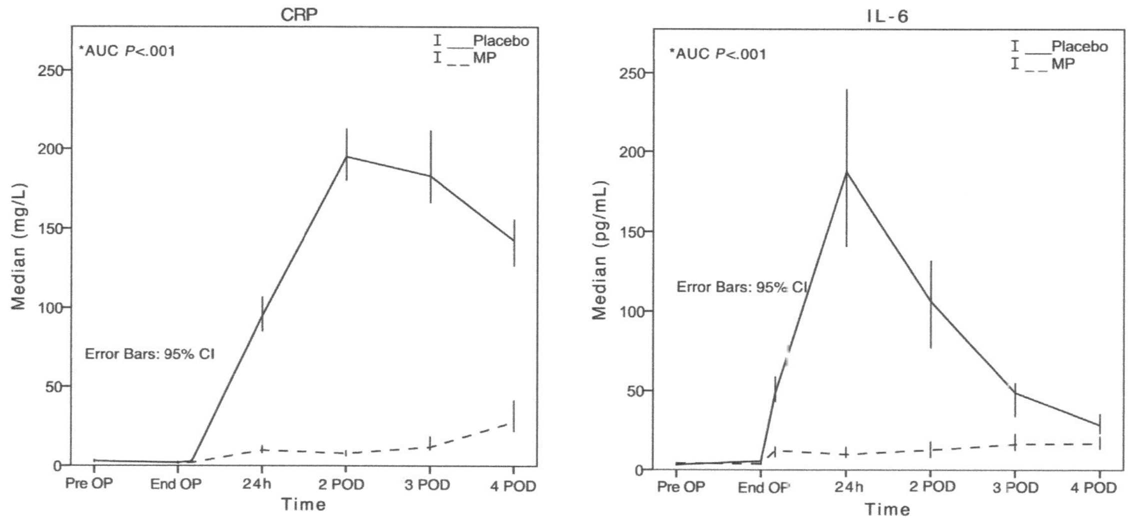

Fig. 3. Antiinflammatory effect of a single preoperative dose of methylprednisolone. Patients undergoing elective endovascular aortic repair (EVAR) were randomized to a single preoperative dose of 30 mg/kg MP or saline administered 2 hours before the procedure. AUC, area under the curve; CRP, C-reactive protein; IL-6, interleukin 6; MP, methylprednisolone; POD, postoperative day. (*Adapted from* de la Motte L, Kehlet H, Vogt K, et al. Preoperative methylprednisolone enhances recovery after endovascular aortic repair: a randomized, double-blind, placebo-controlled clinical trial. Ann Surg 2014;260(3):540–8 [discussion: 548–9]; with permission.)

effects have been shown in biliary and hepatic surgery and colorectal procedures [47,50,70] and also in cardiac surgery regarding postoperative infection, duration of postoperative mechanical ventilation, hyperthermia, and LOS [71,72]. The RCT on preoperative MP in EVAR proved the same reduction in postoperative pain and fever, and attenuation of the increase in plasma IL-6 and C-reactive protein (see Fig. 3) [51]. So far, there seem to be no safety issues [46–50,70–72] related to a single preoperative dose of GC, including specific studies on wound healing [61,73]. The consequences of preoperative high-dose GC for glucose homeostasis requires further evaluation, but so far the transitory hyperglycemic response has not been related to an increase in postoperative complications [51,56].

Apart from the discomfort related to the inflammatory response, speculations exist regarding long-term effects of EVAR on the inflammatory activity in the aneurysm wall and ILT. Thus, during the perioperative course elevated plasma levels of IL-6, IL-8, and other inflammatory markers have been measured [17,18,28,74], and elevated levels of IL-6 and MMP-9 have been reported up to 18 months after the procedure [31,43,44,75]. In particular, MMP-9 has been related to the risk of endoleaks after EVAR [75], whereas the IL-6 response as an independent risk factor for cardiac morbidity [67] could have implications for cardiovascular morbidity after EVAR [31].

High-dose MP may exert its effect for as long as a couple of weeks after administration and could have the potential to halt the ongoing inflammation reported after EVAR. Although the size of the RCT on MP in EVAR [51] was relatively large ($n = 150$), it was not powered adequately to evaluate the effect of MP on the incidence of endoleaks. Some might argue that the PIS reduces endoleaks by enhancing the development of scar tissue; however, it can just as easily be argued that it enhances continued modulation of the aneurysm wall and, thereby, the development of endoleaks and migration of the stent graft. To date, no reports of negative effects on tissue healing after a single preoperative dose of steroids have been published.

Many different regimes of perioperative steroids have been tested and, although the dose of steroids should be the subject of further studies, the timing of administration should aim at achieving the optimal effect, which relies on the pharmacokinetics of steroids. The diverging results on the use of perioperative GC might therefore be owing to the specific GC administered and to the timing of administration.

SUMMARY

Elective EVAR is followed by a pronounced proinflammatory response, which may contribute to delayed recovery and morbidity. Perioperative GC are already used routinely in EVAR in some departments, primarily to attenuate the PIS, stressing the relevance of studying the effects of GC in relation to EVAR in a randomized setting. Owing to the pharmacokinetics of GC, we suggest that GC be administered as a single preoperative dosage approximately 2 hours before surgery. In a recent RCT of EVAR, a single preoperative high-dose GC (30 mg/kg MP 2 hours preoperatively) led to a pronounced reduction of SIRS and inflammatory biomarker responses with enhanced achievement of discharge criteria and without apparent safety issues, which is in accordance with the findings in numerous studies on preoperative GC in other types of operative procedures. However, a general recommendation of GC during EVAR should be sufficiently scientifically based, calling for future large-scale efficacy/safety as well as dose/timing–response studies.

References

[1] Brustia P, Renghi A, Gramaglia L, et al. Mininvasive abdominal aortic surgery. Early recovery and reduced hospitalization after multidisciplinary approach. J Cardiovasc Surg (Torino) 2003;44(5):629–35.
[2] Brustia P, Renghi A, Fassiola A, et al. Fast-track approach in abdominal aortic surgery: left subcostal incision with blended anesthesia. Interact Cardiovasc Thorac Surg 2007;6(1):60–4.
[3] Javerliat I, Capdevila C, Beauchet A, et al. Results of laparoscopic surgery for abdominal aortic aneurysms in patients with standard surgical risk and anatomic criteria compatible with EVAR. Ann Vasc Surg 2013;27(4):412–7.
[4] Lin JC, Kaul SA, Bhandari A, et al. Robotic-assisted aortic surgery with and without minilaparotomy for complicated occlusive disease and aneurysm. J Vasc Surg 2012;55(1):16–22.
[5] Muehling BM, Ortlieb L, Oberhuber A, et al. Fast track management reduces the systemic inflammatory response and organ failure following elective infrarenal aortic aneurysm repair. Interact Cardiovasc Thorac Surg 2011;12(5):784–8.
[6] Mukherjee D, Becker TE. An update on the "fast-track" abdominal aortic aneurysm repair. Int J Angiol 2008;17(2):93–7.
[7] Volodos NL. Historical perspective: the first steps in endovascular aortic repair: how it all began. J Endovasc Ther 2013;20(Suppl 1):I3–23.
[8] Parodi JC, Palmaz JC, Barone HD. Transfemoral intraluminal graft implantation for abdominal aortic aneurysms. Ann Vasc Surg 1991;5(6):491–9.
[9] Mani K, Lees T, Beiles B, et al. Treatment of abdominal aortic aneurysm in nine countries 2005-2009: a vascunet report. Eur J Vasc Endovasc Surg 2011;42(5):598–607.
[10] Lawrence P, Rigberg D. Arterial aneurysms: general considerations. In: Cronenwett JL, Johnston W, editors. Rutherfords vascular surgery. 7th edition. Philadelphia: Saunders Elsevier; 2010. p. 1920–7.
[11] Lederle FA, Freischlag JA, Kyriakides TC, et al. Long-term comparison of endovascular and open repair of abdominal aortic aneurysm. N Engl J Med 2012;367(21):1988–97.
[12] Greenhalgh RM, Brown LC, Powell JT, et al. Endovascular versus open repair of abdominal aortic aneurysm. N Engl J Med 2010;362(20):1863–71.
[13] Jayia P, Constantinou J, Morgan-Rowe L, et al. Are there fewer complications with third generation endografts in endovascular aneurysm repair? J Cardiovasc Surg (Torino) 2013;54(1):133–43.
[14] De la Motte L, Jensen LP, Vogt K, et al. Outcomes after elective aortic aneurysm repair: a nationwide Danish cohort study 2007-2010. Eur J Vasc Endovasc Surg 2013;46(1):57–64.
[15] Schermerhorn ML, O'Malley AJ, Jhaveri A, et al. Endovascular vs open repair of abdominal aortic aneurysms in the Medicare population. N Engl J Med 2008;358(5):464–74.
[16] Bölke E, Jehle PM, Storck M, et al. Endovascular stent-graft placement versus conventional open surgery in infrarenal aortic aneurysm: a prospective study on acute phase response and clinical outcome. Clin Chim Acta 2001;314(1–2):203–7.
[17] Swartbol P, Norgren L, Albrechtsson U, et al. Biological responses differ considerably between endovascular and conventional aortic aneurysm surgery. Eur J Vasc Endovasc Surg 1996;12(1):18–25.
[18] Rowlands TE, Homer-Vanniasinkam S. Pro- and anti-inflammatory cytokine release in open versus endovascular repair of abdominal aortic aneurysm. Br J Surg 2001;88(10):1335–40.

[19] Rowlands TE, Homer-Vanniasinkam S. Paradoxical neutrophil elastase release in endovascular abdominal aortic aneurysm repair. Vasc Endovascular Surg 2007;41(1):48–54.
[20] Sweeney KJ, Evoy D, Sultan S, et al. Endovascular approach to abdominal aortic aneurysms limits the postoperative systemic immune response. Eur J Vasc Endovasc Surg 2002;23(4): 303–8.
[21] Pearson S, Hassen T, Spark JI, et al. Endovascular repair of abdominal aortic aneurysm reduces intraoperative cortisol and perioperative morbidity. J Vasc Surg 2005;41(6): 919–25.
[22] De La Motte L, Vogt K, Panduro Jensen L, et al. Incidence of systemic inflammatory response syndrome after endovascular aortic repair. J Cardiovasc Surg (Torino) 2011;52(1):73–9.
[23] Hassen TA, Pearson S, Cowled PA, et al. Preoperative nutritional status predicts the severity of the systemic inflammatory response syndrome (SIRS) following major vascular surgery. Eur J Vasc Endovasc Surg 2007;33(6):696–702.
[24] American College of Chest Physicians/Society of Critical Care Medicine Consensus Conference: definitions for sepsis and organ failure and guidelines for the use of innovative therapies in sepsis. Crit Care Med 1992;20(6):864–74.
[25] Arnaoutoglou E, Kouvelos G, Milionis H, et al. Post-implantation syndrome following endovascular abdominal aortic aneurysm repair: preliminary data. Interact Cardiovasc Thorac Surg 2011;12(4):609–14.
[26] Aho PS, Niemi T, Piilonen A, et al. Interplay between coagulation and inflammation in open and endovascular abdominal aortic aneurysm repair–impact of intra-aneurysmal thrombus. Scand J Surg 2007;96(3):229–35.
[27] Gabriel EA, Locali RF, Romano CC, et al. Analysis of the inflammatory response in endovascular treatment of aortic aneurysms. Eur J Cardiothorac Surg 2007;31(3):406–12.
[28] Gerasimidis T, Sfyroeras G, Trellopoulos G, et al. Impact of endograft material on the inflammatory response after elective endovascular abdominal aortic aneurysm repair. Angiology 2005;56(6):743–53.
[29] Swartbol P, Truedsson L, Norgren L. Adverse reactions during endovascular treatment of aortic aneurysms may be triggered by interleukin 6 release from the thrombotic content. J Vasc Surg 1998;28(4):664–8.
[30] Voûte MT, Bastos Gonçalves FM, van de Luijtgaarden KM, et al. Stent graft composition plays a material role in the postimplantation syndrome. J Vasc Surg 2012;56(6): 1503–9.
[31] Dawson JA, Choke E, Cockerill GW, et al. The long-term effects of open and endovascular aneurysm repair on circulating interleukin-6. Eur J Vasc Endovasc Surg 2009;37(1):43–5.
[32] Risberg B, Delle M, Lönn L, et al. Management of aneurysm sac hygroma. J Endovasc Ther 2004;11(2):191–5.
[33] Bailey MA, Griffin KJ, Sohrabi S, et al. Plasma thrombin-antithrombin complex, prothrombin fragments 1 and 2, and D-dimer levels are elevated after endovascular but not open repair of infrarenal abdominal aortic aneurysm. J Vasc Surg 2013;57(6):1512–8.
[34] Swartbol P, Truedsson L, Norgren L. The inflammatory response and its consequence for the clinical outcome following aortic aneurysm repair. Eur J Vasc Endovasc Surg 2001;21(5): 393–400.
[35] Arnaoutoglou E, Papas N, Milionis H, et al. Post-implantation syndrome after endovascular repair of aortic aneurysms: need for postdischarge surveillance. Interact Cardiovasc Thorac Surg 2010;11(4):449–54.
[36] Nano G, Occhiuto MT, Stegher S, et al. Postimplantation syndrome after endovascular aortic repair using the AnacondaTM endograft. Ann Vasc Surg 2014;28(6):1409–15.
[37] Alomran F, de Blic R, Mallios A, et al. De novo periaortic fibrosis after endovascular aortic repair. Ann Vasc Surg 2014;28(2):493.e1–3.
[38] Lachat ML, Pecoraro F, Mayer D, et al. Outpatient endovascular aortic aneurysm repair: experience in 100 consecutive patients. Ann Surg 2013;258(5):754–8 [discussion: 758–9].

[39] Dosluoglu HH, Lall P, Blochle R, et al. Ambulatory percutaneous endovascular abdominal aortic aneurysm repair. J Vasc Surg 2014;59(1):58–64.
[40] Pettersson M, Bergbom I, Mattsson E. Health related quality of life after treatment of abdominal aortic aneurysm with open and endovascular techniques — a two-year follow up. Surg Sci 2012;2012:436–44.
[41] Lederle FA, Freischlag JA, Kyriakides TC, et al. Outcomes following endovascular vs open repair of abdominal aortic aneurysm: a randomized trial. JAMA 2009;302(14):1535–42.
[42] Fontaine V, Jacob MP, Houard X, et al. Involvement of the mural thrombus as a site of protease release and activation in human aortic aneurysms. Am J Pathol 2002;161(5):1701–10.
[43] Lorelli DR, Jean-Claude JM, Fox CJ, et al. Response of plasma matrix metalloproteinase-9 to conventional abdominal aortic aneurysm repair or endovascular exclusion: implications for endoleak. J Vasc Surg 2002;35(5):916–22.
[44] Sangiorgi G, D'Averio R, Mauriello A, et al. Plasma levels of metalloproteinases-3 and -9 as markers of successful abdominal aortic aneurysm exclusion after endovascular graft treatment. Circulation 2001;104(12 Suppl 1):I288–95.
[45] Hackmann AE, Rubin BG, Sanchez LA, et al. A randomized, placebo-controlled trial of doxycycline after endoluminal aneurysm repair. J Vasc Surg 2008;48(3):519–26 [discussion: 526].
[46] Holte K, Kehlet H. Perioperative single-dose glucocorticoid administration: pathophysiologic effects and clinical implications. J Am Coll Surg 2002;195(5):694–712.
[47] De Oliveira GS, Almeida MD, Benzon HT, et al. Perioperative single dose systemic dexamethasone for postoperative pain: a meta-analysis of randomized controlled trials. Anesthesiology 2011;115(3):575–88.
[48] Lunn TH, Kehlet H. Perioperative glucocorticoids in hip and knee surgery - benefit vs harm? A review of randomized clinical trials. Acta Anaesthesiol Scand 2013;57(7):823–34.
[49] Sauerland S, Nagelschmidt M, Mallmann P, et al. Risks and benefits of preoperative high dose methylprednisolone in surgical patients: a systematic review. Drug Saf 2000;23(5):449–61.
[50] Srinivasa S, Kahokehr AA, Yu TC, et al. Preoperative glucocorticoid use in major abdominal surgery: systematic review and meta-analysis of randomized trials. Ann Surg 2011;254(2):183–91.
[51] De la Motte L, Kehlet H, Vogt K, et al. Preoperative methylprednisolone enhances recovery after endovascular aortic repair: a randomized, double-blind, placebo-controlled clinical trial. Ann Surg 2014;260(3):540–8 [discussion: 548–9].
[52] Rhen T, Cidlowski JA. Antiinflammatory action of glucocorticoids–new mechanisms for old drugs. N. Engl. J Med 2005;353(16):1711–23.
[53] Rehm M, Bruegger D, Christ F, et al. Shedding of the endothelial glycocalyx in patients undergoing major vascular surgery with global and regional ischemia. Circulation 2007;116(17):1896–906.
[54] Chappell D, Jacob M, Hofmann-Kiefer K, et al. Hydrocortisone preserves the vascular barrier by protecting the endothelial glycocalyx. Anesthesiology 2007;107(5):776–84.
[55] Chappell D, Hofmann-Kiefer K, Jacob M, et al. TNF-alpha induced shedding of the endothelial glycocalyx is prevented by hydrocortisone and antithrombin. Basic Res Cardiol 2009;104(1):78–89.
[56] Abdelmalak BB, Bonilla AM, Yang D, et al. The hyperglycemic response to major noncardiac surgery and the added effect of steroid administration in patients with and without diabetes. Anesth Analg 2013;116(5):1116–22.
[57] Welch WD, Devlin P. Hydrocortisone sodium succinate reversibly inhibits human neutrophil oxidative activity at clinically relevant concentrations. Chem Biol Interact 1983;43(2):239–44.
[58] Kehlet H, Wilmore DW. Evidence-based surgical care and the evolution of fast-track surgery. Ann Surg 2008;248(2):189–98.
[59] Schulze S, Sommer P, Bigler D, et al. Effect of combined prednisolone, epidural analgesia, and indomethacin on the systemic response after colonic surgery. Arch Surg 1992;127(3):325–31.

[60] Schulze S, Møller IW, Bang U, et al. Effect of combined prednisolone, epidural analgesia and indomethacin on pain, systemic response and convalescence after cholecystectomy. Acta Chir Scand 1990;156(3):203–9.
[61] Schulze S, Andersen J, Overgaard H, et al. Effect of prednisolone on the systemic response and wound healing after colonic surgery. Arch Surg 1997;132(2):129–35.
[62] Vignali A, Di Palo S, Orsenigo E, et al. Effect of prednisolone on local and systemic response in laparoscopic vs open colon surgery: a randomized, double-blind, placebo-controlled trial. Dis Colon Rectum 2009;52(6):1080–8.
[63] Liakopoulos OJ, Schmitto JD, Kazmaier S, et al. Cardiopulmonary and systemic effects of methylprednisolone in patients undergoing cardiac surgery. Ann Thorac Surg 2007;84(1): 110–8 [discussion: 118–9].
[64] Mortality results for randomised controlled trial of early elective surgery or ultrasonographic surveillance for small abdominal aortic aneurysms. The UK Small Aneurysm Trial Participants. Lancet 1998;352(9141):1649–55.
[65] Brady AR, Fowkes FG, Thompson SG, et al. Aortic aneurysm diameter and risk of cardiovascular mortality. Arterioscler Thromb Vasc Biol 2001;21(7):1203–7.
[66] Dawson J, Cockerill GW, Choke E, et al. Aortic aneurysms secrete interleukin-6 into the circulation. J Vasc Surg 2007;45(2):350–6.
[67] Ridker PM, Rifai N, Stampfer MJ, et al. Plasma concentration of interleukin-6 and the risk of future myocardial infarction among apparently healthy men. Circulation 2000;101(15): 1767–72.
[68] Delves PJ, Roitt IM. The immune system. Second of two parts. N Engl J Med 2000;343(2): 108–17.
[69] Sapolsky RM, Romero LM, Munck AU. How do glucocorticoids influence stress responses? Integrating permissive, suppressive, stimulatory, and preparative actions. Endocr Rev 2000;21(1):55–89.
[70] Orci LA, Toso C, Mentha G, et al. Systematic review and meta-analysis of the effect of perioperative steroids on ischaemia-reperfusion injury and surgical stress response in patients undergoing liver resection. Br J Surg 2013;100(5):600–9.
[71] Whitlock RP, Chan S, Devereaux PJ, et al. Clinical benefit of steroid use in patients undergoing cardiopulmonary bypass: a meta-analysis of randomized trials. Eur Heart J 2008;29(21): 2592–600.
[72] Dieleman JM, Nierich AP, Rosseel PM, et al. Intraoperative high-dose dexamethasone for cardiac surgery: a randomized controlled trial. JAMA 2012;308(17):1761–7.
[73] Wang AS, Armstrong EJ, Armstrong AW. Corticosteroids and wound healing: clinical considerations in the perioperative period. Am J Surg 2013;206(3):410–7.
[74] Houard X, Touat Z, Ollivier V, et al. Mediators of neutrophil recruitment in human abdominal aortic aneurysms. Cardiovasc Res 2009;82(3):532–41.
[75] Antoniou GA, Georgiadis GS, Antoniou SA, et al. Plasma matrix metalloproteinase 9 levels may predict endoleaks after endovascular aortic aneurysm repair. Angiology 2013;64(1): 49–56.

Advances in Surgery 49 (2015) 185–204

ADVANCES IN SURGERY

Are Higher Hospital Venous Thromboembolism Rates an Indicator of Better Quality?

Evaluation of the Validity of a Hospital Quality Measure

Christina A. Minami, MD, Karl Y. Bilimoria, MD, MS*

Department of Surgery, Surgical Outcomes and Quality Improvement Center, Center for Healthcare Studies, Northwestern Memorial Hospital, Feinberg School of Medicine, Northwestern University, 633 North Saint Clair Street, 20th Floor, Chicago, IL 60611, USA

Keywords

• Venous thromboembolism • Patient safety indicator 12 • Surveillance bias
• SCIP-VTE-2

Key points

- VTE is a clinically important and potentially preventable problem that has deservedly received significant attention on the policy level.
- Surveillance bias is an important issue and the VTE outcomes measure is likely not valid.
- Although there is potentially some room for improvement in PSI-12, and improvements should continually be made as long as this measure remains a part of quality reporting, efforts should be directed more toward developing a new measure reflecting a hospital's ability to prevent VTE.

INTRODUCTION

Venous thromboembolism (VTE), which includes deep vein thrombosis (DVT) and pulmonary embolism (PE), is a common postoperative complication that remains a significant (and potentially preventable) cause of morbidity and mortality [1]. With 300,000 to 600,000 new cases each year and 100,000 to 300,000 deaths per year [2], VTE can occur after 1% of major surgeries [3,4].

The authors have nothing to disclose.

*Corresponding author. *E-mail address*: k-bilimoria@northwestern.edu

0065-3411/15/$ – see front matter
http://dx.doi.org/10.1016/j.yasu.2015.03.002

Although mortality rates from PE are sobering, morbidity in the form of post-thrombotic syndrome (which may manifest as debilitating pain, ulceration, and limb swelling) and pulmonary hypertension are also serious sequelae that complicate 5% to 50% of VTE events [5–8].

The significance of VTE is not only evident in postoperative morbidity and mortality rates, but also in the resultant economic burden. In 2010, total DVT costs were estimated at $7.5 to $26.5 billion, with hospital-acquired and preventable costs figuring at $5 to $26.5 billion and $2.5 to $19.5 billion, respectively [9]. A DVT may add at least a mean cost of $7769 and a PE $9176, to a hospital stay [10]. In addition to direct patient, lost productivity costs to employers have also been found to be significant. Mean short- and long-term disability claims for DVT were estimated at $7400 and $58,000, respectively. For PE, these were estimated to be slightly higher, at approximately $7600 and $48,800 for short- and long-term disability claims, respectively [2].

Major surgery has long been implicated as an important risk factor for VTE [3,11], and early large studies encompassing general surgery and various surgical subspecialties have demonstrated that the postoperative VTE rate ranges from 10% to 40% without prophylaxis [12]. Certain subpopulations of surgical patients have been touted as being at especially high risk, including those who have suffered trauma or burns or who have undergone neurosurgery or orthopedic surgery. The incidence of VTE in the unprophylaxed cancer, trauma, and burn populations varies widely; early studies found that 35% to 65% of these patients suffered from VTE without prophylaxis, and this number seems to largely depend on the type of injury and other risk factors, such as age [13–15]. Death from PE in this population may range from 8% to 15% [12]. Patients undergoing combined cranial/spinal procedures without prophylaxis have a DVT rate of 29% to 43% [16] and studies in the spinal cord surgery population show incidences that vary between 12% and 100% [17]. Incidence in patients who have undergone elective total hip arthroplasty has been reported to range between 45% and 70% when no prophylaxis is given [18].

With chemical and/or mechanical prophylaxis, however, VTE rates can be reduced by as much as 74% to 86% and can reduce all-cause mortality in surgical patients [2,19,20]. Although the use of sequential compression devices, unfractionated heparin, and low-molecular-weight heparin may not eliminate VTE [21], DVT and PE are still preventable events [22,23]. Evidence-based guidelines regarding the appropriate type, duration, and dose of prophylaxis have been provided by the American College of Chest Physicians since 1986 [24]. Despite this, it has been found that thromboprophylaxis was being underused; only 62% of the 18,461 postoperative patients in the Epidemiologic International Day for the Evaluation of Patients at Risk of Venous Thrombosis in the Acute Hospital Care Setting study received the recommended prophylaxis (per the 2004 American College of Chest Physicians guidelines) in the acute care hospital setting [22]. Another study used the US Surgical Care Improvement Project (SCIP) VTE-2 performance measure, which measures the proportion of surgery patients who received appropriate VTE prophylaxis within 24 hours before surgery to 24 hours after surgery, to evaluate patient receipt of timely and appropriate prophylaxis. Only 56.2% received appropriate prophylaxis and only 52.7% of the 149,785 patients in the study were found to receive appropriate and timely prophylaxis [25]. There has been a recent call to arms regarding enforcement of evidence-based prophylaxis guidelines to address this failure of implementation and in more recent studies, VTE prophylaxis adherence rates have been found to be 90% or greater [4,26].

VTE has continually grown in its importance in health care policy and is widely publicly reported and used in pay-for-performance programs. VTE currently has nine main measures, but two have been focused on historically: one process measure and one outcome measure. The VTE process measure is manifested in SCIP-VTE-2, which measures VTE prophylaxis administration. Established in 2003, SCIP is a national partnership of more than 40 organizations whose original goal was to reduce preventable surgical morbidity and mortality by 25% by 2010 [27]. Although initially focused on surgical site infection, VTE measures grew to encompass other areas of quality concern and currently six VTE measures focus on various aspects of care related to VTE prevention and treatment (Table 1) [26].

The outcome measure, Patient Safety Indicator 12 (PSI-12), was developed by the Agency for Healthcare Research and Quality and is a risk-adjusted postoperative VTE rate measure per 1000 surgical discharges [28]. Since its endorsement by the National Quality Forum in 2008, this measure has been integrated into several quality improvement (QI) programs and public reporting initiatives, including the Centers for Medicare and Medicaid Services (CMS) 2015 Value-based Purchase program [29]. In 2008, CMS added DVT and PE after total knee arthroplasty and total hip arthroplasty to their list of "never events" [21] and under current policy, institutions will fail to be reimbursed for VTE events in these populations.

SURVEILLANCE BIAS IN VENOUS THROMBOEMBOLISM MEASUREMENT

Surveillance bias, often discussed in epidemiology, rarely comes into question in clinical studies [30]. It is also called detection bias or ascertainment bias. It is a type of information bias in which fluctuations in outcome may merely reflect variation in screening; in effect, it illustrates "the more you look, the more you find" phenomenon [30,31]. Differences in screening for VTE may be caused by the presence of screening protocols, in which asymptomatic patients undergo routine VTE imaging studies on a set postoperative day. Alternatively, the differences could be caused by differences in clinicians' thresholds for ordering imaging studies in patients with potential signs or symptoms of VTE [4]. For example, although bilateral leg swelling may prompt bilateral venous duplex at one hospital, the finding may be attributed to anasarca and fluid overload at another hospital. Thus, differences in VTE outcomes may be more

Table 1
VTE quality measures

Measure	Description	Calculation
VTE-1: VTE Prophylaxis	Assesses number of patients who received VTE prophylaxis or have documentation why no VTE prophylaxis was given the day of or the day after hospital admission or surgery end date for surgeries that start the day of or the day after hospital admission	$\frac{\text{Patients who received VTE prophylaxis or have no documentation why no VTE prophylaxis was given}}{\text{Patients who developed confirmed VTE during hospitalization}}$
VTE-2: Intensive Care Unit VTE Prophylaxis	Assesses the number of patients who received VTE prophylaxis or have documentation why no VTE prophylaxis was given the day of or the day after the initial admission (or transfer) to the intensive care unit (ICU) or surgery end date for surgeries that start the day of or the day after ICU admission (or transfer)	$\frac{\text{Patients who received VTE prophylaxis or have documentation why no VTE prophylaxis was given}}{\text{Patients directly admitted or transferred to ICU}}$
VTE-3: VTE Patients with Anticoagulation Overlap Therapy	Assesses the number of patients diagnosed with confirmed VTE who receive an overlap of parenteral (intravenous [IV] or subcutaneous) anticoagulation and warfarin therapy For patients who received less than 5 d of overlap therapy, they should be discharged on both medications or have reason for discontinuation of parenteral therapy Overlap therapy should be administered for at least 5 d with an international normalized ratio (INR) greater than or equal to 2 before discontinuation of the parenteral anticoagulation therapy, discharged on both medications or have reason for discontinuation of parenteral therapy	$\frac{\text{Patients who received overall therapy}}{\text{Patients with confirmed VTE who received warfarin}}$

VTE-4: VTE Patients Receiving Unfractionated Heparin (UFH) with Dosages/Platelet Count Monitoring by Protocol or Nomogram	Assesses the number of patients diagnosed with confirmed VTE who received intravenous UFH therapy dosages and had their platelet counts monitored using defined parameters, such as a nomogram or protocol	Patients who have their IV UFH therapy dosages and platelet counts monitored according to defined parameters such as nomogram or protocol / Patients with confirmed VTE discharged on warfarin therapy
VTE-5: VTE Discharge Instructions	Assesses the number of patients diagnosed with confirmed VTE that are discharged to home, home care, court/law enforcement, or home on hospice care on warfarin with written discharge instructions that address all four criteria: compliance issues, dietary advice, follow-up monitoring, and information about the potential for adverse drug reactions/interaction	Patients with documentation that they or their caregivers were given written discharge instructions or other educational material about warfarin / Patients with confirmed VTE discharged on warfarin therapy
VTE-6: Incidence of Potentially Preventable VTE	Assesses the number of patients diagnosed with confirmed VTE during hospitalization (not present at admission) who did not receive VTE prophylaxis between hospital admission and the day before the VTE diagnostic testing order date	Patients who received no VTE prophylaxis prior to the VTE diagnostic test order date / Patients who developed confirmed VTE during hospitalization

(*Adapted from* Joint Commission. http://www.jointcommission.org/specifications_manual_for_national_hospital_inpatient_quality_measures.aspx. In Specifications manual for national hospital inpatient quality measures. 2014.)

attributable to screening preferences rather than serving as an indicator of higher hospital quality.

Pierce and colleagues [31] suggested that this bias may underlie the high DVT rates found at certain trauma centers. After querying the National Trauma Data Bank, they found that hospital DVT rates had a positive association with hospital duplex rates. On average, for every percentage point increase in ultrasound rate, there was a relative increase of 7% in the reported DVT rate. Importantly, they found that VTE rates were significantly higher in the highest imaging quartile, and it turns out these hospitals had screening protocols for all patients, most of whom had no signs or symptoms of VTE. A single-center retrospective study at a Level I trauma center concurred, finding that the implementation of practice management guidelines for DVT prophylaxis and ultrasound surveillance resulted in a significant increase in duplex screening examinations and, as a result, DVT identification rates [32].

The use of screening protocols stems from the theory that early detection of a DVT will lead to early appropriate treatment and avoidance of a fatal PE, but the true utility of this has been hotly debated. Although some studies have found that routine screening of asymptomatic trauma patients may have clinical benefits and is a cost-effective method of preventing PE [33–36], others have suggested that if appropriate prophylaxis is given, routine surveillance has no role in preventing clinically significant VTE [12,37,38]. Opinions among trauma surgeons and trauma centers were recently polled in a survey study. Wide variability in opinions and practice patterns for DVT screening in the high-risk asymptomatic trauma patient was demonstrated, with half of the individual trauma surgeons responding in support of routine surveillance, and one-quarter of the trauma centers reporting having instituted written guidelines for DVT screening. However, it remained questionable as to how high-risk patients should be defined [36]. Given these results, it seems that any effort to institute national screening guidelines in this population would be hamstrung by the fractured opinion of the trauma community. The Eastern Association for the Surgery of Trauma guidelines on screening asymptomatic patients say that serial duplex imaging may be cost-effective and decrease the incidence of PE, but the use of ultrasound suffers from a low sensitivity when compared with venography; this, however, is from 2002, and is based on class III data [39].

Screening protocols are not only an issue in the trauma population, but also in other surgery subspecialty populations. Use of protocols in neurosurgery, orthopedic surgery, and bariatric surgery has been linked to higher VTE rates in these studies [4]. VTE is a common problem in the neurosurgery and orthopedic surgery populations, but to our knowledge, there have not been studies focusing on surveillance bias similar to those performed in the trauma populations.

In the absence of screening protocols, there may be significant variation in ordering of surveillance studies for VTE within and between institutions. Personal practice patterns have been documented to contribute significantly to imaging ordering [40], because each physician has his or her own clinical threshold at which to order a lower extremity duplex or chest computed tomography (CT). Hospital teaching status has also been suggested to be linked with VTE rate. Vartak and colleagues [41] found that there was strong relationship between a hospital's teaching status and VTE rates (major teaching hospitals having notably higher odds of PE and DVT) and Romano and colleagues [42] found similar results, with higher rates of postoperative VTE in urban teaching centers. Although the authors speculated that this and other notably higher rates of postoperative complications in teaching hospitals may be attributed to major teaching centers being more likely to do more complicated surgeries on patients with more comorbidities, it may be that the differences in performance on PSI-12 can be attributed to resident physician imaging ordering patterns and surveillance bias.

Multiple high-profile academic centers are performing poorly on the current VTE measures. A recent paper by our group pointed out that there was no association between VTE processes and outcome [4]. This undercuts the basic assumption that there is causal link between services provided and observed quality measures (ie, that high measured adherence results in better outcomes) [43]. This study chose eight hospital characteristics that had previously been used to indicate a hospital's resources, QI capacity, and general health care quality: bed size, Joint Commission accreditation, Commission on Cancer designation, level 1 trauma center designation, presence of a residency training program approved by the Accreditation Council for Graduate Medical Education, provision of burn care service, provision of transplant surgery services, and whether hospital reports on quality and cost of health care services were disseminated by the hospital to the community. Using 2010 Hospital Compare, American Hospital Association, and Medicare claims data, VTE imaging usage (duplex ultrasonography, chest CT/MRI, and ventilation-perfusion scans) and VTE event rates were calculated in surgical populations. Two main relationships were explored: the association between hospital VTE prophylaxis adherence and risk-adjusted VTE event rates, and the association between a summary score of hospital structural characteristics reflecting quality and performance on VTE prophylaxis and risk-adjusted VTE measures.

First, there was a weak, paradoxic association between greater hospital VTE prophylaxis adherence rates and worse risk-adjusted VTE event rates (r^2 = 4.2%; P = .03). Second, hospitals with higher structural quality scores had higher VTE prophylaxis adherence rates (better performance on the SCIP-VTE-2 process measure) but worse risk-adjusted VTE rates (poorer performance on the PSI-12 VTE outcome measure). Risk-adjusted VTE rates increased significantly with VTE imaging rates (Figs. 1 and 2). Importantly, the hospitals in the highest quartile of imaging usage rates were also the ones with the highest SCIP-VTE-2 prophylaxis adherence rates; this suggests that poor prophylaxis was not the cause of their high VTE rate and high imaging rate. This study was in concordance with other studies that found that better VTE prophylaxis adherence did not result in lower VTE rates [26,44]. There

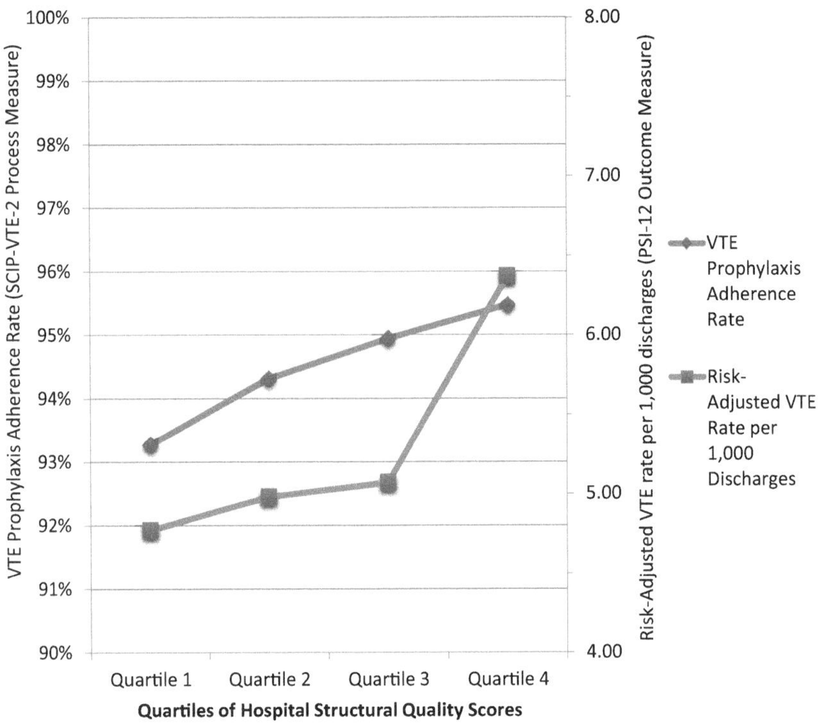

Fig. 1. Hospitals with higher structural quality scores had better VTE prophylaxis adherence rates but paradoxically worse risk-adjusted VTE rates. $P<.001$ for trend and compared with Quartile 4 for VTE prophylaxis adherence rates and risk-adjusted VTE rates. The Hospital Structural Quality Score is the total number of characteristics of a hospital related to structural measures of quality including size, accreditations, and quality initiatives. (*From* Bilimoria KY, Chung J, Ju MH, et al. Evaluation of surveillance bias and the validity of the venous thromboembolism quality measure. JAMA 2013;310:1482–9; with permission.)

was actually a weak association between better VTE prophylaxis adherence (which hospitals with more accreditation and engagement in quality initiatives that typically suggest high-quality care were more successful at achieving) and worse risk-adjusted VTE rates, which indicates that the current measures in use should be re-examined.

The most likely explanation for these results seemed to be that the authors were detecting the effect of surveillance bias on the VTE outcome measure rather than problems inherent to the process measure. The surgical population examined included patients undergoing 1 of 11 major operations: abdominal aortic aneurysm repair, coronary artery bypass graft, craniotomy, colectomy, cystectomy, esophagectomy, gastric bypass, lung resection, pancreatic resection, proctectomy, or total knee arthroplasty. As previously discussed, certain surgical patient populations are unique because of the use (albeit variable) of screening protocols; trauma, orthopedic, neurosurgery, and bariatric

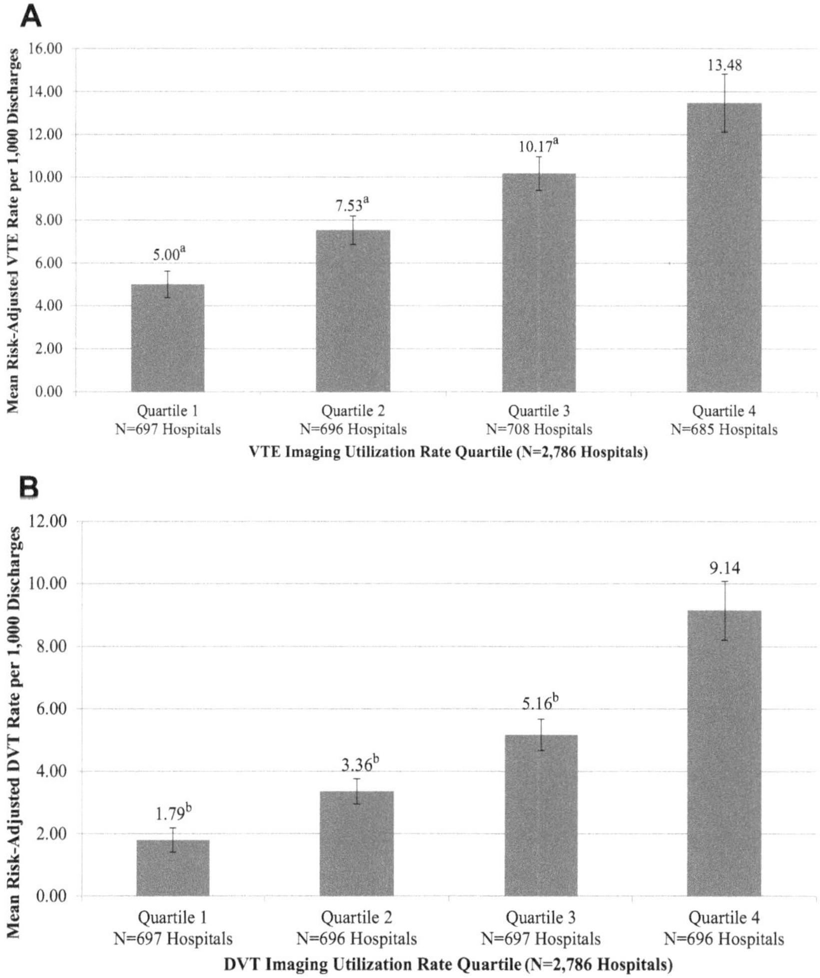

Fig. 2. (*A*) Mean risk-adjusted VTE rate per 1000 discharges by VTE imaging utilization rate quartile. [a] *P*<.001 trend and pairwise. Two-tailed test for differences in mean adjusted VTE rates compared with imaging utilization rate Quartile 4 (highest VTE imaging rate). Error bars indicate 95% confidence intervals around intraquartile means. (*B*) Mean risk-adjusted DVT rate per 1000 discharges by DVT imaging utilization rate quartile. [b] *P*<.001 trend and pairwise. Two-tailed test for differences in mean adjusted DVT rates compared with DVT imaging utilization rate Quartile 4 (highest DVT imaging rate). Error bars indicate 95% confidence intervals around intraquartile means. (*C*) Mean risk-adjusted PE rate per 1000 discharges by PE imaging utilization rate quartile. [c] *P*<.001 trend and pairwise. Two-tailed test for differences in mean adjusted PE rates compared with PE imaging utilization rate Quartile 4 (highest PE imaging rate). Error bars indicate 95% confidence intervals around intraquartile means. (*From* Bilimoria KY, Chung J, Ju MH, et al. Evaluation of surveillance bias and the validity of the venous thromboembolism quality measure. JAMA 2013;310:1482–9; with permission.)

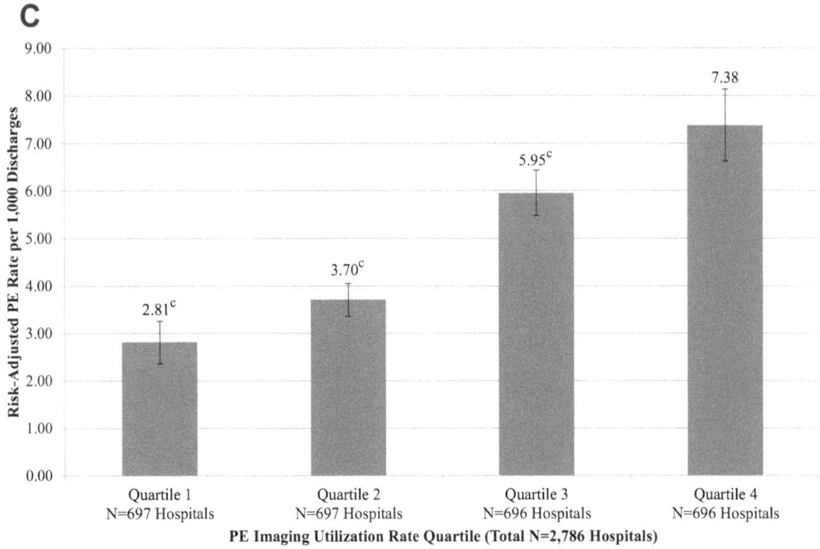

Fig. 2. (*continued*)

populations are usually the ones thought to be subjected to more screening tests with correspondingly higher VTE rates. However, in our group's study, the significant association between surveillance imaging use and higher risk-adjusted VTE rates was seen when evaluating individual procedures, suggesting that this surveillance bias influenced VTE rates for patients and procedures where VTE screening protocols were not generally in use (eg, colorectal surgery) [4]. This likely indicates a difference in threshold for imaging for VTE; that is, hospital culture and practice patterns can influence how often swollen extremities prompt a venous duplex ultrasound and how often tachycardia results in a patient being sent for chest CT.

Before attributing these findings wholly to surveillance bias, however, one must consider alternative explanations. It may be that some hospitals do suffer from higher VTE rates by not providing appropriate postoperative VTE prophylaxis and thus higher VTE rates indicate poorer quality of care; although this was not suggested in our group's study given consistent SCIP-VTE-2 rates across all surveillance quartiles, this possibility should underscore the importance of ensuring quality prophylaxis before writing high VTE event rates off to surveillance bias. In addition, one must be aware that variation in VTE surveillance imaging may be caused by flux at the hospital level in case mix and illness severity. Optimal risk-adjustment may be performed but there is always the possibility of residual confounding from risk-factors that could not be assessed [4]. Our group used administrative data, which are less than ideal for risk adjustment.

Another study from our group examined whether the surveillance bias would persist when using clinical data. The clinically abstracted VTE outcome measure was used, because clinical data are more accurate than administrative data when it comes to postoperative complications [45]. In this study, the association between imaging rates and observed and risk-adjusted postoperative VTE rates were examined using Medicare claims and American College of Surgeons (ACS) National Surgery Quality Improvement Program (NSQIP) data. Hospital characteristics as defined by the American Hospital Association were also examined to assess for other hospital-dependent variables that may be associated with differing event rates. Not only was this study consistent with our group's previous study that found that frequent VTE imaging users had higher rates of inpatient VTE, but it also found, by making use of the 30-day follow-up data in ACS NSQIP database, that the 30-day VTE event rate was associated with hospital volume of VTE imaging. No other hospitals characteristics had significant associations with VTE event rates by hospital [46].

Analysis of potential hospital factors that drive imaging rates has also been examined. In a population of Medicare beneficiaries who underwent 11 major operations between 2009 and 2010, associations between VTE imaging use rates and hospital characteristics, such as case severity, size, ownership, VTE process measure adherence, accreditations, staffing, malpractice environment, and county market factors, were examined using quantile regressions. Hospital teaching status, resident-to-bed ratio, malpractice environment, and local market factors were found to be the drivers of VTE imaging use among hospitals. This suggests that nonclinical forces may be driving imaging practices to a greater extent than purely clinical assessments and judgments [47].

The presence of surveillance bias in PSI-12 thus creates four possible groups: (1) truly poor-quality hospitals, who have poor VTE outcomes because of poor prophylaxis adherence (true-positives); (2) higher-quality hospitals with higher PSI-12 scores caused of high VTE imaging rates (false-positives); (3) high-quality hospitals with low VTE rates (true-negatives); and (4) hospitals with ostensibly low PSI-12 scores caused by inappropriately low imaging rates (false-negatives). Use of this outcome measure can lead to hospital misclassification and several unintended effects. Consumers may be misled and proceed to choose hospitals that have low VTE rates because of inadequate surveillance or reject higher-quality hospitals whose higher PSI-12 rates are caused by keener surveillance. Payers may withhold reimbursements from hospitals that fall into the false-positive category and misdirect payments toward the false-negatives. QI projects aimed at improving hospital performance on PSI-12 may inappropriately consume hospital resources [48]. This measure is thus of little use and needs to be revised or eliminated given the current consumer, hospital, and payer reliance on PSI-12.

MEASURING VENOUS THROMBOEMBOLISM PREVENTION

To measure and improve patient care, there must be effective oversight of the ability of hospitals to prevent VTE. If the outcome measure is not valid, then alternate approaches are needed to assessing VTE quality. Discussions of quality measures require differentiation between process and outcome measures. To a certain extent, the former can be characterized as a means, and the latter as an end, although this is a gross oversimplification of both. Technically, process measures relate to encounters between clinical providers concerning patient interventions [49], whereas outcome measures refer to impact on the health status of the patient [50].

Both have their pros and cons (Table 2). Although the validity and stability of most outcomes (eg, morbidity and mortality rates) seem self-apparent, there are several limitations. First, risk adjustment is required. Second, one must be aware that outcomes are the end result of a multifactorial process and using them as a measure may not necessarily reflect results of controlled medical processes [51]. Third, the time required in outcome data collection is often a significant issue, given that these events may be rare (eg, mortality) or require years to determine (eg, quality of life and functional status). Low event rates, risk-adjustment issues, and long time-horizons can reduce the value of using outcomes as a measurement. The outcomes measurement in the VTE arena is also complicated by the lack of uniformity of the definition of a DVT across institutions. Some hospitals do not deem gastrocnemius or soleal venous thrombosis DVTs, whereas others do. Some vascular laboratories do not even routinely evaluate any below-knee veins, because of the debate regarding whether to treat these DVT and also because of a lack of reimbursement for the additional time required [52]. In addition, the true clinical significance of calf thrombi is debated. Although the simple presence of a gastrocnemius or soleal clot may not be an indication to therapeutically anticoagulate, patients still run the risk of proximal propagation of the clot and subsequent embolic event [53]. The same question has been raised over peripheral rounded PEs, termed "dots" by one set of authors, which may not be associated with detectable extremity clots and which may not justify anticoagulation [54].

Variation in surgical quality is becoming increasingly apparent [55–57]. As such, there is a push to scrutinize existing measures. Clinical validation studies of PSI-12 demonstrated that this measure is prone to inaccuracies given that PSIs rely on International Classification of Diseases (ICD)-9-CM coding [58]. The coding process for VTE may be particularly prone to errors given that objective documentation of a VTE event is neither sufficient nor required for diagnosis (only a health care provider diagnosis is used), and there is a disconnect between commonly used clinical nomenclature and the available ICD-9-CM codes [59–62]. ICD coding and PSI software will have to be adjusted to decrease false-positives and increase positive predictive value. This measure also misses all postdischarge events, an important caveat in a clinical complication that often develops after discharge [63].

This is an important issue to resolve given that VTE measures are still publicly reported. The VTE outcome measure was recently dropped from the *US News and World Report*, University HealthSystem Consortium (UHC), and the ACS

NSQIP based on Bilimoria and coworkers' [4] 2013 study and other clinical evidence. PSI-12, however, is still part of PSI-90 (patient safety for selected indicators) and CMS value-based purchasing; as long as this measure remains an integral part of hospital reporting and reimbursement, there is a continued need to refine and revise it. Higher PSI-12 rates may actually be an indicator of more vigilant care (ie, ordering of more imaging studies to ensure VTE events are not missed), and patients attempting to choose hospitals based on VTE performance metrics may easily be misled. It also hinders poor-performing hospitals in search of improvement; although these institutions may strive to improve their performance on this measure by increasing VTE vigilance, they may find more VTEs, and paradoxically find themselves sliding even further in the ranks.

Process measures may overcome some of these problems inherent to outcomes measures, because process measures are usually generated in a shorter time-frame, are under more direct control by clinicians, act as specific targets for improvement, and lack the need for risk adjustment of patient-related factors [27,64]. Clinicians can demonstrate progress more readily in terms of process measures and the shorter time-frame needed to generate results means that these measures can be used to inform QI initiatives. Process measures, however, often indicate a specific element of care rather than comprehensive processes. The implementation of these measures, however, can be difficult because they require constant updating as science advances. One must also bear in mind that process measures, to be valid, should generally demonstrate a relationship with the outcome measure [65].

The SCIP measures were initially selected because of their purported strong evidence-based linkage with outcomes. Whether compliance with these will actually result in improved outcomes in the long run seems doubtful [64,66]. After all, although the SCIP-VTE measure is arguably more important than devoting efforts to surveillance scanning [12], SCIP-VTE-2 is limited to prophylaxis administration in the 24-hour perioperative period. Moreover, it is a process associated with a rare outcome [44]. Although some data exist that show certain process compliance rates for certain events (eg, acute myocardial infarction) are related to inpatient mortality rate and do reflect other dimensions of quality, there are many well-designed studies in the VTE arena that suggest that increased compliance is not associated with better outcomes and, in fact, can be linked to poorer outcomes [4,64,66]. A poor association between process measure compliance and improved outcomes effectively invalidates the current system of measurement and, thus, the data suggesting this are pivotal to policy changes.

POTENTIAL SOLUTIONS

There are several ways to address the problems displayed by the current VTE measures. The first is to commit more focus to process measures rather than outcomes. Rather than focusing on DVT rates alone, concerted efforts devoted to measuring the process of care (ie, DVT prophylaxis rates) and changing the structure of care (eg, requiring VTE prevention guidelines in high-risk hospital

Table 2
Advantages and disadvantages: comparison of process and outcome measures

	Process measures	Outcome measures
Resources		
Need for updating and maintenance of measures	Require updating and maintenance of guidelines, review criteria, instruments and software according to advances in treatment	Known risk factors and models may require some updating, generally less often than updates to process measures are needed
Need for development of risk-adjustment models and collection of risk data	Most measure do not require the use of extensive risk-adjustment models; however, require good definition of eligible patients	Risk adjustment is difficult; need different models for each outcome
Time needed for measurement	Takes less time to accumulate, smaller sample needed, less observation time needed for processes occurring during provider contact	Because of need for risk adjustment a larger sample is needed; also many outcomes of interest are long-term, such as 5- or 10-y survival requiring long period of observation
Size of population needed for measurement	Can use a smaller sample size because all included patients experience the process and once eligible patients are defined, only descriptive statistics are needed	Because of need for risk adjustment a larger sample is usually needed for comparisons among providers or treatments
Need for additional follow-up tracking of patients for later data collection	Data collection can be done when clinical process is occurring	Requires follow-up for measurement of short- and long-term outcomes at time when routine data collection not occurring
Use of routine collected data	Has the potential to be abstracted from data already recorded for clinical and administrative use, and ultimately to be completely integrated into such data collection	Often requires collection of data elements that are not being recorded for clinical or billing purposes, such as long-term survival or patient-reported health and well-being on standardized scales
Need for advanced statistical consultation for development of measures and analysis of data	Not needed in general	Needed to create risk-adjustment models and evaluated them when analyzing data

Validity		
What patients care about	Often inaccessible to patients who often do not understand the significance of a specific component of care	The generic outcomes of survival, health, and well-being are what patients care about and measures of these can be used to validate process changes; more specific or proxy outcomes may not be accessible to patients
What providers care about	Face validity with providers; relates directly to what the provider is doing	Providers are wary of outcome measures that are influenced by many other things besides what they do; must measure performance of risk-adjustment models
Ease of use		
Ease of specification and identification of population at risk	Difficult to specify population eligible for a process; there can be many exclusions, contraindications, and special outcomes, and many important process measures are specific for a single disease	Easy to define population for which want to measure an outcome; many important outcomes are generic and can be compared across several conditions
Creation of valid summary measures	Difficult to summarize process measures in a valid way because they are rarely comprehensive	Many important outcome measures, such as survival, health, and well-being, are global and generic and can be compared across conditions and processes
Interpretability of feedback for quality improvement	Provides clear and interpretable feedback for quality improvement about what providers are actually doing; easy to benchmark	Most measures cannot be used to give feedback to providers about how to improve what they are doing because rarely is an outcome always a consequence of a particular faulty process; benchmarking is needed for comparisons among groups and adjusted outcomes can be difficult to understand

(*From* Ubin HR, Pronovost P, Diette GB. The advantages and disadvantages of process-based measures of health care quality. Int J Qual Health Care 2001;13:469–74; with permission.)

units or trauma centers) should be made [30]. Design of a new measure may be a more attractive alternative than tinkering with existing ones. A forthcoming study by Kinnier and colleagues compared SCIP-VTE-2 compliance rates at a single institution with a new composite measure that required risk-appropriate ambulation, mechanical prophylaxis, and chemoprophylaxis during patients' hospital stay. Although 99.7% of patients passed SCIP-VTE-2, only 37.8% passed the new VTE prophylaxis composite measure. Although additional evaluation is needed, this may be a step in the right direction in revising the surgery community's approach to VTE quality measures.

Second, if an outcome measure is to be used, then PSI-12 needs to be improved. Fixing this measure, however, is admittedly a tall order given the wide variation in clinicians' threshold to image and the varying factors that drive imaging rates. Unless criteria specifying VTE imaging indications are developed, this measure will remain flawed. However, there are certain adjustments that can be made. Revisions of the ICD-9-CM coding have helped to differentiate between acute embolism and thrombosis of the superficial and deep veins of the upper and lower extremities (previously, there was no way to distinguish superficial thromboses from deep thromboses), but further adjustment of what events are captured in the numerator of reported VTE rates needs to occur. Excluding subclinical VTEs from the numerator should be considered. The point of using this metric is to ensure that patients with clinically significant VTEs are promptly diagnosed and properly treated. However, a quality metric that is colored by surveillance bias may prompt clinicians to decrease their use of surveillance imaging; inappropriately order chemoprophylaxis in patients at low risk of VTE (and unnecessarily increasing their bleeding risk); and increase use of preoperative inferior vena cava filter, which carries its own inherent procedural risks and postoperative complications [30,67]. Hospitals with tendencies toward high-imaging rates, who find themselves with significant rates of otherwise asymptomatic VTE, may in turn suffer from iatrogenic complications from bleeding secondary to anticoagulation or inferior vena cava filter placement. Keeping these incidentally discovered subclinical clots from being including in PSI-12 would help to decrease the effects of surveillance bias.

Third, new SCIP measures may represent an improvement in process measure selection. SCIP-VTE-6 assesses the number of patients diagnosed with confirmed VTE during hospitalization (and which are not present at admission), who did not receive VTE prophylaxis between hospital admission and the day before the VTE diagnostic testing order date [68]. This seeks to act as a measure of preventable harm. It is a complex measure and institutions may struggle to raise awareness among clinicians of its importance. Documentation of a clinicians' reasoning behind either ordering or not ordering VTE prophylaxis and behind ordering diagnostic imaging is paramount if this measure is to be accurate. Further work toward finding process measures that allow for accurate quality of care assessment and timely hospital QI intervention needs to be ongoing.

SUMMARY

VTE is a clinically important and potentially preventable problem that has deservedly received significant attention on the policy level. Surveillance bias, however, is an important issue and the VTE outcomes measure is likely not valid. Although there is potentially some room for improvement in PSI-12 and although improvements should continually be made as long as this measure remains a part of quality reporting, efforts should be directed more toward developing a new measure reflecting a hospital's ability to prevent VTE.

References

[1] Gould MK, Garcia DA, Wren SM, et al. Prevention of VTE in nonorthopedic surgical patients: antithrombotic therapy and prevention of thrombosis, 9th ed: American College of Chest Physicians Evidence-Based Clinical Practice Guidelines. Chest 2012;141: e227S–77S.

[2] Page RL 2nd, Ghushchyan V, Gifford B, et al. Hidden costs associated with venous thromboembolism: impact of lost productivity on employers and employees. J Occup Environ Med 2014;56(9):979–85.

[3] White RH, Zhou H, Romano PS. Incidence of symptomatic venous thromboembolism after different elective or urgent surgical procedures. Thromb Haemost 2003;90:446–55.

[4] Bilimoria KY, Chung J, Ju MH, et al. Evaluation of surveillance bias and the validity of the venous thromboembolism quality measure. JAMA 2013;310:1482–9.

[5] Lefebvre P, Laliberte F, Nutescu EA, et al. All-cause and potentially disease-related health care costs associated with venous thromboembolism in commercial, Medicare, and Medicaid beneficiaries. J Manag Care Pharm 2012;18:363–74.

[6] Goldhaber SZ, Bounameaux H. Pulmonary embolism and deep vein thrombosis. Lancet 2012;379:1835–46.

[7] Kahn SR, Solymoss S, Lamping DL, et al. Long-term outcomes after deep vein thrombosis: postphlebitic syndrome and quality of life. J Gen Intern Med 2000;15:425–9.

[8] Prandoni P, Lensing AW, Cogo A, et al. The long-term clinical course of acute deep venous thrombosis. Ann Intern Med 1996;125:1–7.

[9] Mahan CE, Holdsworth MT, Welch SM, et al. Deep-vein thrombosis: a United States cost model for a preventable and costly adverse event. Thromb Haemost 2011;106:405–15.

[10] Ollendorf DA, Vera-Llonch M, Oster G. Cost of venous thromboembolism following major orthopedic surgery in hospitalized patients. Am J Health Syst Pharm 2002;59:1750–4.

[11] Anderson FA Jr, Spencer FA. Risk factors for venous thromboembolism. Circulation 2003;107:I9–16.

[12] Cipolle MD, Wojcik R, Seislove E, et al. The role of surveillance duplex scanning in preventing venous thromboembolism in trauma patients. J Trauma 2002;52:453–62.

[13] Sevitt S, Gallagher N. Venous thrombosis and pulmonary embolism. A clinico-pathological study in injured and burned patients. Br J Surg 1961;48:475–89.

[14] Freeark RJ, Boswick J, Fardin R. Posttraumatic venous thrombosis. Arch Surg 1967;95: 567–75.

[15] Kudsk KA, Fabian TC, Baum S, et al. Silent deep vein thrombosis in immobilized multiple trauma patients. Am J Surg 1989;158:515–9.

[16] Henwood PC, Kennedy TM, Thomson L, et al. The incidence of deep vein thrombosis detected by routine surveillance ultrasound in neurosurgery patients receiving dual modality prophylaxis. J Thromb Thrombolysis 2011;32:209–14.

[17] Weingarden SI. Deep venous thrombosis in spinal cord injury. Overview of the problem. Chest 1992;102:636s–9s.

[18] Grady-Benson JC, Oishi CS, Hanson PB, et al. Routine postoperative duplex ultrasonography screening and monitoring for the detection of deep vein thrombosis. A survey of 110 total hip arthroplasties. Clin Orthop Relat Res 1994;(307):130–41.

[19] Maynard G, Stein J. Designing and implementing effective venous thromboembolism prevention protocols: lessons from collaborative efforts. J Thromb Thrombolysis 2010;29:159–66.
[20] Collins R, Scrimgeour A, Yusuf S, et al. Reduction in fatal pulmonary embolism and venous thrombosis by perioperative administration of subcutaneous heparin. Overview of results of randomized trials in general, orthopedic, and urologic surgery. N Engl J Med 1988;318:1162–73.
[21] Streiff MB, Haut ER. The CMS ruling on venous thromboembolism after total knee or hip arthroplasty: weighing risks and benefits. JAMA 2009;301:1063–5.
[22] Kakkar AK, Cohen AT, Tapson VF, et al. Venous thromboembolism risk and prophylaxis in the acute care hospital setting (ENDORSE survey): findings in surgical patients. Ann Surg 2010;251:330–8.
[23] Cohen AT, Agnelli G, Anderson FA, et al. Venous thromboembolism (VTE) in Europe. The number of VTE events and associated morbidity and mortality. Thromb Haemost 2007;98:756–64.
[24] Guyatt GH, Akl EA, Crowther M, et al. Executive summary: antithrombotic therapy and prevention of thrombosis, 9th ed: American College of Chest Physicians Evidence-Based Clinical Practice Guidelines. Chest 2012;141:7S–47S.
[25] Deitelzweig SB, Lin J, Hussein M, et al. Are surgical patients at risk of venous thromboembolism currently meeting the Surgical Care Improvement Project performance measure for appropriate and timely prophylaxis? J Thromb Thrombolysis 2010;30:55–66.
[26] Altom LK, Deierhoi RJ, Grams J, et al. Association between Surgical Care Improvement Program venous thromboembolism measures and postoperative events. Am J Surg 2012;204:591–7.
[27] Ingraham AM, Cohen ME, Bilimoria KY, et al. Association of surgical care improvement project infection-related process measure compliance with risk-adjusted outcomes: implications for quality measurement. J Am Coll Surg 2010;211:705–14.
[28] (AHRQ) AfHRaQ. Patient safety indicators #12, technical specifications. Postoperative pulmonary embolism or deep vein thrombosis Rate. Available at: http://www.qualityindicators.ahrq.gov/Downloads/Modules/PSI/V50/TechSpecs/PSI_12_Perioperative_Pulmonary_Embolism_or_Deep_Vein_Thrombosis_Rate.pdf. Accessed April 21, 2015.
[29] CMS. Centers for Medicare & Medicaid Services: hospital-acquired conditions (HAC) in acute inpatient prospective payment system (IPPS) Hospitals. Available at: http://www.cms.gov/Outreach-and-Education/Medicare-Learning-Network-MLN/MLNProducts/downloads/Hospital_VBPurchasing_Fact_Sheet_ICN907664.pdf. Accessed April 21, 2015.
[30] Haut ER, Pronovost PJ. Surveillance bias in outcomes reporting. JAMA 2011;305:2462–3.
[31] Pierce CA, Haut ER, Kardooni S, et al. Surveillance bias and deep vein thrombosis in the national trauma data bank: the more we look, the more we find. J Trauma 2008;64:932–6 [discussion: 936–7].
[32] Haut ER, Noll K, Efron DT, et al. Can increased incidence of deep vein thrombosis (DVT) be used as a marker of quality of care in the absence of standardized screening? The potential effect of surveillance bias on reported DVT rates after trauma. J Trauma 2007;63:1132–5 [discussion: 1135–7].
[33] Burns GA, Cohn SM, Frumento RJ, et al. Prospective ultrasound evaluation of venous thrombosis in high-risk trauma patients. J Trauma 1993;35:405–8.
[34] Brasel KJ, Borgstrom DC, Weigelt JA. Cost-effective prevention of pulmonary embolus in high-risk trauma patients. J Trauma 1997;42:456–60 [discussion: 460–2].
[35] Napolitano LM, Garlapati VS, Heard SO, et al. Asymptomatic deep venous thrombosis in the trauma patient: is an aggressive screening protocol justified? J Trauma 1995;39:651–7 [discussion: 657–9].
[36] Haut ER, Schneider EB, Patel A, et al. Duplex ultrasound screening for deep vein thrombosis in asymptomatic trauma patients: a survey of individual trauma surgeon opinions and current trauma center practices. J Trauma 2011;70:27–33 [discussion: 33–4].

[37] Meyer CS, Blebea J, Davis K Jr, et al. Surveillance venous scans for deep venous thrombosis in multiple trauma patients. Ann Vasc Surg 1995;9:109–14.
[38] Satiani B, Falcone R, Shook L, et al. Screening for major deep vein thrombosis in seriously injured patients: a prospective study. Ann Vasc Surg 1997;11:626–9.
[39] Rogers FB, Cipolle MD, Velmahos G, et al. Practice management guidelines for the prevention of venous thromboembolism in trauma patients: the EAST practice management guidelines work group. J Trauma 2002;53:142–64.
[40] Sistrom C, McKay NL, Weilburg JB, et al. Determinants of diagnostic imaging utilization in primary care. Am J Manag Care 2012;18:e135–44.
[41] Vartak S, Ward MM, Vaughn TE. Do postoperative complications vary by hospital teaching status? Med Care 2008;46:25–32.
[42] Romano PS, Geppert JJ, Davies S, et al. A national profile of patient safety in U.S. hospitals. Health Aff (Millwood) 2003;22:154–66.
[43] Powell AE, Davies HT, Thomson RG. Using routine comparative data to assess the quality of health care: understanding and avoiding common pitfalls. Qual Saf Health Care 2003;12: 122–8.
[44] Nicholas LH, Osborne NH, Birkmeyer JD, et al. Hospital process compliance and surgical outcomes in Medicare beneficiaries. Arch Surg 2010;145:999–1004.
[45] Lawson EH, Louie R, Zingmond DS, et al. A comparison of clinical registry versus administrative claims data for reporting of 30-day surgical complications. Ann Surg 2012;256: 973–81.
[46] Ju MH, Chung JW, Kinnier CV, et al. Association between hospital imaging use and venous thromboembolism events rates based on clinical data. Ann Surg 2014;260:558–66.
[47] Chung JW, Ju MH, Kinnier CV, et al. Evaluation of hospital factors associated with hospital postoperative venous thromboembolism imaging utilisation practices. BMJ Qual Saf 2014;23(11):947–56.
[48] Chung JW, Ju MH, Kinnier CV, et al. Postoperative venous thromboembolism outcomes measure: analytic exploration of potential misclassification of hospital quality due to surveillance bias. Ann Surg 2014;261(3):443–4.
[49] Brook RH, McGlynn EA, Cleary PD. Quality of health care. Part 2: measuring quality of care. N Engl J Med 1996;335:966–70.
[50] Kupersmith J. Quality of care in teaching hospitals: a literature review. Acad Med 2005;80: 458–66.
[51] Donabedian A. Evaluating the quality of medical care. 1966. Milbank Q 2005;83: 691–729.
[52] Lautz TB, Abbas F, Walsh SJ, et al. Isolated gastrocnemius and soleal vein thrombosis: should these patients receive therapeutic anticoagulation? Ann Surg 2010;251: 735–42.
[53] Agnelli G, Piovella F, Buoncristiani P, et al. Enoxaparin plus compression stockings compared with compression stockings alone in the prevention of venous thromboembolism after elective neurosurgery. N Engl J Med 1998;339:80–5.
[54] Suh JM, Cronan JJ, Healey TT. Dots are not clots: the over-diagnosis and over-treatment of PE. Emerg Radiol 2010;17:347–52.
[55] Khuri SF, Daley J, Henderson W, et al. Risk adjustment of the postoperative mortality rate for the comparative assessment of the quality of surgical care: results of the National Veterans Affairs Surgical Risk Study. J Am Coll Surg 1997;185:315–27.
[56] Birkmeyer JD, Siewers AE, Finlayson EV, et al. Hospital volume and surgical mortality in the United States. N Engl J Med 2002;346:1128–37.
[57] Birkmeyer JD, Stukel TA, Siewers AE, et al. Surgeon volume and operative mortality in the United States. N Engl J Med 2003;349:2117–27.
[58] Henderson KE, Recktenwald AJ, Reichley RM, et al. Clinical validation of the AHRQ postoperative venous thromboembolism patient safety indicator. Jt Comm J Qual Patient Saf 2009;35:370–6.

[59] White RH, Sadeghi B, Tancredi DJ, et al. How valid is the ICD-9-CM based AHRQ patient safety indicator for postoperative venous thromboembolism? Med Care 2009;47: 1237–43.
[60] Weller WE, Gallagher BK, Cen L, et al. Readmissions for venous thromboembolism: expanding the definition of patient safety indicators. Jt Comm J Qual Saf 2004;30:497–504.
[61] White RH, Romano PS, Zhou H, et al. Incidence and time course of thromboembolic outcomes following total hip or knee arthroplasty. Arch Intern Med 1998;158:1525–31.
[62] Huber O, Bounameaux H, Borst F, et al. Postoperative pulmonary embolism after hospital discharge. An underestimated risk. Arch Surg 1992;127:310–3.
[63] Merkow RP, Bilimoria KY, McCarter MD, et al. Post-discharge venous thromboembolism after cancer surgery: extending the case for extended prophylaxis. Ann Surg 2011;254: 131–7.
[64] Werner RM, Bradlow ET, Asch DA. Does hospital performance on process measures directly measure high quality care or is it a marker of unmeasured care? Health Serv Res 2008;43: 1464–84.
[65] Rubin HR, Pronovost P, Diette GB. The advantages and disadvantages of process-based measures of health care quality. Int J Qual Health Care 2001;13:469–74.
[66] Werner RM, Bradlow ET. Relationship between Medicare's hospital compare performance measures and mortality rates. JAMA 2006;296:2694–702.
[67] Baker DW, Qaseem A. Evidence-based performance measures: preventing unintended consequences of quality measurement. Ann Intern Med 2011;155:638–40.
[68] (AHRQ) AfHRaQ. Measure summary. In National Quality Measures Clearinghouse. 2014. Available at: http://www.qualitymeasures.ahrq.gov/content.aspx?id=48118. Accessed April 21, 2015.

Advances in Surgery 49 (2015) 205–220

ADVANCES IN SURGERY

Fluid Restriction During Pancreaticoduodenectomy

Is It Effective in Reducing Postoperative Complications?

Timothy I. Carter, MD[a], Charles J. Yeo, MD[b], Harish Lavu, MD[c,*]

[a]Department of Surgery, SUNY Downstate Medical Center, 450 Clarkson Avenue Brooklyn, New York, NY 11203, USA; [b]Department of Surgery, The Jefferson Pancreas Biliary and Related Cancer Center, Thomas Jefferson University, 1015 Walnut Street, Curtis Building, Suite 620, Philadelphia, PA 19107, USA; [c]Department of Surgery, The Jefferson Pancreas Biliary and Related Cancer Center, Thomas Jefferson University, 1025 Walnut Street, College Building, Suite 605, Philadelphia, PA 19107, USA

Keywords

• Fluid restriction • Hypertonic saline • Pancreaticoduodenectomy
• Whipple operation • Pancreatic cancer

Key points

- Perioperative fluid restriction has been shown to reduce complications in patients undergoing a wide variety of operative procedures.
- Hypertonic saline is an effective means of maintaining appropriate hemodynamic parameters among surgical patients, while contributing to overall fluid restriction.
- The use of hypertonic saline within a moderately restrictive fluid regimen is effective in reducing postoperative complications in patients undergoing pancreaticoduodenectomy.

INTRODUCTION

Nearly 50 years ago, Moore and Shires [1] published an editorial in the *Annals of Surgery* entitled "Moderation," detailing the quandary of fluid resuscitation as it relates to both trauma and elective surgery. Despite their prescient commentary, in the interval to contemporary times, fluid restriction has not been

The authors have nothing to disclose.

*Corresponding author. *E-mail address*: Harish.Lavu@jefferson.edu

0065-3411/15/$ – see front matter
http://dx.doi.org/10.1016/j.yasu.2015.03.004

widely practiced, with much of the focus in the care of surgical patients being directed to the avoidance of under-resuscitation. Only in recent years has there been a renewed interest in restricted resuscitation practices in the surgical literature, and fluid management is gaining a more prominent role in modern surgical thinking. Today, there are data from several surgical disciplines that have suggested that overzealous resuscitation may be linked to a wide variety of complications, including increased rates of paralytic ileus, delayed gastric emptying (DGE), cardiopulmonary incidents, and blood transfusions, as well as wound and anastomotic complications [2–7]. Likewise, in the care of patients with trauma, excessive resuscitation has been shown to have equally damaging effects, leading to a worsening of coagulopathy, pulmonary dysfunction, and increased rates of abdominal compartment syndrome [8–10]. Restricted fluid administration has begun to play a role in many enhanced surgical recovery pathways, with evidence that it reduces the overall rate of surgical complications [3].

As the search for the ideal resuscitation strategy continues, pancreatic surgery may serve as the perfect model for examination. Pancreaticoduodenectomy (PD) is often a long and complex operation that is associated with significant fluid shifts in the perioperative period. PD is also associated with one of the highest morbidity rates in all of surgery, ranging from 40% to 60% [11,12]. Fluid restriction may be a means to help reduce the rate of complications and improve outcomes in patients undergoing PD. To concentrate on the optimal amount of fluid for an individual patient, many surgeon-authors have rightly adopted the terminology of goal-directed fluid resuscitation [13–17]. This concept may be particularly well adapted to patients having PD, given the physiologic impact sustained by these patients through the development of a systemic inflammatory response syndrome (SIRS). Patients having PD are particularly predisposed to an aggressive inflammatory response, possibly related to dissection around and transection of the pancreas. Combined with post-PD pancreatitis, this contributes to the large fluid shifts that may occur in this unique patient population [18,19].

This article discusses the specific aspects of fluid resuscitation that pertain to patients having PD, and also discusses the underlying physiology and approach to fluid restriction.

PHYSIOLOGY AND APPROACH TO FLUID RESTRICTION

Early surgical research (much attributed to Walter Cannon in Boston and Alfred Blalock, first at Vanderbilt and then at Johns Hopkins) focused extensively on the extracellular fluid compartment, fluid shifts between compartments, and the appropriateness of crystalloid administration [20]. In the Vietnam War era, radiolabeled sulfur studies described contraction of the extracellular space, with loss of fluid into the so-called third space (eg, ascites, alveoli,) [21–23]. Although the methods and conclusions of many of these studies have been called into question, it seems clear that the inflammatory response to surgery results in a systemic capillary leak reaction, sequestering and depleting the intravascular space [24]. The physiology of perioperative surgical patients leads to a contraction of the intravascular volume, which, if not accounted for and corrected, reduces cardiac output and results in dysoxia at the tissue level, which produces membrane dysfunction, cellular swelling, and cyclic inflammation, resulting in the capillary leak phenomenon [25]. Low levels of tissue oxygen tension lead to reduced collagen deposition and inhibition of wound healing, with the potential for increased rates of infection [26,27]. These issues of under-resuscitation are well characterized and have been the primary hallmarks of surgical teaching for generations. However, in recent years, the harmful effects of over-resuscitation have begun to be more carefully evaluated, with evidence suggesting that the consequent hemodilution and tissue edema can in their own right lead to a reduction in tissue oxygen delivery, potentially resulting in the same complications as under-resuscitation [9,28].

The timing of fluid administration may also play a significant role. Indicators of malperfusion at the cellular level, such as serum lactate, blood urea nitrogen, and creatinine, can be helpful in identifying patients who may be under-resuscitated [13,29]. However, these indicators are late markers, and a significant accumulation of oxygen debt in the tissues may have already occurred by the time the abnormality is detected. There is evidence to suggest that tissue hypoxia may further drive inflammation. Hypoxia induction factor allows a cell to sense low oxygen tension and respond by the transcription of multiple genes, among them nuclear factor kB and toll-like receptors, perpetuating the SIRS response [30].

Estimates of cardiac output (and therefore oxygen delivery), such as blood pressure, heart rate, central venous pressure (CVP), pulse pressure variation, and central venous oxygen saturation, are helpful, but remain imperfect, leaving room for interpretation by experienced clinicians. If a patient shows evidence of volume depletion in the perioperative setting, these modalities allow the practitioner to administer the fluid needed to correct this deficit. However, the traditional approach of a default 1-L bolus of saline is outmoded. If a patient requires only 250 mL to correct a volume deficit then a 1-L bolus will result in 750 mL of excessive fluid administration. This fluid has the potential to rapidly extravasate from the intravascular space into the third space, and will not prevent the development of a future intravascular volume deficit. With this model in mind, the importance of volume timing can be easily seen because many wasteful and potentially harmful liters of administered excess fluid may be avoided in a given patient in the perioperative setting.

The colorectal field was one of the earliest to support the enhanced recovery pathway movement, and contains the largest body of literature studying fluid restriction (Table 1). In this patient population, conservative fluid administration has been shown to improve the return of bowel function and reduce the rate of DGE and cardiopulmonary complications [3,31]. Using a goal-directed approach to fluid administration with intraoperative transesophageal echocardiography in patients having colorectal surgery, researchers found a

Table 1
Clinical trials of fluid restriction and hypertonic saline use in surgery

Author/year	Procedure/design	Arms	Findings
Brandstrup et al [3], 2003	Colorectal RCT (intraoperative/ postoperative)	Restricted (69 patients): 500 mL 6% HAES bolus; 7 mL/kg/h (first hour), 5 mL/kg/h (second hour), 3 mL/kg/h (remaining hour); blood loss 2–3:1 with 0.9% Liberal (72 patients): no bolus or continuous, blood replace with 6% HAES if <1500 mL, >1500 mL replace with blood Postoperative: Target preoperative weight with Lasix	Intention to treat: complications 33% vs 51%; cardiopulmonary 7% vs 24%; no difference in mortality
Nisanevich et al [2], 2005	Mixed GI RCT (intraoperative)	Restricted (75 patients): 4 mL/kg/h Liberal (77 patients): 10 mg/kg bolus + 12 mL/kg/h	↓LOS (1 d); ↓Total complications Earlier bowel function
Noblett et al [32], 2006	Colorectal RCT (intraoperative)	Restricted (52 patients): intraoperative TEE-guided bolus fluids to optimize stroke volume (HAES used) Liberal (51 patients): anesthesia discretion without TEE data	↓LOS (9 vs 7 d) ↓Complication rate ↓Interleukin-6 level ↓Vasopressor support Earlier diet initiation
Futier et al [37], 2010	Abdominal RCT (intraoperative)	Restricted (36 patients): 6 mL/kg/h with guided prn bolus Liberal (34 patients): 12 mL/kg/h with guided prn bolus	↑Complications ↓$ScVo_2$ Restricted: ↑sepsis and anastomotic leaks
Shackford et al [48], 1983	AAA RCT (intraoperative)	Hypertonic (30 patients): balanced hypertonic solution to target CVP Control (28 patients): LR to target CVP	↓Intraoperative fluid (5L less) ↓Intrapulmonary shunt
Bulger et al [56], 2011	Trauma RCT	Hypertonic (269 patients): initial resuscitation with 250 mL 7.5% Control (395 patients): initial resuscitation with 250 mL 0.9%	No mortality benefit Concluded for futility

Abbreviations: AAA, abdominal aortic aneurysm; HAES, hydroxyethyl starch; LOS, length of stay; LR, lactated Ringer; prn, as needed; RCT, randomized controlled trial; $ScVo_2$, central venous oxygen saturation; TEE, transesophageal echocardiography.

reduction in complications, postoperative hospital length of stay (LOS), and interleukin-6 levels [32]. These findings have been supported by other investigators, noting reduced complications and LOS [14,15,33,34]. In addition, in liver surgery, low CVP targets and hemodilution have been found to reduce overall blood loss and rates of transfusion [5,35]. However, many of the data remain ambiguous, as does the concept of tissue oxygen delivery, with some investigators finding that tissue oxygen saturation correlates directly with fluid administration [36,37]. The targets and methods of practice in each of these studies are highly variable and range from simply reducing crystalloid infusion rates, to the administration of plasma volume expanders (such as hetastarch), to the performance of isovolumetric hemodilution.

HYPERTONIC THEORY AND EVIDENCE

In keeping with the goal of appropriate fluid administration, one highly effective mechanism for achieving this objective is with 3% hypertonic saline (HYS). HYS may serve as a means to redirect the net movement of fluid back to the intravascular space and maintain a buffer between fluid overload and under-resuscitation. Because of its narrow volume of distribution or high osmotic load (>3 times that of 0.9% normal saline) equilibration of the blood to physiologic tonicity requires a 3-fold volume equivalent of free water to enter the vascular space. Although similar to other colloids, this mechanism has the benefit of easy elimination. The added salt load can be excreted via the kidneys, without the tendency of albumin or starch to remain sequestered in the tissues. HYS excretion is carefully regulated by the renal tubules and the renin-angiotensin-aldosterone system, making it physiologically appropriate (in contrast with an agent such as mannitol, the excretion of which is not physiologically managed). What is notable about this HYS model is the requirement of sufficient substrate water from which the hypertonic saline (or other colloid) can draw, to autotransfuse the intravascular compartment. Theoretically this requirement may in part explain the mixed results seen by hetastarch and hydroxyethyl starch, particularly with respect to renal dysfunction [38]. Without substrate fluid to draw into the vascular space, hyperosmolar therapies are, at best, ineffective. High-chloride solutions have been linked to poor outcomes in patients with trauma and sepsis and cause decreased renal cortical perfusion and urine output [39–41]. This outcome has not been identified in elective surgical patients. In well-managed, adequately resuscitated patients with acceptable cardiac output, the renal effects of high-chloride solutions are unclear. Adequate tissue oxygen delivery and maintenance of euvolemia through reduced urine output could conceivably be beneficial.

The intravenous use of HYS solutions dates back to the early twentieth century, with some of the first experiments focused on reducing intracranial pressure and limiting postoperative ileus [42,43]. HYS has become more relevant in recent times as the search for the ideal resuscitation fluid has continued: one that stays in the vascular space, serving the hemodynamic and metabolic needs of the patient. During fluid resuscitation, tissue edema accumulates in the organs and there is evidence that this plays a role in end-organ dysfunction [44–46]. HYS administration has been tested as a means to reduce this phenomenon of tissue edema [47]. Renewed interest in the use of HYS was seen in the early to mid 1980s, with an increased awareness of the damage caused by massive resuscitation and the abdominal compartment syndrome (see Table 1). Ruptured aortic aneurysm, a life-threatening condition often giving rise to abdominal compartment syndrome, prompted vascular surgeons to investigate small-volume resuscitation with HYS [48]. Trauma surgeons have also committed extensive study to the use of HYS for resuscitation, with reports of decreased resuscitation volumes, fewer complications, and a blunted immune response, but no impact on survival [39,49–56]. With respect to elective surgery, a Cochrane Review was completed in 2010 identifying HYS as a means to achieve end-organ perfusion with a smaller volume of fluid, although no significant clinical impact was identified [57].

Complications specifically related to the administration of HYS are predominantly electrolyte related. Severe hypernatremia may cause central pontine myelinolysis if the serum sodium level increases too abruptly. Hyperchloremia may result in a non–anion gap metabolic acidosis; independently less damaging but, when paired with other forms of acidosis, it can further decrease blood pH and impair enzyme function. These issues can be circumvented and easily corrected with appropriate monitoring of serum electrolytes and attention to the patient's starting sodium level.

PANCREAS-SPECIFIC EVIDENCE

The data on fluid restriction in pancreatic surgery are sparse, with variable conclusions. Five articles address (directly or indirectly) the relationship between fluid administration in the perioperative period and complications following pancreatic resection. The first trial by Fischer and colleagues [58] from Memorial Sloan Kettering was designed to evaluate the effect of acute normovolemic hemodilution on the rate of blood transfusion during and following pancreatic resection (the investigators had previous success with this method during liver resection) [35]. The trial found no reduction in the rate of blood transfusion, but there was an increase in pancreas-specific complications. These complications were attributed to an increase in intraoperative fluid administration.

Second, Melis and colleagues [59] divided patients into those who had received greater than or less than 6 L of fluid in the operating room. Fluid administration was related to the length of the procedure but did not have a bearing on the rate of complications, or LOS, highlighting the need to control for operative time. Third, following their work on hemodilution, the Memorial Sloan Kettering group conducted a retrospective review of their experience with pancreatectomy, examining the relationship between intraoperative fluid administration and complications [60]. They found a trend but no statistically significant relationship between complications and LOS in relation to fluid administration.

Fourth, another retrospective review, by Eng and colleagues [61], examined 124 patients over a 5-year period, finding a direct correlation between increased intraoperative fluid administration and complications when controlling for patient weight and length of surgery. They also identified an albumin level of less than 3.0 g/dL as a marker for increased intraoperative fluid administration. This finding may be one reason for the well-described association between low albumin levels and increased rates of complication following elective surgery. Fifth, their findings were confirmed by Weinberg and colleagues [62], who found not only increased intraoperative fluid administration but also a positive fluid balance in the early postoperative period to correlate directly with an increased rate of complications. What become difficult to decipher in these retrospective series are the parameters that have guided the resuscitation and whether the increased fluid administration is a marker for higher-risk patients or a more complex operation. This finding highlights the need for prospective trials in pancreatic surgery, and was the motivation for our group to conduct our own study on fluid resuscitation in patients having PD.

The HYSLAR (A Prospective Randomized Controlled Trial of the Use of a Restrictive Fluid Regimen With 3% Hypertonic Saline vs Lactated Ringers in Patients Undergoing Pancreaticoduodenectomy) trial [7] was designed to determine whether a restrictive fluid regimen using HYS could reduce postoperative complications in patients undergoing PD. This trial was a single-center, prospective, randomized, controlled, parallel design study (NCT 01428050). Patients undergoing PD at Thomas Jefferson University Hospital (TJUH) from May 2011 to November 2013 were deemed eligible for enrollment. Study subjects were stratified by pancreatic gland texture (hard or soft) and were randomized in a 1:1 fashion to either the lactated Ringer (LAR) or HYS arms. The fluid protocols for each group were developed by a multidisciplinary group of pancreatic surgeons, anesthesia staff, and critical care staff, and were based on institutional experience, standard fluid paradigms, and the literature on HYS administration.

The control arm (LAR) of the study involved the administration of 15 mL/kg/h of LAR during the PD procedure, with blood loss replaced with LAR in a 3:1 ratio (Fig. 1). Patients were continued on LAR in the immediate postoperative period, at a rate of administration of 2 mL/kg/h. The experimental arm (HYS) consisted of the administration of 9 mL/kg/h of LAR and 1 mL/kg/h of HYS during surgery, with blood loss replaced with LAR at a ratio of 1:1. Postoperatively, patients were maintained solely on HYS at a rate of 1 mL/kg/h. At 8 AM on the morning of postoperative day (POD) 1, patients in both groups were switched to 0.45% saline solution with 5% dextrose and 20 mEq of potassium chloride per liter at a rate of 1 mL/kg/h. In patients receiving HYS, fluid administration was performed via a central line, and serum sodium and chloride levels (which can increase rapidly) were monitored every 2 hours. HYS was discontinued if the serum sodium level increased to more than 150 mEq/L or more than 10 mEq/L above the preoperative sodium level, which occurred in less than 10%

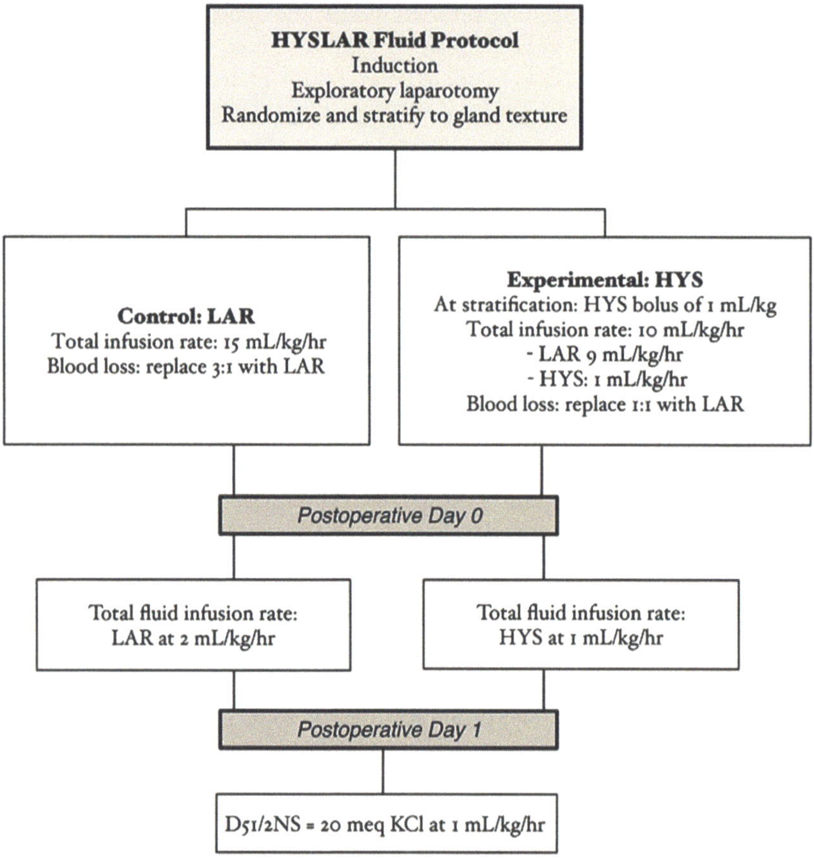

Fig. 1. Fluid administration schema for the HYSLAR trial. Low urine output or hypotension receives a 500-mL bolus. Low urine output is defined as less than 0.3 to 0.5 mL/kg/h. Blood pressure maintained within 20% of preinduction pressure. HYS, 3% hypertonic saline; LAR, lactated Ringer.

of patients, and when it did occur they were switched to LAR. Chloride levels frequently increased but rarely enough to cause acidemia. The study subjects were monitored carefully via standard hemodynamic parameters such as blood pressure, pulse pressure variation, CVP, and urine output. Patients who did not meet the appropriate parameters (typically low hourly urine output defined as <0.5 mL/kg/h) were given 500-mL boluses of LAR as deemed necessary. All of the surgeons who participated in the study followed a standardized post-PD clinical pathway [63]. The primary outcome for this study was the overall postoperative complication rate, and all of the common complications associated with PD were tracked [64–67]. The secondary outcomes for the study were the total number of complications in each group, estimated intraoperative blood loss, fluid boluses, postoperative hospital LOS, readmission rate, and mortality.

Four-hundred patients were evaluated for eligibility from May 2011 to November 2013 (Fig. 2). Of those 400, 264 underwent randomization and 5 were excluded, leaving a total of 259 patients evaluable at the conclusion of enrollment (128 LAR, 131 HYS). Clinical parameters and demographics were comparable between groups with the exception of preoperative weight, which was greater in the HYS group (78.2 vs 72.3 kg) (Table 2). Serum albumin was measured preoperatively, with no difference between the HYS and LAR groups (4.1 vs 4.2 g/dL), respectively. Periampullary malignancy (71%) was the most common indication for PD. There were no significant differences between the groups in terms of estimated intraoperative blood loss or procedure length, and most patients underwent pylorus-preserving PD (75% HYS and 80% LAR). Portal venous resection was performed in 4% of patients overall (2% HYS and 5% LAR). Notably, there were no additional complications or difficulties specific to this subgroup.

The HYS group received significantly less fluid during the operation, through the remainder of POD 0, on POD 1, and over the entire hospital admission (see Table 2). During surgery the urine output was significantly greater in the LAR group (2.5 mL/kg/h vs 1.8 mL/kg/h; $P = .008$). There were no significant differences between groups with respect to blood transfusion (the median number of transfused units per group was zero), or vasopressor use. In the postoperative period there was no significant difference in

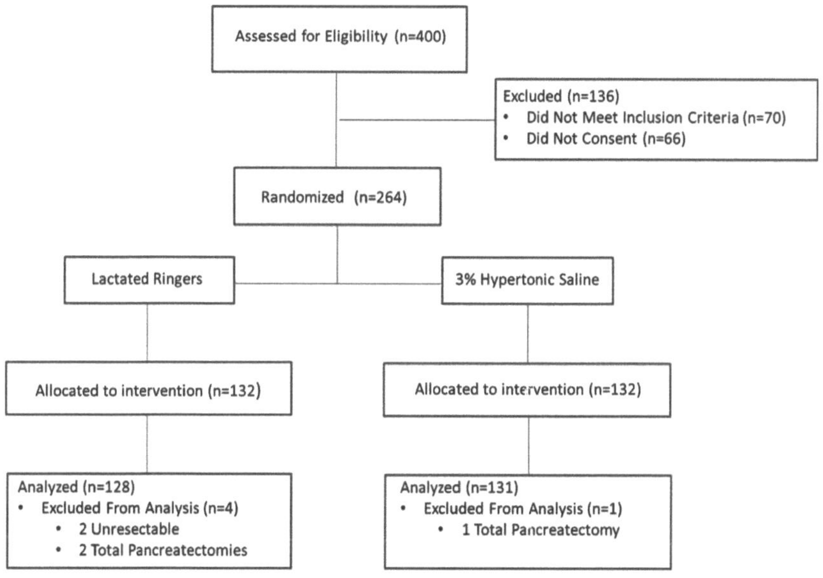

Fig. 2. Patient enrollment flowchart for the HYSLAR trial.

Table 2
HYSLAR demographic, operative, and fluid data

Total (n = 259)	Lactated ringers (n = 128)	Hypertonic saline (n = 131)	*P*
Demographics			
Age (y)[a]	68.3 (25–91)	66.6 (25–91)	NS
Weight (kg)	72.3 (46–126)	78.2 (44.9–125)	NS
Operative Data			
EBL (mL)	400 (50–6900)	350 (45–2250)	NS
Procedure length (min)	386 (247–674)	414 (265–686)	NS
Gland texture			
Hard, n (%)	67 (52)	69 (53)	NS
Soft, n (%)	61 (48)	62 (47)	NS
Fluid Data			
Intraoperative intake (mL/kg/h)	14.7 (4.7–45)	11.0 (2.8–26.5)	<.001
Remainder POD 0 (mL/kg)	19.3 (7.6–64)	13.1 (2–131)	<.001
POD 1 (mL/kg)	46.3 (20–152)	39.3 (14.3–639)	.002
Total intake (mL/kg)	315 (139–2022)	278 (130–2751)	.017
Total admission balance (mL/kg)	93.1 (−51 to 617)	64.8 (−120 to 881)	.019

Total intake is the cumulative inputs for the entire hospital admission; total admission balance is the cumulative inputs subtracted from cumulative outputs for the entire hospital admission.

Abbreviations: EBL, estimated blood loss; NS, nonsignificant; POD, postoperative day.

[a]Procedure length, EBL, and fluid data reported as means (ranges).

urine output between groups. Fluid boluses for hypotension or oliguria were not significantly different between groups in the postoperative period (1250 mL HYS, 1000 mL LAR), which resulted in a net fluid balance that was significantly reduced in the HYS group over the total hospital admission (HYS, 64.8 mL/kg vs LAR, 93.1 mL/kg; $P = .019$).

The results of the study (Table 3) showed that the HYS group had a lower overall rate of complications, at 43%, compared with 54% in the LAR group; when adjusted for pancreas texture, age, and weight using Poisson regression, this resulted in a relative risk of 0.75 (95% confidence interval [CI], 0.58–0.96; $P = .023$ (Table 4). The HYS group also had a significant reduction in the total number of complications (counting multiple complications per patient) compared with the LAR group (93 vs 123; $P = .027$). When adjusted for differences in pancreas texture, age, and weight, this amounted to an incident rate ratio of 0.69 (95% CI, 0.52–0.90; $P = .0068$), or a 31% reduction in complications per patient in the HYS cohort compared with the LAR cohort.

There were nonsignificant trends toward increased infectious (intra-abdominal abscess, wound infection, urinary tract infection) and cardiopulmonary (myocardial infarction, pneumonia, reintubation) complications in the LAR group. There were nonsignificant trends toward increased DGE in the LAR group (18% vs 11%) and increased hepaticojejunostomy/duodenojejunostomy (HJ/DJ) leak in the HYS group (6% vs 2%). The rate of pancreatic fistula was equivalent between groups at 16% with a similar grade distribution: HYS: 43% grade A, 48% grade B, 9% grade C. LAR: 43% grade A, 57% grade

Table 3
Postoperative outcomes and complications

Total (n = 259)	Lactated ringers (n = 128)	Hypertonic saline (n = 131)	*P*
Subjects with at least 1 complication, n (%)	69 (54)	56 (43)	.073[a]
Hard texture, n (%)	32 of 67 (48)	27 of 69 (39)	—
Soft texture, n (%)	37 of 61 (61)	29 of 62 (47)	—
Total number of complications	123	93	.027[b]
Individual Complications			
Pancreatic fistula, n (%)	21 (16)	21 (16)	NS
DGE, n (%)	23 (18)	15 (11)	NS
Intra-abdominal abscess, n (%)	20 (16)	12 (9)	NS
Wound infection, n (%)	14 (11)	9 (7)	NS
UTI, n (%)	11 (9)	7 (5)	NS
Cardiac, n (%)	6 (5)	4 (3)	NS
Pulmonary, n (%)	5 (4)	2 (2)	NS
Renal, n (%)	1 (1)	0 (0)	NS
DVT, n (%)	0 (0)	2 (2)	NS
HJ/DJ leak, n (%)	3 (2)	8 (6)	NS
Other, n (%)	17 (13)	13 (10)	NS
Pancreas-specific complications, n (%)	50 (39)	41 (31)	NS
Median LOS, days (range)	7 (4–41)	7 (5–61)	NS
Readmission, n (%)	13 (10)	16 (12)	NS
Reoperative rate, n (%)	1 (1)	5 (4)	NS
30-d mortality, n (%)	1 (1)	0 (0)	NS
90-d mortality, n (%)	3 (2)	4 (3)	NS

Pancreas-specific complications: pancreatic fistula, DGE, abscess, wound infection, hepaticojejunostomy/duodenojejunostomy leak.

Abbreviations: DVT, deep vein thrombosis; HJ/DJ, hepaticojejunostomy/duodenojejunostomy; UTI, Urinary tract infection.

[a]Cochran-Mantel-Haenszel test with pancreas texture as a covariate.

[b]Poisson regression with pancreas texture as covariate.

Table 4
Multivariate regression analysis: factors affecting complications

Variable	Risk ratio	95% Risk ratio confidence limits	*P*
Age (y)	1.007	0.997, 1.018	.16
Preoperative weight (kg)[a]	1.011	1.004, 1.017	.004
Pancreas texture (hard vs soft)	0.83	0.65, 1.07	.15
Complication rate[b] (HYS vs LAR)	0.75	0.58, 0.96	.023
Total number of complications (HYS vs LAR)	0.69	0.52, 0.90	.0068

Abbreviations: HYS, 3% hypertonic saline; LAR, lactated Ringer.

[a]Preoperative weight analyzed as a continuous variable.

[b]Percentage of patients with at least 1 complication.

B, 0% grade C. For the combined rate of pancreas-specific complications (ie, pancreatic fistula, DGE, intra-abdominal abscess, wound infection, and HJ/DJ leak) there was a trend toward reduced rates in the HYS arm, although this did not reach statistical significance. The lack of significant findings among these individual complications is not surprising because the trial was powered to the overall complication rate. There were no significant differences in postoperative hospital LOS, readmission rates, or mortality. One death occurred in the LAR group during the first 30 days after a massive aspiration event. The 90-day mortalities were 2% and 3% in the LAR and HYS groups respectively.

The HYSLAR trial had several limitations. It was a single-center study, and the investigators were not blinded to the study arms once the treatment assignment was made. The groups were not equal with respect to preoperative weight (greater in the HYS arm), which is a known risk factor for complications following PD. In addition, no objective physiologic measures were used, such as an assessment of peripheral edema levels or tissue oxygen tension. The trial was powered to detect a 33% reduction in complication rate, with a starting complication rate that was already in the lowest decile of National Surgical Quality Improvement Program data (Altimark R, and Lavu H, MD, personal communication, 2014). It is likely that this target was overly ambitious.

SUMMARY

Based on our findings in the HYSLAR trial, which showed a 25% reduction in the complication rate and a 31% reduction in the cumulative number of complications for patients receiving a moderately restrictive fluid regimen with HYS, we recommend this approach as the standard of care for perioperative fluid management in patients undergoing PD. This recommendation is concordant with our review of the literature on fluid management in abdominal surgery and its relationship to complications. We have altered our practice at TJUH since the conclusion of the HYSLAR trial to routinely use HYS at the study's prescribed rates in our patients having PD.

There is clearly a need for continued research in this area. Newer studies evaluating lower rates of fluid administration should be carefully randomized and controlled to adjust for such variables as patient weight and operative time, and should also include early postoperative fluid administration levels to avoid patients leaving the operating room under-resuscitated and then being given massive volumes of fluid in the early postoperative period. The concept that all patients can be maintained on the same golden rate of fluid administration is clearly facile, because many factors come into play for individual patients. Although we have shown that an intraoperative fluid administration rate of 10 mL/kg/h with a small component of HYS is superior to 15 mL/kg/h (without HYS), other investigators may suggest that further improvements in outcomes may occur with an even greater reduction to 8 or 6 mL/kg/h. Given some of the negative findings associated with ultrarestricted fluid regimens, a goal-directed approach as the next step in the evolution of PD resuscitation strategies seems prudent. Furthermore, objective data regarding tissue edema and oxygenation would be informative, to add to the understanding of the underlying physiology. A multi-institutional trial in pancreatectomy and other procedures is warranted to further study this question.

References

[1] Moore FD, Shires G. Moderation. Ann Surg 1967;166(2):300–1.

[2] Nisanevich V, Felsenstein I, Almogy G, et al. Effect of intraoperative fluid management on outcome after intraabdominal surgery. Anesthesiology 2005;103(1):25–32.

[3] Brandstrup B, Tønnesen H, Beier-Holgersen R, et al. Effects of intravenous fluid restriction on postoperative complications: comparison of two perioperative fluid regimens: a randomized assessor-blinded multicenter trial. Ann Surg 2003;238(5):641–8.

[4] Lobo DN, Bostock KA, Neal KR, et al. Effect of salt and water balance on recovery of gastrointestinal function after elective colonic resection: a randomised controlled trial. Lancet 2002;359(9320):1812–8.

[5] Melendez JA, Arslan V, Fischer ME, et al. Perioperative outcomes of major hepatic resections under low central venous pressure anesthesia: blood loss, blood transfusion, and the risk of postoperative renal dysfunction. J Am Coll Surg 1998;187(6):620–5.

[6] Matot I, Paskaleva R, Eid L, et al. Effect of the volume of fluids administered on intraoperative oliguria in laparoscopic bariatric surgery: a randomized controlled trial. Arch Surg 2012;147(3):228–34.

[7] Lavu H, Sell NM, Carter TI, et al. The HYSLAR trial: a prospective randomized controlled trial of the use of a restrictive fluid regimen with 3% hypertonic saline versus lactated ringers in patients undergoing pancreaticoduodenectomy. Ann Surg 2014;260(3):445–55.

[8] Gryth D, Rocksén D, Drobin D, et al. Effects of fluid resuscitation with hypertonic saline dextrane or Ringer's acetate after nonhemorrhagic shock caused by pulmonary contusion. J Trauma 2010;69(4):741–8.

[9] Wang CH, Hsieh WH, Chou HC, et al. Liberal versus restricted fluid resuscitation strategies in trauma patients: a systematic review and meta-analysis of randomized controlled trials and observational studies. Crit Care Med 2014;42(4):954–61.

[10] Pawelczyk NS, Huby MD, Salsbury JR, et al. Association of hemodilution and blood pressure in uncontrolled bleeding. J Surg Res 2013;184(2):959–65.

[11] Huang JJ, Yeo CJ, Sohn TA, et al. Quality of life and outcomes after pancreaticoduodenectomy. Ann Surg 2000;231(6):890–8.

[12] Sohn TA, Yeo CJ, Cameron JL, et al. Resected adenocarcinoma of the pancreas-616 patients: results, outcomes, and prognostic indicators. J Gastrointest Surg 2000;4(6):567–79.

[13] Hu BY, Laine GA, Wang S, et al. Combined central venous oxygen saturation and lactate as markers of occult hypoperfusion and outcome following cardiac surgery. J Cardiothorac Vasc Anesth 2012;26(1):52–7.

[14] Corcoran T, Rhodes JE, Clarke S, et al. Perioperative fluid management strategies in major surgery: a stratified meta-analysis. Anesth Analg 2012;114(3):640–51.

[15] Pearse R, Dawson D, Fawcett J, et al. Early goal-directed therapy after major surgery reduces complications and duration of hospital stay. A randomized, controlled trial [ISRCTN38797445]. Crit Care 2005;9(6):R687–93.

[16] Rivers E, Nguyen B, Havstad S, et al. Early goal-directed therapy in the treatment of severe sepsis and septic shock. N Engl J Med 2001;345(19):1368–77.

[17] ARISE Investigators, ANZICS Clinical Trials Group, Peake SL, et al. Goal-directed resuscitation for patients with early septic shock. N Engl J Med 2014;371(16):1496–506.

[18] Misawa T, Shiba H, Usuba T, et al. Systemic inflammatory response syndrome after hand-assisted laparoscopic distal pancreatectomy. Surg Endosc 2007;21(8):1446–9.

[19] Assifi MM, Lindenmeyer J, Leiby BE, et al. Surgical Apgar score predicts perioperative morbidity in patients undergoing pancreaticoduodenectomy at a high-volume center. J Gastrointest Surg 2012;16(2):275–81.

[20] Maier RV. Scudder oration on trauma. A century of evolution in trauma resuscitation. J Am Coll Surg 2014;219(3):335–45.
[21] Shires T, Williams J, Brown F. Acute change in extracellular fluids associated with major surgical procedures. Ann Surg 1961;154:803–10.
[22] Shires T, Williams J, Brown F. Simultaneous measurement of plasma volume, extracellular fluid volume, and red blood cell mass in man utilizing I-131, S-35-labeled sulfate, and Cr-51. J Lab Clin Med 1960;55:776–83.
[23] Kragelund E. Changes of the apparent 3HOH, 82Br, 125I human albumin and 51Cr red blood cell dilution volumes before, during and after operation in human subjects. Ann Surg 1970;172(1):116–24.
[24] Brandstrup B, Svensen C, Engquist A. Hemorrhage and operation cause a contraction of the extracellular space needing replacement–evidence and implications? A systematic review. Surgery 2006;139(3):419–32.
[25] Gross SD. A system of surgery: pathological, diagnostic, therapeutic, and operative. Philadelphia: HC Lea; 1882.
[26] Kulemann B, Timme S, Seifert G, et al. Intraoperative crystalloid overload leads to substantial inflammatory infiltration of intestinal anastomoses–a histomorphological analysis. Surgery 2013;154(3):596–603.
[27] Funk W, Baldinger V. Microcirculatory perfusion during volume therapy. A comparative study using crystalloid or colloid in awake animals. Anesthesiology 1995;82(4):975–82.
[28] Chan ST, Kapadia CR, Johnson AW, et al. Extracellular fluid volume expansion and third space sequestration at the site of small bowel anastomoses. Br J Surg 1983;70(1):36–9.
[29] Meregalli A, Oliveira RP, Friedman G. Occult hypoperfusion is associated with increased mortality in hemodynamically stable, high-risk, surgical patients. Crit Care 2004;8(2): R60–5.
[30] Schwartz RS, Eltzschig HK, Carmeliet P. Hypoxia and inflammation. N Engl J Med 2011;364(7):656–65.
[31] Lomivorotov VV, Fominskiy EV, Efremov SM, et al. Hypertonic solution decreases extravascular lung water in cardiac patients undergoing cardiopulmonary bypass surgery. J Cardiothorac Vasc Anesth 2013;27(2):273–82.
[32] Noblett SE, Snowden CP, Shenton BK, et al. Randomized clinical trial assessing the effect of Doppler-optimized fluid management on outcome after elective colorectal resection. Br J Surg 2006;93(9):1069–76.
[33] Holte K, Kehlet H. Fluid therapy and surgical outcomes in elective surgery: a need for reassessment in fast-track surgery. J Am Coll Surg 2006;202(6):971–89.
[34] Rahbari NN, Zimmermann JB, Schmidt T, et al. Meta-analysis of standard, restrictive and supplemental fluid administration in colorectal surgery. Br J Surg 2009;96(4):331–41.
[35] Jarnagin WR, Gonen M, Maithel SK, et al. A prospective randomized trial of acute normovolemic hemodilution compared to standard intraoperative management in patients undergoing major hepatic resection. Ann Surg 2008;248(3):360–9.
[36] Arkiliç CF, Taguchi A, Sharma N, et al. Supplemental perioperative fluid administration increases tissue oxygen pressure. Surgery 2003;133(1):49–55.
[37] Futier E, Constantin JM, Petit A, et al. Conservative vs restrictive individualized goal-directed fluid replacement strategy in major abdominal surgery: a prospective randomized trial. Arch Surg 2010;145(12):1193–200.
[38] Kashy BK, Podolyak A, Makarova N, et al. Effect of hydroxyethyl starch on postoperative kidney function in patients having noncardiac surgery. Anesthesiology 2014;121(4): 730–9.
[39] Huang PP, Stucky FS, Dimick AR, et al. Hypertonic sodium resuscitation is associated with renal failure and death. Ann Surg 1995;221(5):543–54.
[40] Shaw AD, Bagshaw SM, Goldstein SL, et al. Major complications, mortality, and resource utilization after open abdominal surgery: 0.9% saline compared to Plasma-Lyte. Ann Surg 2012;255(5):821–9.

[41] Chowdhury AH, Cox EF, Francis ST, et al. A randomized, controlled, double-blind crossover study on the effects of 2-L infusions of 0.9% saline and Plasma-Lyte® 148 on renal blood flow velocity and renal cortical tissue perfusion in healthy volunteers. Ann Surg 2012;256(1):18–24.
[42] Ross JW. Hypertonic saline in adynamic ileus. Can Med Assoc J 1926;16(3):241–4.
[43] Cohen H. The use of hypertonic saline solutions in increased intracranial tension. Br Med J 1924;1(3297):420–1.
[44] Moon PF, Hollyfield-Gilbert MA, Myers TL, et al. Fluid compartments in hemorrhaged rats after hyperosmotic crystalloid and hyperoncotic colloid resuscitation. Am J Physiol 1996;270(1 Pt 2):F1–8.
[45] Desai KV, Laine GA, Stewart RH, et al. Mechanics of the left ventricular myocardial interstitium: effects of acute and chronic myocardial edema. Am J Physiol Heart Circ Physiol 2008;294(6):H2428–34.
[46] Radhakrishnan RS, Xue H, Weisbrodt N, et al. Resuscitation induced intestinal edema decreases the stiffness and residual stress of the intestine. Shock 2005;24(2):165.
[47] Ing RD, Nazeeri MN, Zeldes S, et al. Hypertonic saline/dextran improves septic myocardial performance. Am Surg 1994;60(7):505–7.
[48] Shackford SR, Sise MJ, Fridlund PH, et al. Hypertonic sodium lactate versus lactated Ringer's solution for intravenous fluid therapy in operations on the abdominal aorta. Surgery 1983;94(1):41–51.
[49] Junger WG, Coimbra R, Liu FC, et al. Hypertonic saline resuscitation: a tool to modulate immune function in trauma patients? Shock 1997;8(4):235.
[50] Coimbra R, Hoyt DB, Junger WG, et al. Hypertonic saline resuscitation decreases susceptibility to sepsis after hemorrhagic shock. J Trauma Acute Care Surg 1997;42(4):602.
[51] Deitch EA, Shi HP, Feketeova E, et al. Hypertonic saline resuscitation limits neutrophil activation after trauma-hemorrhagic shock. Shock 2003;19(4):328.
[52] Harvin JA, Mims MM, Duchesne JC, et al. Chasing 100%: the use of hypertonic saline to improve early, primary fascial closure after damage control laparotomy. J Trauma Acute Care Surg 2013;74(2):426–30.
[53] Duchesne JC, Simms E, Guidry C, et al. Damage control immunoregulation: is there a role for low-volume hypertonic saline resuscitation in patients managed with damage control surgery? Am Surg 2012;78(9):962–8.
[54] Oliveira RP, Velasco I, Soriano FG, et al. Clinical review: hypertonic saline resuscitation in sepsis. Crit Care 2002;6(5):418–23.
[55] Gunn ML, Hansbrough JF, Davis JW, et al. Prospective, randomized trial of hypertonic sodium lactate versus lactated Ringer's solution for burn shock resuscitation. J Trauma 1989;29(9):1261–7.
[56] Bulger EM, May S, Kerby JD, et al. Out-of-hospital hypertonic resuscitation after traumatic hypovolemic shock: a randomized, placebo controlled trial. Ann Surg 2011;253(3):431–41.
[57] McAlister V, Burns KE, Znajda T, et al. Hypertonic saline for peri-operative fluid management. Cochrane Database Syst Rev 2010;(1):CD005576.
[58] Fischer M, Matsuo K, Gonen M, et al. Relationship between intraoperative fluid administration and perioperative outcome after pancreaticoduodenectomy: results of a prospective randomized trial of acute normovolemic hemodilution compared with standard intraoperative management. Ann Surg 2010;252(6):952–8.
[59] Melis M, Marcon F, Masi A, et al. Effect of intra-operative fluid volume on peri-operative outcomes after pancreaticoduodenectomy for pancreatic adenocarcinoma. J Surg Oncol 2012;105(1):81–4.
[60] Grant FM, Protic M, Gonen M, et al. Intraoperative fluid management and complications following pancreatectomy. J Surg Oncol 2013;107(5):529–35.
[61] Eng OS, Goswami J, Moore D, et al. Intraoperative fluid administration is associated with perioperative outcomes in pancreaticoduodenectomy: a single center retrospective analysis. J Surg Oncol 2013;108(4):242–7.

[62] Weinberg L, Wong D, Karalapillai D, et al. The impact of fluid intervention on complications and length of hospital stay after pancreaticoduodenectomy (Whipple's procedure). BMC Anesthesiol 2014;14(1):35.
[63] Kennedy EP, Rosato EL, Sauter PK, et al. Initiation of a critical pathway for pancreaticoduodenectomy at an academic institution–the first step in multidisciplinary team building. J Am Coll Surg 2007;204(5):917–23.
[64] Wente MN, Bassi C, Dervenis C, et al. Delayed gastric emptying (DGE) after pancreatic surgery: a suggested definition by the International Study Group of Pancreatic Surgery (ISGPS). Surgery 2007;142(5):761–8.
[65] Horan TC, Andrus M, Dudeck MA. CDC/NHSN surveillance definition of health care-associated infection and criteria for specific types of infections in the acute care setting. Am J Infect Control 2008;36(5):309–32.
[66] Thygesen K, Alpert JS, White HD. Joint ESC/ACCF/AHA/WHF Task Force for the Redefinition of Myocardial Infarction. Universal definition of myocardial infarction. Eur Heart J 2007;28(20):2525–38.
[67] Bellomo R, Ronco C, Kellum JA, et al. Acute Dialysis Quality Initiative workgroup. Acute renal failure - definition, outcome measures, animal models, fluid therapy and information technology needs: the second international consensus conference of the Acute Dialysis Quality Initiative (ADQI) Group. Crit Care 2004;8:R204–12.

Advances in Surgery 49 (2015) 221–233

ADVANCES IN SURGERY

ELSEVIER
MOSBY

Is There a Relationship Between Patient Satisfaction and Favorable Surgical Outcomes?

Sarah E. Tevis, MD, Gregory D. Kennedy, MD, PhD, K. Craig Kent, MD*

Department of Surgery, University of Wisconsin School of Medicine and Public Health, Highland Avenue, Madison, WI 53792, USA

Keywords

• Patient satisfaction • HCAHPS • Outcomes

Key points

- Patient satisfaction continues to gain importance in health care with public reporting of scores along with ties between satisfaction scores and Medicare reimbursement.
- High hospital and surgical volume and low risk-adjusted mortality rates are associated with high overall patient satisfaction.
- More traditional measures of outcome as well as markers of hospital quality and safety are not consistently associated with high patient satisfaction.
- The focus on patient satisfaction is here to stay; a multidisciplinary, surgeon-led effort dedicated to improving patients' perceptions of their care is essential.

INTRODUCTION

The Hospital Consumer Assessment of Healthcare Providers and Systems (HCAHPS) survey was developed by the Centers for Medicare & Medicaid Services (CMS) and the Agency for Healthcare Research and Quality. The HCAHPS survey is the first standardized survey of patient satisfaction and is designed to compare hospitals across the nation. The 3 main goals driving survey development were (1) to motivate hospitals to improve their quality of care with regard to patient

The authors have no conflicts of interest to declare. Support for this study was provided by the NIH T32 training grant (CA090217).

*Corresponding author. Department of Surgery, University of Wisconsin, 650 Highland Avenue, Madison, WI 53792. *E-mail address:* kent@surgery.wisc.edu

0065-3411/15/$ – see front matter
http://dx.doi.org/10.1016/j.yasu.2015.03.006

satisfaction, (2) to provide transparent public reporting of survey results, and (3) to allow consumers to objectively compare hospitals [1]. The temporal sequence leading to the creation of the HCAHPS survey is outlined in Fig. 1. Survey development began in 2002 with an extensive review of the literature, assessment of available survey tools, and cognitive testing [2]. Over a 15-month period, the survey was piloted in 3 states: Maryland, Arizona, and New York. The National Quality Forum endorsed the survey in May 2005, and the Office of Management and Budget approved the survey for national use in December 2005.

The HCAHPS survey consists of 10 measures including 6 summary measures, 2 individual items, and 2 items evaluating overall patient satisfaction [1]. There are a total of 32 questions of which 25 assess patients' perception of their care and 7 collect demographic information. Fig. 2 demonstrates the HCAHPS questions pertaining to overall patient satisfaction [3]. The survey is administered to medical, surgical, and maternity care patients within 6 weeks of hospital discharge. Hospitals may individually collect data or use approved vendors. Multiple attempts are made to connect with patients using any of the 4 available survey modes: mail, telephone, mail with telephone follow-up, and active interactive voice recognition. Hospitals are required to collect at least 300 surveys annually for the inpatient prospective payment system, and surveys must be collected on a monthly basis [1]. A case-mix adjustment using the variables self-reported health status, educational attainment, service line, age, admission from emergency department, interaction between service line and age, and primary language other than English is applied to survey scores to allow for reliable comparisons across hospitals with differing patient populations [4–7]. In addition, scores are adjusted based on the mode of survey.

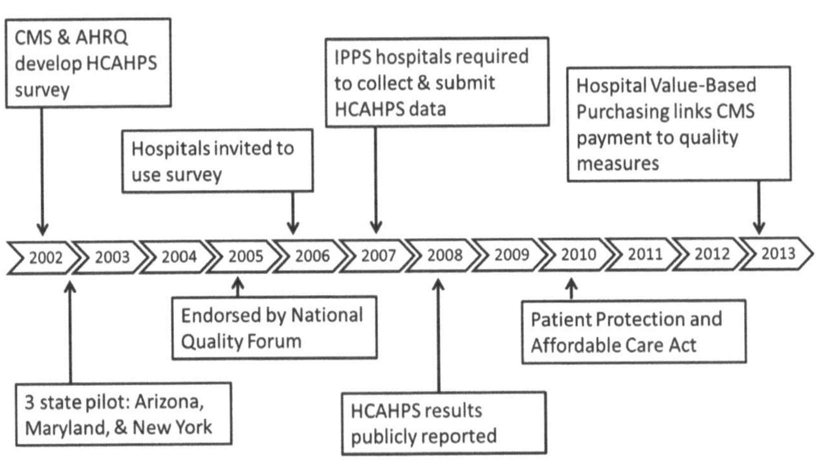

Fig. 1. Sequence for the development and implementation of the HCAHPS survey. CMS, Centers for Medicare & Medicaid Services; AHRQ, Agency of Healthcare Research and Quality; IPPS, Inpatient Prospective Payment System. (*From* Tevis ST, Schmocker RK, Kennedy GD. Can patients reliably identify safe, high quality care? Hosp Admin, 2014;5(3):150–60.)

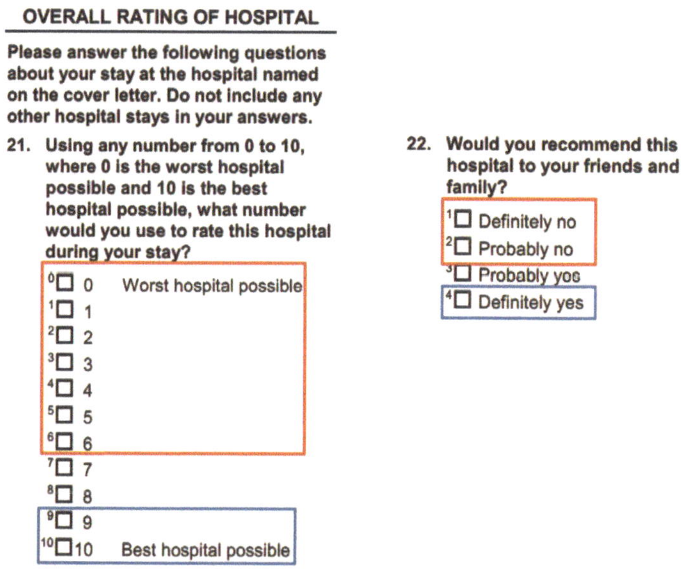
OVERALL RATING OF HOSPITAL

Please answer the following questions about your stay at the hospital named on the cover letter. Do not include any other hospital stays in your answers.

21. Using any number from 0 to 10, where 0 is the worst hospital possible and 10 is the best hospital possible, what number would you use to rate this hospital during your stay?
- 0 Worst hospital possible
- 1
- 2
- 3
- 4
- 5
- 6
- 7
- 8
- 9
- 10 Best hospital possible

22. Would you recommend this hospital to your friends and family?
- Definitely no
- Probably no
- Probably yes
- Definitely yes

Fig. 2. Overall satisfaction HCAHPS domains. "Top box" responses are outlined in blue, while "bottom box" responses are outlined in red. (*From* HCAHPS Survey. Available at: www.hcahpsonline.org/files/HCAHPS V9.0 Appendix A - Mail Survey Materials (English) March 2014.pdf. Accessed February 13, 2014.)

Results of the case-mix adjusted HCAHPS survey scores are publicly reported 4 times each year on the Hospital Compare Web site [8]. Scores are characterized as "top box" and "bottom box" percentiles for each HCAHPS domain. As demonstrated in Fig. 2, top box scores represent the most favorable responses and bottom box scores are the least positive responses [1].

NATIONAL IMPACT OF SATISFACTION SURVEYS

The goals for the development of the HCAHPS survey were to motivate hospitals to improve the quality of care and to publicly provide information regarding patient satisfaction. Publicly reported HCAHPS scores are easily accessible to all consumers and are presented in a way that is simple to interpret. It is reasonable to assume that savvy consumers, if given the choice, choose to have their care at hospitals with higher reported patient satisfaction scores. While narrow networks have limited access to some patients, when choice is possible, patients tend to select providers and hospitals with higher ratings, including HCAHPS satisfaction scores [9,10]. In addition, Medicare reimbursement has been linked to performance on the HCAHPS surveys. This process began in 2005 when the Deficit Reduction Act mandated public reporting of HCAHPS scores in order for hospitals to receive full Medicare payment [1]. The recent enactment of the Patient Protection and Affordable Care Act in 2010 includes HCAHPS measures in the Value-Based Purchasing (VBP) program. The VBP program ties the hospital payments to clinical processes of care and patient experience. Top box HCAHPS scores are used to determine the patient experience domain of VBP, comparing hospitals to the national median and assessing the improvement of individual hospitals in each domain. HCAHPS scores encompass 30% of VBP performance (which by 2017 will account for 2% of overall Medicare reimbursement) [1].

CORRELATING HOSPITAL CHARACTERISTICS AND SURGICAL OUTCOME MEASURES WITH PATIENT SATISFACTION

With increasing pressure on hospitals and providers to improve performance on HCAHPS surveys, the authors thought it important within the surgical realm to identify those variables that influence patient satisfaction. Surgeons for years have focused on outcomes such as mortality, rate of complication, or specific assessments of surgical success (such as pain relief or bypass patency). Whether achievement of favorable surgical outcomes is at all correlative with satisfied patients is not clear. At present, a few studies in the literature assess predictors of patient satisfaction. To this end, the authors recently evaluated patient satisfaction as determined by HCAHPS and correlated this to hospital characteristics as well as more traditional surgical outcomes derived from the University Health Systems Consortium database. The findings were surprising and provocative and overall suggest very little correlation between traditional surgical outcomes and patient satisfaction. The only factors that correlated with enhanced patient satisfaction were high hospital and surgical volume and low risk-adjusted mortality. Multiple other outcomes including rate of surgical complications, readmissions, and process measures did not correlate. These relationships are demonstrated in Figs. 3 and 4 and are summarized in the paragraphs that follow.

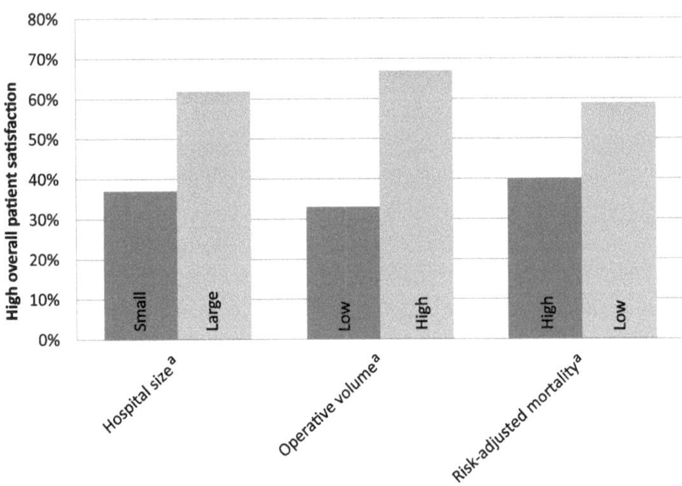

Fig. 3. Predictors of overall patient satisfaction. [a] $P<.001$. Overall Satisfaction = Definitely Recommend Hospital.

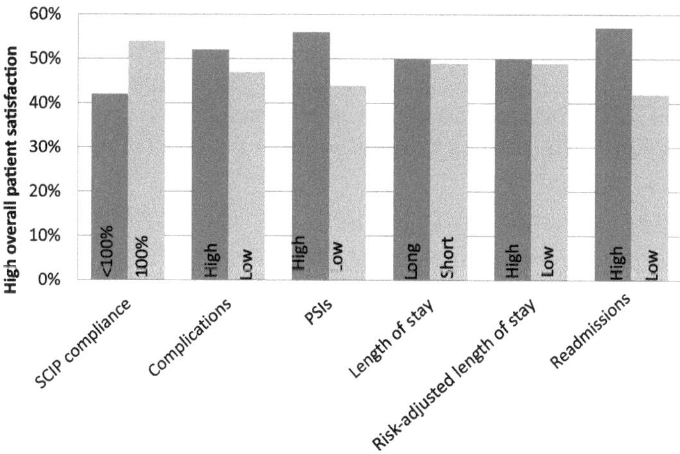

Fig. 4. Nonpredictors of overall patient satisfaction. None of these variables reached statistical significance. Overall Satisfaction = Definitely Recommend Hospital.

Measures that correlate with patient satisfaction

Hospital and surgical volume

Both hospital and surgical volume were found to significantly correlate with high overall patient satisfaction ($P<.001$). Tsai and colleagues [11] recently identified a similar association between larger hospitals and the likelihood of recommending a hospital ($P<.001$). Alternatively, in another study of medical and surgical patients, small hospitals were most likely to score in the top quartile for patient satisfaction [12]. The difference in these findings may be related to the HCAHPS domains used for the analysis. The study correlating patient satisfaction with small hospitals used a broader HCAHPS composite score for comparison (including factors such as a clean and quiet room and food service). Smaller hospitals may be more capable of achieving quiet, clean rooms and an attentive nursing staff, whereas larger hospitals seem to score better on the summative HCAHPS domain "would you recommend this hospital to friends and family." When using the summative HCAHPS measures as the sole outcome, there seems to be a clear relationship between large hospital size as well as high surgical volume and patient satisfaction.

Risk-adjusted mortality

The authors were particularly interested in determining if patient satisfaction correlated with hospital mortality. They found that patients at hospitals with low risk-adjusted mortality were significantly more likely on HCAHPS to recommend the hospital (see Fig. 3, $P<.001$). Tsai and colleagues [11] also found an association between low risk-adjusted mortality in surgical patients and high satisfaction scores on HCAHPS. However, Sheetz and colleagues [13] in an evaluation of the Michigan Surgical Quality Collaborative registry did not find a significant difference in risk-adjusted mortality between hospitals with high and low HCAHPS total performance scores (4% mortality in the lowest quintile vs 3.3% mortality in the highest quintile). Elliott and colleagues [14] similarly showed no correlation between patient satisfaction and 1-year mortality. The difference in findings of the various studies may again be related to the variable domains used to measure patient satisfaction and the types of surgical patients evaluated.

Nonpredictors of patient satisfaction

Surprisingly, the remainder of the surgical outcomes that the authors evaluated had no correlation with overall patient satisfaction.

Clinical process measure compliance

Compliance with Surgical Care Improvement Project (SCIP) measures was not significantly associated with higher overall satisfaction ($P = .122$, see Fig. 4). Lyu and colleagues [15] also evaluated SCIP process measure compliance and consistent with the authors' findings found no significant association between SCIP compliance and patient satisfaction. In contrast, several additional studies have demonstrated a positive relationship between compliance with SCIP and higher satisfaction scores [11,12,16,17]. Thus, the relationship between SCIP compliance and patient satisfaction on HCAHPS is inconsistent. One of the possible reasons for this inconsistency is that over time hospitals have performed increasingly well on SCIP, with the majority achieving near 100% compliance. Therefore differences in SCIP compliance rates nationwide are small making any correlation between process measure compliance and patient satisfaction difficult to establish.

Postoperative complications

Interestingly, the authors identified an unexpected trend of higher patient satisfaction in hospitals with higher rates of in-hospital complications, although this finding was not statistically significant ($P = .49$). Similarly, Sheetz and colleagues [13] showed no correlation between risk-adjusted complication rates and satisfaction on the HCAHPS survey (25% morbidity in lowest quintile vs 25% morbidity in highest quintile). Gurland and colleagues [18] also found that patients with postoperative complications had no diminution in the overall patient satisfaction ranking domains. This finding is a surprising one; one possible explanation is that surgical patients are forewarned and anticipate complications and factor these into their overall care process.

Patient safety indicators

The authors also found numerically but not statistically that the greater the number of patient safety events, the higher the patient satisfaction. In others studies, Patient Safety Indicators (PSIs) have had a mixed association with patient satisfaction. In an evaluation of hospitals in the National CAHPS Benchmarking Database, Isaac and colleagues [17] found no correlation with overall patient satisfaction for most PSIs. PSIs are rare and as such are unlikely to affect overall patient satisfaction.

Length of stay

The authors found no significant correlation between hospital length of stay (observed $P = .819$, risk adjusted $P = .939$) and patients' perceptions of their care. Their findings conflict with those of a previous study in which shorter risk-adjusted length of hospital stay was associated with improved performance on the "recommendation of hospital" HCAHPS domain (7.1 days in high satisfaction group vs 7.7 days in low satisfaction group) [11]. The difference in findings may be related to differences in the surgical populations studied. The authors evaluated all patients discharged by general surgery, while Tsai and colleagues [11] only evaluated patients undergoing the following 6 procedures: coronary artery bypass grafting, pulmonary lobectomy, endovascular aneurysm repair, open abdominal aortic aneurysm repair, colectomy, and hip replacement.

Postoperative readmissions

Given the increasing emphasis on readmission reduction, the authors wished to evaluate whether readmission might produce a negative impact on patient satisfaction. Although one might assume that hospitals with higher rates of readmission would have lower patient satisfaction, the authors actually found the opposite trend ($P = .252$). This finding contrasts with previous studies in medical patients in which investigators found low readmission rates to be associated with higher overall patient satisfaction. An evaluation of 30-day readmission rates in patients with myocardial infarction, congestive heart failure, and pneumonia revealed an association with higher overall satisfaction. Thus in chronic medical conditions, readmission leads to diminished patient satisfaction, but this is not the case, at least in our analysis, for surgical patients.

Correlation between patient outcomes and provider, hospital systems, and environmental hospital consumer assessment of healthcare providers and systems domains

The authors evaluated 8 HCAHPS domains that addressed provider services as well as hospital systems and environment and attempted to correlate these to patient outcomes. The relationship was essentially random (Table 1). The 2 HCAHPS domains that best correlated with patient outcomes were a clean room and pain control. These findings underscore the complexity of comparing multiple patient satisfaction domains to multiple quality outcome measures. The overall conclusion from this evaluation, however, is that there is essentially no meaningful correlation between traditional surgical outcomes and patient satisfaction.

ADDITIONAL PATIENT AND HOSPITAL FACTORS THAT INFLUENCE PATIENT SATISFACTION

Proxy and nonresponse bias

The methods used to survey patients have been shown to affect patient satisfaction scores. Although survey scores are adjusted for mode of administration,

Table 1
Correlation of patient satisfaction in the provider, hospital system, and environmental domains with surgical outcomes

	Nursing communication	Physician communication	Received help	Pain controlled	Medications explained	Cleanliness of room	Quietness of room	Discharge instructions
Hospital size	—	—	—	—	—	—	—	—
Surgical volume	—	—	—	—	—	—	—	—
SCIP compliance	.039	—	—	.01	.022	—	—	—
Complications	—	—	—	—	—	—	—	—
PSIs	—	—	.018	.03	—	<.001	—	—
LOS (observed)	—	—	.005	—	—	.001	—	—
LOS (risk adjusted)	—	—	.007	.011	—	<.001	—	.012
Readmission	—	—	—	—	—	.016	—	—
Mortality (observed)	—	.002	.012	<.001	.005	.002	—	—
Mortality (risk adjusted)	.012	.027	.005	.001	.027	<.001	—	.003

P values denote significant relationships, whereas blanks represent lack of significance.

Abbreviation: LOS, length of stay.

Adapted from Kennedy GD, Tevis ST, Kent KC. Is there a relationship between patient satisfaction and favorable outcomes? Ann Surg 2014;260(4):593; with permission.

other variables such as proxy response and assistance of a proxy in preparing the response have been found to influence satisfaction scores [19]. Almost 20% of HCAHPS surveys are completed by or with the assistance of a proxy. Life partners or spouses usually respond in a manner similar to patients, whereas other family members and nonfamily members often provide a less-favorable response. Nonresponders have also been evaluated and are more likely to be racial minorities, patients leaving against medical advice, or obstetric or medical patients (vs surgical patients) [20–22].

Health care use

With increasing pressure to provide high-quality and efficient care, studies have assessed health care use and patient satisfaction. Patients who are less likely to use the emergency department are more satisfied [23]. Alternatively, there is a positive relationship between satisfied patients and those more likely to accrue higher total health expenditures.

Hospital characteristics

Various hospital factors have been identified as predictors of patient satisfaction, including staffing, teaching status, and use of health information technology (HIT). Higher nurse to patient ratios are more likely to produce higher overall satisfaction (66% top box scores in high nurse to patient day ratio hospitals vs 61% in low nurse to patient day ratio hospitals) [11,16]. Mixed results have been reported regarding the relationship between hospital teaching status and patient satisfaction on HCAHPS with some studies reporting no difference [16], whereas others finding teaching hospitals to be associated with higher satisfaction scores [11,12]. With health care evolving to greater use of the electronic medical record (EMR), little is known about the effect of the EMR on patient satisfaction. One study assessed the relationship between HIT and patient satisfaction scores in groups of patients seeing specialists and primary care providers [24]. The following 4 factors were found to be highly associated with favorable scores on the physician communication domain: ability to have questions answered in a timely manner through e-mail, ability to an make appointments by e-mail, physician use of a computer, and a provider Web site.

The value of feedback in improving patient satisfaction scores

A study by Elliott and colleagues [25] demonstrated statistically significant improvement in patient satisfaction scores (8 of 9 satisfaction domains) in the first year after survey results were publicly reported. It seems that hospitals have embraced these surveys as well as their findings and are identifying ways to change culture and improve systems to enhance patient satisfaction. Many quality improvement projects have been implemented in an effort to improve patient satisfaction scores. Projects have focused on pain management, communication, or provider incentives; however, the modest success of these individual initiatives suggests that tackling patient satisfaction is a complex undertaking.

Pain management

A study of the rating of the pain intensity for surgical, trauma, and oncology patients revealed no association between pain and satisfaction scores [26]. Although these investigators did identify a trend between higher pain scores and decreased satisfaction, this difference did not reach statistical significance.

Communication training

Given the increasing emphasis on improving HCAHPS scores, improving provider communication has become an area of interest. One group implemented a communication skills training program on a nonteaching hospitalist service. The program consisted of three 90-minute sessions and provided education about patient satisfaction and communication skills, a simulation based communication exercise, and coaching sessions during clinical encounters. Only 40% of physicians completed all 3 training sessions, and after training there were no significant differences in overall or physician communication satisfaction scores. The findings were similar when a relationship-based care (RBC) model was implemented for nursing at a single institution [27]. RBC models focused on collaboration and patient-centered care. Average nursing satisfaction scores were unchanged (91% vs 91%) after the implementation of this model. Thus, efforts to enhance physician and staff communication have not yet yielded positive results.

Provider incentives

The effect of monetary incentives to enhance patient satisfaction has been investigated. It would seem that incentivizing providers with monetary rewards might have a positive effect on their efforts toward patient satisfaction. In one study, emergency department residents could earn discount cards for espressos or a monetary bonus as patient satisfaction scores increased (ie, $50 for the 50th percentile and $200 for the 80th percentile). Unfortunately, these monetary incentives had no overall effect on resident performance in the realm of patient satisfaction.

Patient and team communication

Several studies have demonstrated success in improving patient satisfaction by addressing communication and rewarding compassion. In one study, physicians with high communication scores were interviewed to determine what common practices they used when providing patient care [28]. Participating physicians stressed the importance of hiring staff with excellent people skills and involving office staff in patient visits. High-scoring physicians also valued the use of nonverbal communication, providing clear explanations for patients, asking patients personal questions and recalling the information later, and developing an agreed upon plan at the end of each interaction. In-depth interviews with 30 patients on a hospitalist service provided additional insight with regard to patient satisfaction. Areas that were emphasized by these patients were physician behavior, team communication, and systems issues [29]. Patients valued interactions in which physicians displayed a caring attitude and allowed patients to participate in medical decision making. Satisfaction with specialists was based on perceived competence and continuity of care. Major themes of dissatisfied patients included the perception that physicians were not communicating with each other or lacked understanding of the responsibility of each of the individual members of the team. Any disorganized care, inclusive of food services or housekeeping, produced a decrement in physician HCAHPS scores.

Devotion of additional hospital resources

Bastani and colleagues [30] were able to improve patient satisfaction in the emergency department by using a scribe in the setting of an EMR to improve efficiency of care and physician communication. The investigators found an improvement in overall emergency department satisfaction (58% to 75%) and physician satisfaction (62% to 92%) after implementation of a scribe program. Similarly, the addition of a physician partner, who acted as a scribe and performed administrative duties in a medical clinic, led patients to report high satisfaction by increasing the amount physician contact [31]. Guss and colleagues [32] implemented a telephone call to patients after discharge from the emergency department in an effort to improve patient satisfaction. Patients who received a postdischarge phone call were more likely to recommend the hospital compared with those who did not receive a phone call (89% vs 56%). Of note, the cost associated with these interventions can be substantial and may limit broad implementation. These successes aside, programs aimed at changing only 1 aspect of patient care have had variable results in improving patient satisfaction scores. It has become clear that increased patient satisfaction requires simultaneously changing multiple variables or a significant cultural change.

SURGEONS AS LEADERS IN PATIENT SATISFACTION

To consistently provide high-quality patient-centered care, a patient-centered multidisciplinary team approach is required. This team should include physicians, nurses, residents, pharmacists, students, patients, and families. Expansion of the health care team to include staff from other areas including environmental services, information technology, food service, facilities, and administrative personnel is essential. Given the dominant role that surgeons play in the care of their patients, it is incumbent on surgeons to take the lead in organizing and supporting this caregiver team. High patient satisfaction correlates with effective communication, personalization of care, patient education, and continuity of care. Surgeons are uniquely positioned to lead this complex multidisciplinary team to provide patient-centered care that results in highly satisfied patients. A previous study by Banki and colleagues [33] demonstrated improved patient satisfaction scores after the development of a multidisciplinary surgeon-led team. This improvement project consisted of staff education and standardization of care in patients who underwent laparoscopic fundoplication and Heller myotomy. The surgeon-led team participated in monthly teaching sessions and multidisciplinary conferences, team leaders attended weekly meetings, and the surgeon led daily multidisciplinary bedside rounds. An emphasis was also placed on weekly review of issues, concerns, and processes that required improvement. Patients reported higher satisfaction in the following domains after implementation of the surgical team: overall rating, communication with nurses, communication about medications, and discharge instructions. In addition, after the implementation of a surgeon-led team, operative times, length of stay, and costs all significantly decreased. An organizational change to a team-based, mindful, approach to patient care will result in patients who are highly satisfied with their surgical outcomes and hospital experience.

SUMMARY

Patients' perceptions have become an important measure of hospital care. Patient satisfaction scores are now available publicly and are tied to Medicare reimbursement incentivizing hospitals to improve patients' perceptions of their care. Although higher hospital and surgical volumes and low risk-adjusted mortality have been found to translate into increased patient satisfaction on HCAHPS, many other variables are likely in play. A collaborative team-based approach is needed to continuously improve the quality of care and to improve patients' perceptions of their care. Surgeons are uniquely poised to lead organizational change aimed at providing exceptional team-based patient service.

References

[1] HCAHPS Fact Sheet. Available at: http://www.hcahpsonline.org/files/August%202013%20HCAHPS%20Fact%20Sheet2.pdf. Accessed February 13, 2014.

[2] Goldstein E, Farquhar M, Crofton C, et al. Measuring hospital care from the patients' perspective: an overview of the CAHPS Hospital Survey development process. Health Serv Res 2005;40(6 Pt 2):1977–95.

[3] HCAHPS Survey. Available at: http://www.hcahpsonline.org/files/HCAHPS%20V10.0%20Appendix%20A%20-%20HCAHPS%20Mail%20Survey%20Materials%20(English)%20March%202015.pdf. Accessed February 13, 2014.

[4] Morales LS, Elliott MN, Weech-Maldonado R, et al. Differences in CAHPS adult survey reports and ratings by race and ethnicity: an analysis of the National CAHPS benchmarking data 1.0. Health Serv Res 2001;36(3):595–617.

[5] Elliott MN, Swartz R, Adams J, et al. Case-mix adjustment of the National CAHPS benchmarking data 1.0: a violation of model assumptions? Health Serv Res 2001;36(3):555–73.

[6] Elliott MN, Zaslavsky AM, Goldstein E, et al. Effects of survey mode, patient mix, and nonresponse on CAHPS hospital survey scores. Health Serv Res 2009;44(2 Pt 1):501–18.

[7] Weech-Maldonado R, Morales LS, Elliott M, et al. Race/ethnicity, language, and patients' assessments of care in Medicaid managed care. Health Serv Res 2003;38(3):789–808.

[8] Hospital Compare. Available at: www.medicare.gov/hospitalcompare/search.html. Accessed February 13, 2014.

[9] Faber M, Bosch M, Wollersheim H, et al. Public reporting in health care: how do consumers use quality-of-care information? A systematic review. Med Care 2009;47(1):1–8.

[10] Kolstad JT, Chernew ME. Quality and consumer decision making in the market for health insurance and health care services. Med Care Res Rev 2009;66(1 Suppl):28S–52S.

[11] Tsai TC, Orav EJ, Jha AK. Patient satisfaction and quality of surgical care in US hospitals. Ann Surg 2015;261:2–8.

[12] Lehrman WG, Elliott MN, Goldstein E, et al. Characteristics of hospitals demonstrating superior performance in patient experience and clinical process measures of care. Med Care Res Rev 2010;67(1):38–55.
[13] Sheetz KH, Waits SA, Girotti ME, et al. Patients' perspectives of care and surgical outcomes in Michigan: an analysis using the CAHPS hospital survey. Ann Surg 2014;260(1):5–9.
[14] Elliott MN, Haviland AM, Cleary PD, et al. Care experiences of managed care Medicare enrollees near the end of life. J Am Geriatr Soc 2013;61(3):407–12.
[15] Lyu H, Wick EC, Housman M, et al. Patient satisfaction as a possible indicator of quality surgical care. JAMA Surg 2013;148(4):362–7.
[16] Jha AK, Orav EJ, Zheng J, et al. Patients' perception of hospital care in the United States. N Engl J Med 2008;359:1921–31.
[17] Isaac T, Zaslavsky AM, Cleary PD, et al. The relationship between patients' perception of care and measures of hospital quality and safety. Health Serv Res 2010;45(4):1024–40.
[18] Gurland BH, Merlino J, Sobol T, et al. Surgical complications impact patient perception of hospital care. J Am Coll Surg 2013;217(5):843–9.
[19] Elliott MN, Beckett MK, Chong K, et al. How do proxy responses and proxy-assisted responses differ from what Medicare beneficiaries might have reported about their health care? Health Serv Res 2008;43(3):833–48.
[20] Elliott MN, Edwards C, Angeles J, et al. Patterns of unit and item nonresponse in the CAHPS Hospital Survey. Health Serv Res 2005;40(6 Pt 2):2096–119.
[21] Klein DJ, Elliott MN, Haviland AM, et al. Understanding nonresponse to the 2007 Medicare CAHPS survey. Gerontologist 2011;51(6):843–55.
[22] Zaslavsky AM, Zaborski LB, Cleary PD. Factors affecting response rates to the Consumer Assessment of Health Plans Study survey. Med Care 2002;40(6):485–99.
[23] Fenton JJ, Jerant AF, Bertakis KD, et al. The cost of satisfaction: a national study of patient satisfaction, health care utilization, expenditures, and mortality. Arch Intern Med 2012;172(5):405–11.
[24] McInnes DK, Brown JA, Hays RD, et al. Development and evaluation of CAHPS questions to assess the impact of health information technology on patient experiences with ambulatory care. Med Care 2012;50:S11–9.
[25] Elliott MN, Lehrman WG, Goldstein EH, et al. Hospital survey shows improvements in patient experience. Health Aff (Millwood) 2010;29(11):2061–7.
[26] Phillips S, Gift M, Gelot S, et al. Assessing the relationship between the level of pain control and patient satisfaction. J Pain Res 2013;6:683–9.
[27] Cropley S. The relationship-based care model: evaluation of the impact on patient satisfaction, length of stay, and readmission rates. J Nurs Adm 2012;42(6):333–9.
[28] Quigley DD, Martino SC, Brown JA, et al. Evaluating the content of the communication items in the CAHPS((R)) clinician and group survey and supplemental items with what high-performing physicians say they do. Patient 2013;6(3):169–77.
[29] Wild DM, Kwon N, Dutta S, et al. Who's behind an HCAHPS score? Jt Comm J Qual Patient Saf 2011;37(10):461–8.
[30] Bastani A, Shaqiri B, Palomba K, et al. An ED scribe program is able to improve throughput time and patient satisfaction. Am J Emerg Med 2013;32(5):399–402.
[31] Reuben DB, Knudsen J, Senelick W, et al. The effect of a physician partner program on physician efficiency and patient satisfaction. JAMA Intern Med 2014;174:1190–3.
[32] Guss DA, Gray S, Castillo EM. The impact of patient telephone call after discharge on likelihood to recommend in an academic emergency department. J Emerg Med 2013;46(4):560–6.
[33] Banki F, Ochoa K, Carrillo ME, et al. A surgical team with focus on staff education in a community hospital improves outcomes, costs and patient satisfaction. Am J Surg 2013;206(6):1007–14 [discussion: 1014–5].

Advances in Surgery 49 (2015) 235–245

ADVANCES IN SURGERY

ELSEVIER
MOSBY

Does Volume Affect Outcome with Severe Trauma?

Jordan A. Weinberg, MD*, Timothy C. Fabian, MD

Department of Surgery, University of Tennessee Health Science Center, 910 Madison Avenue, 2nd Floor, Memphis, TN 38163, USA

Keywords

• Volume • Outcomes • Trauma • Trauma systems • Quality

Key points

- The relationship between surgical volume and outcome goes beyond relative experience, and the relationship between volume and outcome is unlikely a simple reflection of the old adage "practice makes perfect."
- The association between trauma case volume and outcome is not entirely clear, and the direction of support for the volume-outcome hypothesis with respect to trauma care may be strongly influenced by study design.
- Although the optimal case volume threshold for Level 1 trauma center accreditation remains unknown, it is important to recognize that a minimum threshold is necessary to facilitate a hospital's ability to maintain the resources necessary for trauma care.

INTRODUCTION

The association between case volume and outcome has been a focus of research for nearly 4 decades. Although it is intuitive that better outcomes would be associated with more experience, both at the level of hospital and individual practitioner, the relationship between higher case volumes and better outcomes has been demonstrated to be strong for some specific disease states or surgical procedures while weak or nonexistent for others. Nonetheless, the volume-outcome relationship has been used to justify regionalization of care for specific procedures and disease states.

The authors have nothing to disclose.

*Corresponding author. 910 Madison Avenue, #218, Memphis, TN 38163. *E-mail address*: jaw@uthsc.edu

0065-3411/15/$ – see front matter
http://dx.doi.org/10.1016/j.yasu.2015.03.009

The volume-outcome connection, as it pertains to the care of the injured patient, has been of specific interest to those in the discipline of trauma care. Stressing the perceived importance of case volume, the American College of Surgeons Committee on Trauma (ACSCOT) requires that a Level 1 designated trauma center should care for an annual minimum of 1200 patients, or alternatively at least 240 patients per year having what is considered to be severe injury (Injury Severity Score >15) [1]. Whether a veritable positive association between trauma patient volume and good outcomes exists remains a matter of debate, as studies that both support and refute this association have been published in recent years.

IS CASE VOLUME RELATED TO OUTCOME IN HEALTH CARE?

Despite it being a surrogate marker at best, surgical volume has become, in recent years, a de facto quality indicator. While higher case volumes have been demonstrated to be associated with lower mortality for several specific procedures, case volume, in and of itself, has developed into a popular and prevalent measure of quality. The Leapfrog group, a large coalition of public and private health care purchasers, has recommended that high-risk cancer procedures be performed in high-volume centers [2]. The minimum volume standards for designation of centers of excellence for specific procedures, such as bariatric surgery, along with minimum case volume standards for Level 1 trauma center accreditation as described earlier, are further examples. In the absence of alternative reliable measures of quality, case volume remains an easily accessible metric. As cautioned by Halm and colleagues [3], however, the wisdom of using volume as a quality metric depends critically on the strength of the association between volume and outcome.

Over the past 4 decades, a growing body of research has demonstrated that surgical outcomes are better when performed at centers with a relatively larger case volume. In 1979, Luft and colleagues [4] analyzed mortality rates for 12 surgical procedures in 1498 hospitals to determine the relationship between a hospital's surgical volume and its surgical mortality. The mortality of open heart surgery, vascular surgery, transurethral resection of the prostate, and coronary bypass decreased with increasing numbers of operations. For other procedures, the mortality curve flattened at lower volumes. Some procedures, such as cholecystectomy, showed no relation between volume and mortality.

These observations have proved to be durable over time. In 2002, Birkmeyer and colleagues [5] examined the mortality associated with cardiovascular procedures and major cancer resections, using the national Medicare claims database and the Nationwide Inpatient Sample as their study base. The investigators observed that mortality decreased as volume increased for all 14 procedures studied, but the relative importance of volume varied markedly according to the type of procedure. With respect to the 8 types of cancer resections studied, the effect of volume was most pronounced for esophagectomy and pancreatic resection, and was relatively small for colectomy and nephrectomy (Fig. 1).

The so-called volume-outcome hypothesis has led to enthusiasm for policies that restrict certain procedures to high-volume hospitals, a strategy often described as regionalization [6]. Although regionalization on the surface seems to be good policy, backed up by clinical research demonstrating an association between case volume and outcome, it is important to acknowledge both the specific limitations of this body of research and the general complexity of the volume-outcome relationship.

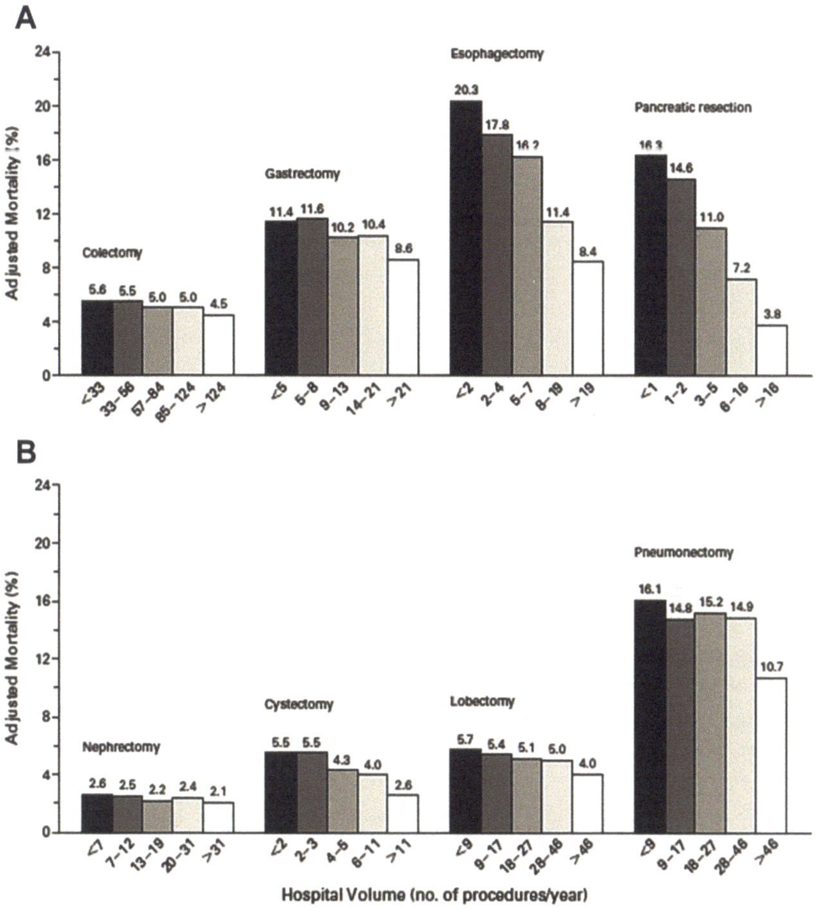

Fig. 1. Adjusted in-hospital or 30-day mortality among Medicare patients (1994–1999), according to quintile of total hospital volume for resections of gastrointestinal cancer (*A*) and resections of other cancers (*B*). (*Adapted from* Birkmeyer JD, Siewers AE, Finlayson EV, et al. Hospital volume and surgical mortality in the United States. N Engl J Med 2002;346:1136; with permission.)

Halm and colleagues [3] performed a systematic review of the volume-outcome relationship, and although they concluded that high volume was associated with better outcomes across a range of procedures and conditions, the magnitude of the association varied greatly, and much of the data used in the studies under review had significant shortcomings, particularly related to adjustment for case mix and processes of care. Of note, they observed that hospital volume-outcome studies that performed risk adjustment with clinical data were less likely to report significant associations than were analyses that were risk adjusted using data derived from administrative sources.

It is also clear that the relationship between case volume and outcome goes beyond relative experience, and the relationship between volume and outcome is unlikely a simple reflection of the old adage "practice makes perfect." Although relative experience with specific medical problems or surgical procedures certainly must contribute on some level to improved outcomes, the relationship between volume and outcome is confounded by case mix, selective referral (whereby patients seek out centers perceived to have good outcomes, thereby increasing those centers' case volumes), and resource allocation. As noted by Halm and colleagues [3], few studies have tracked changes in individual institutional volume over time, and those that did observed that fluctuating numbers of cases within the same institution had a minimal effect on outcome. This finding suggests the possibility that volume-outcome relationships may in part reflect static differences in overall quality between high-volume and low-volume providers, rather than relative experience.

Given the prevalent models and systems of health care delivery in the developed world, it would be uncommon to find a hospital that has a high case volume for only 1 or 2 specific procedures. Instead, the opposite is true: most hospitals with a high case volume for a particular procedure will likely be high-volume centers in general. With this concept in mind, Urbach and Baxter [7] sought to study whether the improved outcome observed in high-volume hospitals was unique to the volume of the procedure for which the outcome was being assessed. In addition to evaluating the relationship between the volume and outcome of specific surgical procedures, they also evaluated the outcomes of specific procedures as related to the volume of other procedures performed at the same hospital. It was observed that the volume-outcome relationship persisted across procedures; for example, outcomes for pancreaticoduodenectomy were better at hospitals with relatively higher case volumes of colorectal resections. The investigators' findings highlight that the outcome disparity by volume may be better explained by a resource differential between large institutions and smaller hospitals, rather than a "practice makes perfect" effect.

The recognition that volume is linked to outcomes has not occurred in a vacuum, but rather in an environment where focus on quality and safety in medicine has been a prominent focus of both research and policy. The study of volume and outcome has uncovered previously unrecognized variations in hospital performance, and a subsequent effort to improve quality, including implementation of checklists and best practice algorithms, has followed suit. Noting that surgical mortality rates have significantly declined over the past decade, Reames and colleagues [8] sought to reevaluate the volume-outcome relationship in light of the focus on safety and improved outcomes of recent years. Using Medicare claims data from 2000 through 2009, the investigators evaluated outcome among more than 3 million patients who underwent 1 of 8 operations. Throughout the 10-year period, a significant inverse relationship between each procedure and mortality was observed, depending on the institutional volume of each procedure. Although the quality of the procedures in place at the institutions studied was not specifically addressed, it is apparent from these results that the volume-outcome relationship has persisted despite the recent institutional focus on quality. The investigators concluded that the issue is not whether a volume-outcome relationship exists but how to use this information to benefit patients, balancing the potential benefits of regionalization against limits to access that could be most pronounced in disadvantaged populations.

IS CASE VOLUME RELATED TO OUTCOME IN TRAUMA CARE?

While acknowledging that the same mechanisms pertaining to the volume-outcome relationship, including relative experience, should apply to the treatment of the injured, it is important to recognize that trauma care has its own inherent characteristics that differentiate it from the performance of elective procedures. These differences may explain why some studies have demonstrated strong relationships between trauma case volume and outcomes while others have not. As noted by Nathens and colleagues [9], care of the trauma patient poses challenges not encountered in other aspects of medicine. In trauma care, time to treatment is a critical parameter influencing both patient survival and functional outcome. The priority of time can affect outcome in opposing manners with respect to volume. On the one hand, it would be expected that institutions that see a relatively large trauma case volume will be adept at delivering trauma care in a prompt, streamlined manner. On the other hand, time may be of the essence in the prehospital setting, and transport over a long distance to a higher-volume center may negate the benefit of earlier treatment initiated at a closer, though smaller center. If critically injured patients truly have a greater chance of survival at a high-volume rather than a low-volume center, the benefit to the patient must outweigh the risk of lengthy transport time, particularly in rural areas where transport times are expected to be relatively long. The impact of time to treatment within the context of the volume-outcome connection has yet to be discerned, given the complexity of the interaction and the inherent limitations of available data sets.

In addition, both the mix and relative severity of injuries sustained by the polytrauma patient further challenge the analysis of outcome with respect to volume or, for that matter, any other variable of interest. Adjustment by Injury Severity Score (ISS) has typically been performed to account for differences in injury severity between patients. It is problematic, however, that patients may have significantly different injuries with disparate prognoses, and yet have similar ISS when all injuries are aggregated. This particular issue makes the nature of the volume-outcome relationship in trauma care not as clear as in other areas of medicine where patient cohorts would be expected to be relatively more or less heterogeneous, and may contribute in part to the contradictory findings reported in the literature to date concerning the volume-outcome relationship.

One of the first studies to address the volume-outcome relationship in trauma concerned the network of Level 1 trauma centers in the city of Chicago in 1987 and 1988 [10]. The investigators evaluated mortality in 1600 seriously injured patients treated at 1 of 7 Level 1 centers, with patient volume ranging from 64 to 459 patients over the 2-year period. The adjusted odds of death were 1.3 times greater at low-volume centers (<140 patients over 2 years) than at high-volume centers (>200 patients over 2 years). However, risk adjustment was limited to stratification to 1 of 2 groups: those with immediately life-threatening injuries and those with a Trauma Score of 12 or less.

Over the same time period (1988-1989), Konvolinka and colleagues [11] analyzed mortality across trauma centers in the state of Pennsylvania. Trauma center volume was defined as the number of patients per institution or surgeon with ISS greater than 13 or a severe head injury. Trauma cases were assumed to be evenly distributed among the individual surgeons within each institution. The investigators found that the annual number of seriously injured patients per surgeon was in fact associated with mortality. The volume threshold determined to meet average rates of mortality was 35 patients per surgeon per annum.

Nathens and colleagues [9], using a retrospective cohort design, evaluated the association between volume and outcome among 31 academic trauma centers in the United States from November 1997 to the end of 1998. Two cohorts were defined by injury characteristics: patients with isolated penetrating abdominal injury and patients with blunt multisystem trauma (minimum of lower extremity long bone fracture and head injury). The investigators observed that mortality rates were inversely associated with hospital volume once case volume exceeded 650 per year (ie, patients with ISS >15). This mortality benefit was evident in both cohorts, but restricted to patients at the highest risk of death. In the penetrating cohort the benefit was limited to those presenting with shock, and in the blunt multisystem cohort the benefit was limited to those with severe head injury (Glasgow Coma Scale <9).

More recent publications have also demonstrated associations between case volume and outcomes. Tepas and colleagues [12] identified trauma patients with severe traumatic brain injury managed at 1 of 7 state-designated Level 1 trauma centers in Florida over an 11-year period. The relatively higher traumatic brain injury case volumes (>40 cases per quarter) were associated with improved survival, namely a 9% lower mortality risk after adjustment for severity of injury, demographics, and insurance status. The investigators also observed that lower-volume hospitals were more likely to discharge brain-injured patients to skilled nursing facilities, rather than to home or rehabilitation facilities.

Noting that much of the trauma volume-outcome literature has been based on administrative data sets or registries wherein accuracy and validity of data have been questioned, Minei and colleagues [13] explored the volume-outcome association within the context of prospectively collected data from multicenter clinical trials. The Resuscitation Outcomes Consortium (ROC) recently performed 2 randomized controlled trials to study prehospital hypertonic saline resuscitation: one trial for patients with presumed hypovolemic shock and the other for patients with severe traumatic brain injury. Minei and colleagues [13] performed a secondary analysis of the patients enrolled in these trials to determine whether an association between volume and survival was present. Their observations demonstrated that as trauma center volume increased, the odds of 24-hour and 28-day mortality decreased. Specifically, there were reduced odds of both all-patient 24-hour and 28-day mortality of 5% and 6%, respectively, for every increase of 500 trauma patients to a trauma center. With stratification by the groups from the initial randomized trials (shock and severe brain injury), the association held for the brain-injured cohort, but lost statistical significance for the shock cohort (Table 1).

Evidence from other studies has refuted the volume-outcome argument for trauma patients. Cooper and colleagues [14] were unable to find any relationship between trauma center volume and mortality rates in an analysis concerning centers in the New York State trauma system. Regardless of the stratification parameters used in their analyses (patients with ISS >9, patients with ISS >15, or volume criteria recommendations of the ACSCOT), risk-adjusted mortality rates were not significantly associated with institutional case volume. Some limitations of this study include the exclusion of deaths in the emergency room, and the exclusion of patients transferred from one institution to another.

Table 1
28-day and 24-hour mortality for all patients, shock cohort, and brain injury cohort

Volume (per 500 patient increase)	28-d mortality		24-h mortality	
	OR (95% CI)	*P*	OR (95% CI)	*P*
All patients	0.93 (0.89–0.97)	.002	0.93 (0.88–0.99)	.027
TBI cohort	0.93 (0.89–0.98)	.003	0.94 (0.88–1.01)	.068
Shock cohort	0.94 (0.88–1.01)	.100	0.94 (0.88–1.02)	.132

Abbreviations: CI, confidence interval; OR, odds ratio; TBI, traumatic brain injury.

Adapted from Minei JP, Fabian TC, Guffey DM, et al. Increased trauma center volume is associated with improved survival after severe injury: results of a Resuscitation Outcomes Consortium study. Ann Surg 2014;260:460.

Glance and colleagues [15], noting the methodological limitations of prior studies of the volume-outcome relationship in trauma, evaluated the volume-outcome relationship with data from the National Trauma Databank (NTDB) for the year 1999. Patients were stratified by mechanism of injury. The investigators did not observe an association between trauma center volume and mortality for either the blunt or penetrating cohort after adjusting for injury severity. The statistical modeling used included corrections or adjustments for analytical concerns not well addressed in prior work, including accounting for the fact that patients from the same trauma center are not independent observations, avoidance of arbitrary cutoffs for groups according to hospital volume, and assessment of model performance. Despite these refinements, the investigators noted that their findings could be applied to the volume-outcome question for centers where case volume exceeded 600 patients (with ISS >15) per year because such centers fell outside of the volume range used to develop their final statistical models. It is possible that centers with the highest volumes for trauma might influence a volume-outcome effect that is not captured in their analysis.

Demetriades and colleagues [16], cognizant of the significant heterogeneity with respect to injuries among trauma patient cohorts, analyzed the volume-outcome effect with respect to a subset of specific injuries that included major vascular injury, cardiac injury, high-grade liver injury, quadriplegia, and complex pelvic fractures. Patients with at least 1 of these injuries along with ISS greater than 15 were compared among Level 1 and Level 2 trauma centers from the NTDB from 1996 through 2003. In this large study of more than 12,000 patients, significantly lower adjusted mortality and disability at hospital discharge was associated with Level 1 centers when compared with Level 2 centers. The volume of trauma admissions, stratified by ACSCOT criteria (240 cases per year) had no effect on outcome in either Level 1 or Level 2 centers.

OUTCOME FOLLOWING SEVERE TRAUMA: DOES CASE VOLUME MATTER?

From the summaries of studies presented here (along with additional studies not discussed [17–20]), it is clear that the relationship between case volume and outcome is not clear cut, and the direction of support for the volume-outcome hypothesis may be strongly influenced by study design. The underlying mechanism for the hypothesis also remains unclear. Is a positive correlation between volume and good outcome a result of relative hospital or individual provider experience, or is it in fact a result of selective referral, whereby patients are attracted to hospitals with better outcomes, and the larger volume is a result of patient migration to these institutions? As noted by Nathens and colleagues [9], this argument may not hold for trauma care, as patients largely have no choice in the matter as to where they are taken for trauma care [21]. Nonetheless, the prehospital care providers do have some control over where they deliver their patients (particularly in trauma systems that are underdeveloped or not centralized), and may be likely to deliver such patients to hospitals they perceive to be superior for trauma care.

Despite the shortcomings and discordant findings in the trauma studies published to date, along with the complex layers of the volume-outcome relationship as described, it is important to appreciate that case volume is requisite to the ongoing existence of a trauma center. It is the economic reality that the resources required to provide modern trauma care (emergency access to imaging, large volumes of blood products, multidisciplinary care, and so forth) cannot be sustained over time in the absence of reasonable utilization. The need for a certain minimum patient volume to maintain adequate experience and expertise for the delivery of effective trauma care has long been recognized by ACSCOT. As described earlier, ACSCOT certification for Level 1 trauma centers includes admission volume requirements of 1200 patients per annum (or 240 patients with ISS >15) [1]. These volume requirements arose from consensus and have not been established from clinical research (as evident from the conflicting body of published studies). So although there is ongoing argument about what the optimum cutoff for volume should be for Level 1 accreditation, it is important to recognize that a minimum threshold is necessary to facilitate a hospital's ability to maintain the resources necessary for trauma care.

It is often the case that clinical research leads to more questions than answers. Given the concept of a minimum case volume threshold to achieve reasonable outcomes, for example, it follows that there may be a point at which volume overwhelms the resources of a trauma center. Bennett and colleagues [22] performed a retrospective analysis of patients with ISS greater than 15 treated at United States Level 1 trauma centers from 2001 through 2006, using the NTDB as their study base. Their findings demonstrated a parabolic relationship between case volume and mortality, whereby mortality decreased as case volume increased, up to an inflection point at approximately 500 patients per annum (with ISS >15), whereby mortality began to increase as volume increased further (Fig. 2). Of note, this relationship applied only to Level 1 centers that had not been ACSCOT verified. Level 1 trauma centers with ACSCOT verification demonstrated a linear relationship between case volume and mortality, whereby mortality consistently decreased with increased case volume. Another question requiring further exploration is whether the outcome of specific subgroups in the trauma patient population may be differentially affected by case volume. Pandya and colleagues [23] and Matsushima and colleagues [24] independently evaluated the outcomes of geriatric trauma patients as related to the volume of patients treated in Pennsylvania and New York State, respectively. The findings of these studies were remarkably similar: survival for geriatric patients was positively associated with geriatric trauma case volume but, interestingly, survival for geriatric patients was paradoxically negatively associated with nongeriatric case volume. Studies such as these add further layers of complexity to the volume-outcome question pertaining to the care of the injured, and warrant further exploration.

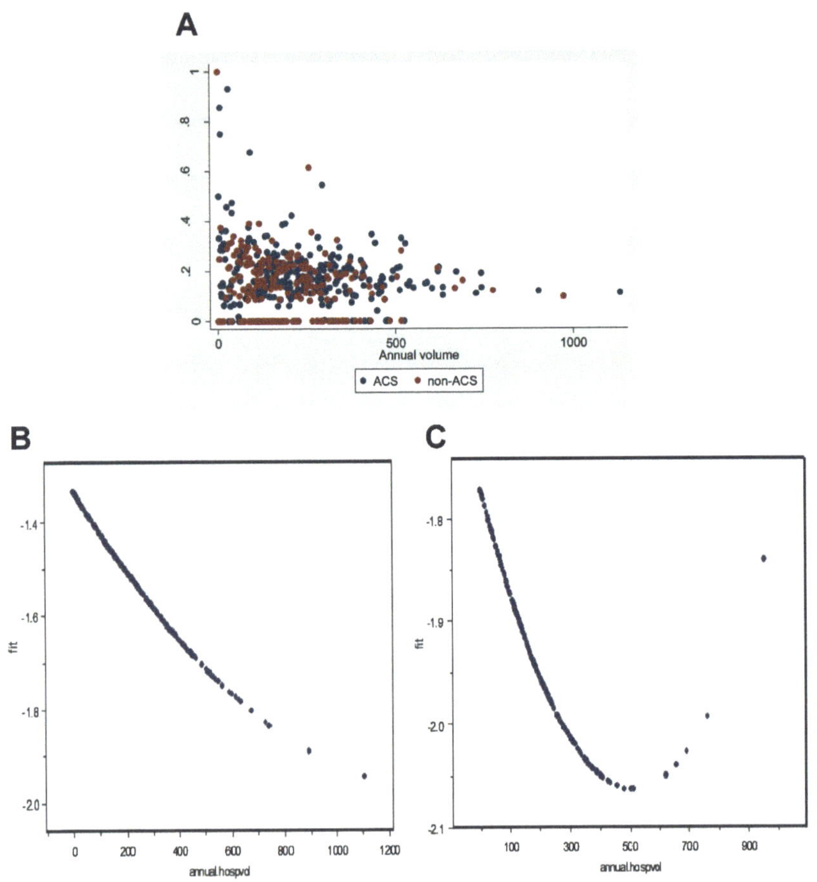

Fig. 2. (*A*) Relationship between center volume (x-axis) and unadjusted mortality (y-axis) for Level I trauma centers. (*B*) Relationship between center volume (x-axis) and fitted mortality (y-axis) for Level I trauma centers with ACSCOT verification. (*C*) Relationship between center volume (x-axis) and fitted mortality (y-axis) for Level I trauma centers without ACSCOT verification. (*Adapted from* Bennett KM, Vaslef S, Pappas TN, et al. The volume-outcomes relationship for United States Level I trauma centers. J Surg Res 2011;167:22, with permission.)

References

[1] American College of Surgeons. Resources for optimal care of the injured patient. Chicago: American College of Surgeons; 2006.
[2] Birkmeyer JD, Finlayson EV, Birkmeyer CM. Volume standards for high-risk surgical procedures: potential benefits of the Leapfrog initiative. Surgery 2001;130:415–22.
[3] Halm EA, Lee C, Chassin MR. Is volume related to outcome in health care? A systematic review and methodologic critique of the literature. Ann Intern Med 2002;137:511–20.
[4] Luft HS, Bunker JP, Enthoven AC. Should operations be regionalized? The empirical relation between surgical volume and mortality. N Engl J Med 1979;301:1364–9.
[5] Birkmeyer JD, Siewers AE, Finlayson EV, et al. Hospital volume and surgical mortality in the United States. N Engl J Med 2002;346:1128–37.

[6] Epstein AM. Volume and outcome—it is time to move ahead. N Engl J Med 2002;346: 1161–3.
[7] Urbach DR, Baxter NN. Does it matter what a hospital is "high volume" for? Specificity of hospital volume-outcome associations for surgical procedures: analysis of administrative data. BMJ 2004;328:737–40.
[8] Reames BN, Ghaferi AA, Birkmeyer JD, et al. Hospital volume and operative mortality in the modern era. Ann Surg 2014;260:244–51.
[9] Nathens AB, Jurkovich GJ, Maier RV, et al. Relationship between trauma center volume and outcomes. JAMA 2001;285:1164–71.
[10] Smith RF, Frateschi L, Sloan EP, et al. The impact of volume on outcome in seriously injured trauma patients: two years' experience of the Chicago trauma system. J Trauma 1990;30: 1066–76.
[11] Konvolinka CW, Copes WS, Sacco WJ. Institution and per-surgeon volume versus survival outcome in Pennsylvania's trauma centers. Am J Surg 1995;170:333–40.
[12] Tepas JJ III, Pracht EE, Orban BL, et al. High-volume trauma centers have better outcomes treating traumatic brain injury. J Trauma Acute Care Surg 2013;74:143–8.
[13] Minei JP, Fabian TC, Guffey DM, et al. Increased trauma center volume is associated with improved survival after severe injury: results of a Resuscitation Outcomes Consortium study. Ann Surg 2014;260:456–64.
[14] Cooper A, Hannan EL, Bessey PQ, et al. An examination of the volume-mortality relationship for New York State trauma centers. J Trauma 2000;48:16–23.
[15] Glance LG, Osler TM, Dick A, et al. The relation between trauma center outcome and volume in the National Trauma Databank. J Trauma 2004;56:682–90.
[16] Demetriades D, Martin M, Salim A, et al. The effect of trauma center designation and trauma volume on outcome in specific severe injuries. Ann Surg 2005;242:512–9.
[17] Margulies DR, Cryer HG, McArthur DL, et al. Patient volume per surgeon does not predict survival in adult level 1 trauma centers. J Trauma 2001;50:597–603.
[18] Marx WH, Simon R, O'Neill P, et al. The relationship between annual hospital volume of trauma patients an in-hospital mortality in New York State. J Trauma 2011;71:339–46.
[19] Sava J, Kennedy S, Jordan M, et al. Does volume matter? The effect of trauma surgeons' caseload on mortality. J Trauma 2003;54:829–34.
[20] London JA, Battistella FD. Is there a relationship between trauma center volume and mortality? J Trauma 2003;54:16–24.
[21] Nathens AB, Maier RV. The relationship between trauma center volume and outcome. Adv Surg 2001;35:61–75.
[22] Bennett KM, Vaslef S, Pappas TN, et al. The volume-outcomes relationship for United States Level I trauma centers. J Surg Res 2011;167:19–23.
[23] Pandya SR, Yelon JA, Sullivan TS, et al. Geriatric motor vehicle collision survival: the role of institutional trauma volume. J Trauma 2011;70:1326–30.
[24] Matsushima K, Schaefer EW, Won EJ, et al. Positive and negative volume-outcome relationships in the geriatric trauma population. JAMA Surg 2014;149:319–26.

Advances in Surgery 49 (2015) 247–262

ADVANCES IN SURGERY

ELSEVIER
MOSBY

Hyperparathyroidism

What Preoperative Imaging Is Necessary?

Rachel R. Kelz, MD, MSCE, FACS*, Douglas L. Fraker, MD, FACS

Division of Endocrine & Oncologic Surgery, Hospital of the University of Pennsylvania, 3400 Spruce Street, 4 Silverstein, Philadelphia, PA 19104, USA

Keywords

• Hyperparathyroidism • Preoperative imaging • Parathyroidectomy • Ultrasonography

Key points

- Imaging should be used to guide surgical decision making; it should not be used to make or confirm the diagnosis of hyperparathyroidism.
- Positive imaging does not exclude the possibility of multigland disease, and, to date, small glands (<300 mg), ectopic glands, and multigland disease remain challenging to detect by all imaging modalities.
- It is important that surgeons consider the use of additional intraoperative tools when operating on a patient with primary hyperparathyroidism regardless of the findings of the preoperative evaluation.
- Primary hyperparathyroidism is a surgical disease for which there is no approved medical therapy; the morbidity of the operation with current strategies is minimal, and the benefits for the patient are tremendous.

The classic 4-gland exploration used to treat primary hyperparathyroidism has been challenged by the routine use of image-guided surgery. The successful use of preoperative localization studies to identify abnormal parathyroid gland(s) [1] has resulted in the frequent use of the minimally invasive approach to parathyroid surgery [2,3]. Surgeons and referring physicians encountering patients with hyperparathyroidism are now challenged to order radiographic studies to localize de novo disease.

Testing, in this case, preoperative imaging studies (Box 1), should be considered only when it would alter the clinical decision making of the treating

The authors have nothing to disclose.

*Corresponding author. *E-mail address*: rachel.kelz@uphs.upenn.edu

0065-3411/15/$ – see front matter
http://dx.doi.org/10.1016/j.yasu.2015.03.011

Box 1: Imaging studies for preoperative evaluation, de novo primary hyperparathyroidism

Noninvasive first-line studies

High-resolution neck ultrasonography

Technetium 99m sestamibi scan

Noninvasive second-line studies

MRI

Computed tomography (CT) scan

Single-photon emission computed tomography/CT scan

Four-dimensional CT scan[a]

Invasive second-line study

Ultrasound-guided jugular venous sampling

[a] Inappropriate for young patients or those with a history of well differentiated thyroid cancer or kidney dysfunction.

physician. More invasive testing may be appropriate for recurrent or reoperative disease than for de novo disease (Box 2). In the case of a patient presenting with a new diagnosis of hyperparathyroidism (de novo), imaging studies should be ordered by or in consultation with the treating surgeon. The results of the preoperative testing should be used to determine the surgical approach, not to decide on the appropriateness of surgical exploration. The decision to refer to a surgeon and to undergo the surgery should be based on the clinical scenario using evidence-based guidelines and clinical expertise [4].

Box 2: Imaging studies for preoperative evaluation, recurrent or persistent primary hyperparathyroidism

Noninvasive

High-resolution neck ultrasonography

Technetium 99m sestamibi scan

MRI

Computed tomography (CT) scan

Single-photon emission computed tomography/CT scan

Four-dimensional CT scan*

Invasive

Selective venous sampling

Angiogram

Ultrasound-guided fine-needle aspiration

* Inappropriate for young patients or those with a history of well differentiated thyroid cancer or kidney dysfunction.

The decision to perform a classic 4-gland exploration as opposed to a minimally invasive parathyroidectomy (MIP) varies across surgeons and can be influenced by the patient's preferences. Parathyroid exploration by an experienced surgeon results in cure rates exceeding 95%, regardless of the surgical approach. Complication rates and long-term cure are believed to be comparable across the 2 groups [5–8]. Because of the excellent cure rates achieved in the setting of negative imaging findings, some experts still criticize the use of extensive preoperative localization studies in patients presenting for an initial operation on the parathyroid glands [9,10]. Moreover, the use of additional intraoperative tools, like intraoperative parathyroid hormone monitoring, may further influence the success of the operation [11]. Preoperative imaging practices should reflect the surgical approach, because multiple localization studies are not necessary, or cost effective, if the surgeon prefers a routine 4-gland exploration.

ULTRASONOGRAPHY

All patients undergoing parathyroid exploration, regardless of the cause of the disease, should have a preoperative neck ultrasound scan. The presence of a goiter, history of neck irradiation, or history of familial thyroid cancer may influence the decision to perform a simultaneous thyroid operation. The neck ultrasound scan is performed for 2 reasons: (1) to identify the presence of concomitant thyroid disease (and perform fine-needle aspiration, if indicated) and (2) to localize the abnormal parathyroid gland(s) when an MIP is being considered. When a simultaneous thyroid operation is planned, neck ultrasonography can also help by examining the lateral neck for evidence of lymph node metastases in case an occult malignancy is identified.

Ultrasonography is the gold standard examination for evaluation of the thyroid gland. Guidelines exist to facilitate the appropriate use of image-guided biopsy when a nodule is identified. All suspicious nodules should be evaluated before neck exploration for hyperparathyroidism to minimize the need for reoperative surgery. Several studies have examined the use of preoperative thyroid imaging in patients referred for hyperparathyroidism, and the identification of occult thyroid disease has been estimated at 30% or more, with approximately 10% representing thyroid malignancy [12–14].

Ultrasonographic findings are influenced by the experience of the operating technician and interpreting physician. However, in experienced hands, the sensitivity is similar for radiologists and surgeons [15]. Moreover, the performance of ultrasonography as a test varies by the indication for the study. Most centers are comfortable with the examination of the thyroid using ultrasonography; however, not all extend the same level of expertise to the identification of parathyroid glands.

Some radiologists are less familiar with the use of ultrasonography for the localization of abnormal parathyroid glands. The sensitivity of ultrasonography for the detection of abnormal parathyroid glands varies from 70% to 100% in most modern cohorts [16]. These estimates are often based on the ability to lateralize an abnormal gland, not the ability to localize the gland to the correct side and position (Table 1).

Table 1
Ultrasonography test characteristics for localization of abnormal parathyroid gland(s)

Author, year	Notes	Number of patients	Sensitivity, % (95% confidence interval)	Specificity, % (95% confidence interval)	Positive predictive value, %	Negative predictive value, %	Accuracy, % (95% confidence interval)	Additional findings
Attie et al [17], 1988	—	40	73	98	90	93	91	—
Whelan et al [18], 1989	—	16	50	75			59	—
Kohri et al [19], 1992	—	28	35	95	71	79	78	—
Kohri et al [19], 1992	—	12	77	91	77	91	87	—
Kohri et al [19], 1992	Secondary hyperparathyroid patients	22	67	100	100	10	68	—
Kohri et al [19], 1992	All patients	68	58	94	92	64	74	—
Gilat et al [20], 2005	—	77	89	33	98	—	—	Not limited by nodular thyroid disease
Rodgers et al [21], 2006	Laterality	75	57 (47–67)	94 (88–99)	—	—	—	—
Rodgers et al [21], 2006	Location[a]	75	29 (20–38)	86 (82–90)	—	—	—	—
Starker et al [22], 2011	Laterality	87	71	—	87	—	—	—
Starker et al [22], 2011	Location[a]	87	48	—	82	—	—	—
Agha et al [23], 2012	—	30	74	—	—	—	—	Cost $56 Time 10 (8–15)[b]
Agha et al [23], 2012	Contrast enhanced	30	100	—	—	—	—	Cost $112 Time 15 (13–20)[b]
Kwon et al [13], 2013	—	105	93 (88–98)	—	97 (94–100)	—	91 (85–96)	—

[a]Location is defined as laterality and position.
[b]Values for median (range) in minutes.

Normal parathyroid glands are seldom visualized on ultrasonographic examination, because of the small size and relatively hypoechoic characteristic (Fig. 1). The most common reasons for false-positive examination results include enlarged lymph nodes and exophytic thyroid nodules [13]. Parathyroid glands are difficult to see on preoperative ultrasonography when they are located behind the thyroid gland or in ectopic locations. Furthermore, substernal visualization is not possible, so true thymic parathyroid adenomas are never shown on ultrasonography. Because ultrasonography cannot image behind the airfield trachea, superior parathyroid adenomas located in the tracheoesophageal groove are frequently missed by ultrasonography as well. This location is particularly challenging for patients with a large body habitus. When concomitant thyroid disease exists, the sensitivity of ultrasonography has been reported to decrease to 47% to 84% [2,20]. For patients with persistent or recurrent hyperparathyroidism, the sensitivity is reported between 36% and 63% [24,25]. Overall, high-resolution ultrasonography, a cost-effective and noninvasive test, is helpful for operative planning.

SESTAMIBI SCAN

The most common nuclear test used for the preoperative localization of abnormal glands(s) is the sestamibi scan. The use of nuclear scanning was popularized for the detection of abnormal parathyroid glands in the 1980s. The most common nuclear study used to identify the parathyroid gland(s) is the technetium 99m (Tc 99m) sestamibi scan [26]. The study uses Tc 99m–labeled methoxyisobutyl isonitrile (sestamibi). The mitochondria in the parathyroid cells sequester the tracer. In hyperfunctioning parathyroid glands, the washout of the tracer is delayed, resulting in the ability to identify the parathyroid gland(s) as distinct from the thyroid gland.

The 2 most common techniques to differentiate between the thyroid and parathyroid gland(s) are the dual-phase or double-phase, single-contrast method (washout) and the dual-tracer or double-tracer, single-phase method

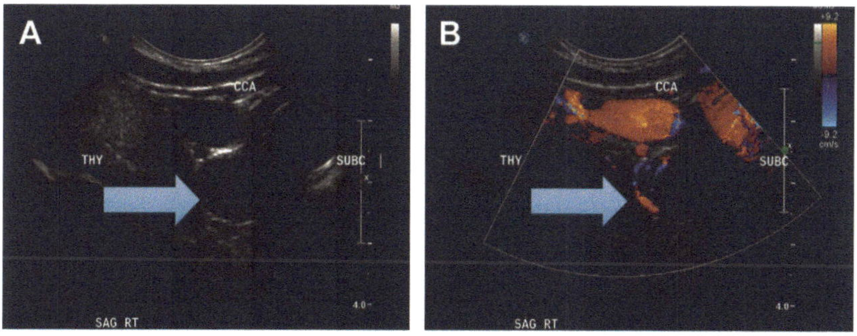

Fig. 1. Ultrasonographic images of right inferior parathyroid adenoma. (*A*) Without color flow; (*B*) with color flow. The blue arrow indicates the parathyroid adenoma. CCA, common carotid artery; SUBC, subclavian artery; THY, thyroid.

(subtraction). The washout method relies on the strong uptake and longer retention of the tracer by the parathyroid gland when compared with the thyroid. Initial images are acquired, and then, delayed images are taken to capitalize on the kinetics of sestamibi sequestration. The presence of concomitant thyroid disease is a major limitation to the washout method. This imaging method does not allow the visualization of the thyroid alone. The dual-phase method achieves better results when combined with an anatomic scan such as concurrent ultrasonography or single-photon emission computed tomography (SPECT) (Tables 2 and 3).

The subtraction method uses 2 agents: one to highlight the thyroid and the other the parathyroid glands. To highlight the thyroid gland by promoting uptake of a tagged isotope specific for the thyroid gland, thyroid hormone replacement is typically stopped 2 to 3 weeks in advance, adding to the morbidity of the procedure. Using digital subtraction, the parathyroid glands are more easily illuminated. Historically, the patient had to lie still to make sure that the images were well superimposed, thus making this method less comfortable for the patient. Now, the agents can be given simultaneously, so the inconvenience of immobility has been curtailed.

The sestamibi scan has a reported sensitivity of 30% to 92%. Sestamibi is less accurate in multigland disease, when concomitant thyroid disease exists, and for glands that are located superiorly. Metabolic conditions can also affect the test performance. The sensitivity can be affected by vitamin D deficiency and thyroid suppression.

Most patients with primary hyperparathyroidism undergo sestamibi imaging before surgery. The added usefulness of sestamibi scanning after ultrasonographic examination is not clear. The location in which ultrasonographic examination is most limited includes inferior parathyroid adenomas in the thymus and superior parathyroid adenomas in the tracheoesophageal groove behind the trachea. In these 2 areas, sestamibi scanning is particularly helpful, with high sensitivity, because they are some distance from the thyroid gland and not obscured by thyroid disease. One study suggested that sestamibi after ultrasonography added additional information in only 8% of patients [29]. These results may not be generalizable. Moreover, the additional information gained may dramatically influence the surgical approach when an ectopic gland is identified. It is unclear how many hyperparathyroid patients undergo sestamibi imaging overall, because many are not referred for surgery if an abnormal gland cannot be localized. This strategy may be a mistake because most cases can be cured by surgical exploration, regardless of the imaging findings.

The role of sestamibi scanning in patients with secondary and tertiary hyperparathyroidism is less clear. Some advocate for sestamibi scanning to identify supernumerary glands and ectopic glands preoperatively. The dual-tracer method has a reported sensitivity of 30% to 90% in this population [19,30]. A recent meta-analysis found the pooled sensitivity to be 58% (95% confidence interval [CI], 52%–65%)and the pooled specificity to be 93% (95% CI, 85%–100%) [30]. Because of the known limitations, especially in detecting small

Table 2
Scintigraphy test characteristics for localization of abnormal parathyroid gland(s)

Author, year	Technique	Number of patients	Sensitivity, % (95% confidence interval)	Specificity, % (95% confidence interval)	Positive predictive value, %	Negative predictive value, %	Accuracy, % (95% confidence interval)	Additional outcomes
Attie et al [17], 1988	Subtraction	62	59	98	94	88	88	—
Kohri et al [19], 1992	Subtraction	24	40	92	67	80	77	—
Kohri et al [19], 1992	Subtraction	12	53	94	80	81	80	—
Kohri et al [19], 1992	Subtraction	20[a]	34	100	100	6	36	—
Kohri et al [19], 1992	Subtraction	62[b]	37	93	88	52	61	—
Agha et al [23], 2012	Washout	30	81	—	—	—	—	Cost $448 Time 180 (150–200)[c]
Kwon et al [13], 2013	Washout	105	92 (87–97)	—	97 (94–100)	—	90 (84–95)	—

[a]Only patients with secondary hyperparathyroidism.
[b]All patients.
[c]Values are median (range) in minutes.

Table 3
Tc 99m–Sestamibi-SPECT test characteristics for localization of abnormal parathyroid gland(s)

Author, year	Condition	Number of patients	Information	Sensitivity, % (95% confidence interval)	Specificity, % (95% confidence interval)	Positive predictive value, %	Negative predictive value, %
Rodgers et al [21], 2006	—	75	Laterality	65 (55–75)	88 (80–96)	—	—
Rodgers et al [21], 2006	—	75	Location[a]	33 (24–42)	83 (79–87)	—	—
Witteveen et al [27], 2011	Primary	23	Laterality	67	100	100	75
Witteveen et al [27], 2011	Reoperative	19	Laterality	33	80	63	53
Starker et al [22], 2011	—	87	Laterality	62	—	84	—
Starker et al [22], 2011	—	87	Location[a]	40	—	79	—
Ciappuccini et al [28], 2012	—	54	Location[a]	92 (80–98)	83 (36–100)	—	—

[a]Location is defined as laterality and position.

glands and along with frequent thyroid disease in the renal cohort, the usefulness of sestamibi in this cohort requires additional study.

Sestamibi is often used after failed parathyroid exploration and in the case of recurrent disease. Before reoperation, imaging should be obtained, because the scar tissue increases the surgical risk. Because nuclear scanning alone does not provide detailed anatomic information, sestamibi scans are typically combined with cross-sectional imaging for patients with recurrent or persistent disease.

SINGLE-PHOTON EMISSION COMPUTED TOMOGRAPHY

SPECT images can be superimposed on sestamibi images to permit the use of 2 localizing agents in the detection of a parathyroid adenoma. Occasionally, multigland disease can be seen using SPECT (Fig. 2). The cross-sectional images enhance understanding of the anatomic location of the adenoma when compared with the scintigraphic images from the sestamibi scan. Using this technique, the reported sensitivity of the study is generally increased compared with scintigraphy alone, and in 1 report, the sensitivity increased from 54% for sestamibi alone to 79% when combined with SPECT [2]. The test does not perform so well in the reoperative setting when compared with the de novo assessment (see Table 3) [27].

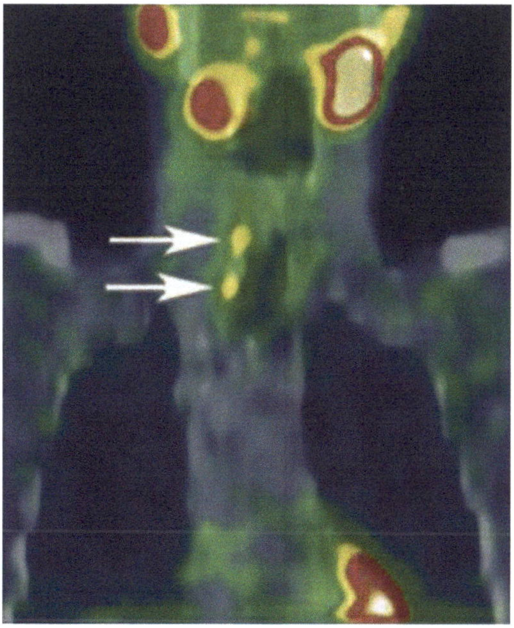

Fig. 2. Two abnormal parathyroid glands identified on SPECT in the right paratracheal region (*white arrows*).

MAGNETIC RESONANCE IMAGING

The sensitivity of MRI varies from 50% to 82% in published studies (Table 4) MRI is not widely used in the imaging algorithm for de novo primary hyperparathyroidism. MRI can be used to identify abnormal parathyroid glands in the setting of persistent or recurrent disease. As a cross-sectional imaging modality, MRI is often preferred to computed tomography (CT) in patients with normal renal function, because of the lack of ionizing radiation exposure. The hyperfunctioning parathyroid gland is generally hypointense on unenhanced T1-weighted images and hyperintense on contrast-enhanced T2-weighted images and T1-weighted images. MRI is expensive relative to some of the other studies and also depends on the radiologist's level of expertise in the identification of parathyroid gland(s). MRI scans do not typically distinguish cervical lymph nodes from similar sized parathyroid adenomas, both of which are located in the same area inferolateral to the thyroid gland. Ultrasonography, on the other hand, distinguishes lymph node anatomy better by looking at the architecture, such as a fatty hilum, as well as the echogenicity of the parathyroids. Sestamibi scans distinguish lymph nodes from parathyroid glands by physiologic uptake of the isotope.

COMPUTED TOMOGRAPHY

Traditional CT scans rely on the vascularity of the parathyroid glands for identification of abnormal glands. Therefore, the use of contrast material increases the yield of the study. The addition of contrast and exposure to ionizing radiation makes the risk of the procedure less desirable than the alternative imaging modalities for patients with de novo hyperparathyroidism. Thin-cut scans are a helpful adjunct positive venous sampling after a failed exploration or suspected ectopic gland. CT scans can also be helpful in visualizing ectopic glands in the chest (Fig. 3). However, in some centers, interpreting physicians have reported that streak artifact and adenopathy make ectopic substernal glands difficult to identify. As with ultrasonography, the results are dependent on the radiologist's experience.

FOUR-DIMENSIONAL COMPUTED TOMOGRAPHY SCAN

More recently four-dimensional (4D) CT scans have been used to identify the location of the parathyroid glands in patients with de novo hyperparathyroidism as well as in those patients presenting for recurrent or persistent disease. The sensitivity of the study ranges from 70% to 94% (Table 5). This study uses time as the fourth dimension in addition to the three-dimensional reconstructions. Over time, the rapid uptake and washout of the contrast material from the hyperfunctioning parathyroid gland(s) add additional information that is not readily available when using the more traditional protocols for CT of the neck. The 4D CT scan is more sensitive and specific in locating the correct quadrant for the abnormal gland than ultrasonography or sestamibi alone. However, its performance in multigland disease is inferior to that in single-gland disease. The study requires exposure to low-dose ionizing

Table 4
MRI test characteristics for localization of abnormal parathyroid gland(s)

Author, year	Specified patient population	Number of patients	Sensitivity, % (95% confidence interval)	Specificity, % (95% confidence interval)	Positive predictive value, %	Negative predictive value, %	Accuracy, %	Additional outcomes
Attie et al [17], 1988	—	60	82	97	90	94	93	—
Whelan et al [18], 1989	—	16	65	66	—	—	66	—
Kohri et al [19], 1992	Primary	12	73	90	79	88	85	—
Kohri et al [19], 1992	Secondary	23	54	50	96	5	54	—
Kohri et al [19], 1992	All	35	57	86	92	41	64	—
Agha et al [23], 2012	—	30	71					Cost $672 Time 60 (50–70)[a]

[a]Values are median (range) in minutes.

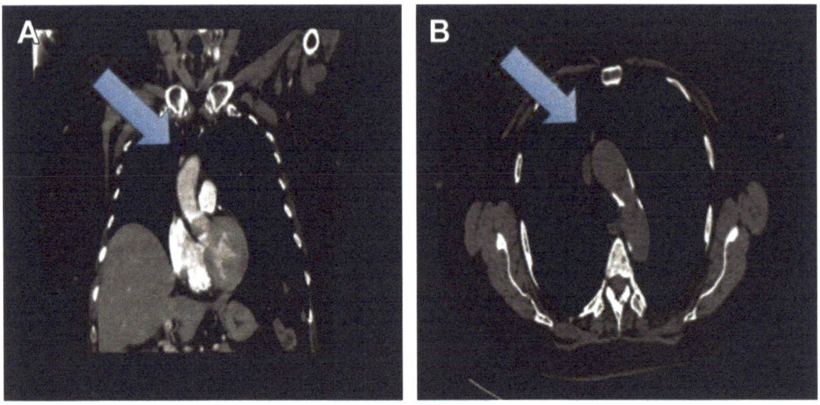

Fig. 3. Sestamibi scanning showed an ectopic gland in the chest. Follow-up CT scan showed the intrathymic adenoma seen here (*blue arrows*). (*A*) Coronal image and (*B*) axial image. The patient underwent a curative transcervical thymectomy.

radiation and iodinated contrast material, and therefore is not recommended for young patients or those with well-differentiated thyroid cancer or impaired kidney function [22]. This study is not yet widely available for use.

VENOUS SAMPLING

Venous sampling is invasive. For bilateral jugular venous sampling, blood is aspirated from bilateral jugular veins to measure parathyroid hormone levels. The gradient is used to determine the side of the suspected adenoma. Bilateral jugular venous sampling can be performed intraoperatively before incision in the case of nonlocalization by imaging or under direct visualization to lateralize the hyperfunctioning gland in the case of a missing adenoma. In 1 series, preoperative aspiration after failed imaging had a sensitivity of 52% and a positive predictive value of 65% [33]. More recently, bilateral jugular vein sampling as an ultrasound-guided office-based procedure has been reported to facilitate a minimally invasive approach after inconclusive ultrasonographic findings. In the case of inconclusive ultrasonographic results, the office-based procedure has been shown in a single study to have an accuracy of 81% [34].

Historically, selective venous sampling for parathyroid hormone levels was considered a helpful adjunct after failed neck exploration. In this invasive test, using catheters inserted through the deep venous system, successive venous samples are obtained from the neck and upper chest veins for parathyroid hormone levels. The samples direct the attention of the radiologist to an area of increased suspicion based on a spike in the parathyroid hormone (PTH) level. An angiogram can then be performed to identify the adenoma, because of its increased vascularity. Alternatively, thin-cut cross-sectional imaging can be performed across the area of suspicion to identify the affected parathyroid gland.

Table 5
Four-dimensional CT scan test characteristics for localization of abnormal parathyroid gland(s)

Author, year	Technique	Number of patients	Accuracy, %	Sensitivity, % (95% confidence interval)	Specificity, % (95% confidence interval)	Positive predictive value, %
Rodgers et al [21], 2006	Laterality	75	—	88 (81–95)	88(80–96)	—
Rodgers et al [21], 2006	Location[a]	75	—	70 (59–81)	89 (85–93)	—
Starker et al [22], 2011	Laterality	87	—	94	—	94
Starker et al [22], 2011	Location[a]	87	—	86	—	84
Hunter et al [31], 2012	Laterality	143	94	—	—	—
Hunter et al [31], 2012	Location[a]	134	87	—	—	—
Kelly et al [32], 2014	De novo	90	78	—	—	86
Kelly et al [32], 2014	Reoperative	36	84	—	—	73

[a]Location is defined as laterality and position.

Because of the invasive nature of the study, it is not used in the case of de novo hyperparathyroidism.

SUMMARY

Imaging should be used to guide surgical decision making. Imaging should not be used to make or confirm the diagnosis of hyperparathyroidism. Positive imaging does not exclude the possibility of multigland disease. Small glands (<300 mg), ectopic glands, and multigland disease remain challenging to detect by all imaging modalities. These are the same challenges that surgeons face during neck exploration. Therefore, it is important that surgeons consider the use of additional intraoperative tools when operating on a patient with primary hyperparathyroidism, regardless of the findings of the preoperative evaluation.

Parathyroid surgery can now be performed safely using a 4-gland approach or minimally invasive technique. The imaging obtained in the preoperative setting should be determined by the clinical condition and planned operative strategy. Local talent and resources play a role in the test ordering strategies, given the important role of the interpreting physician in the test performance. Ultrasonography should always be performed and reviewed before surgery for the treatment of hyperparathyroidism to exclude simultaneous thyroid disease necessitating concomitant thyroid surgery. Additional studies should be ordered judiciously to avoid unnecessary costs. The use of intraoperative aids in conjunction with preoperative testing results yields exceptional cure rates.

One important consideration regarding imaging for hyperparathyroidism is that negative results of imaging should never influence referral for potential surgical cure of this disease. Primary hyperparathyroidism is a surgical disease for which there is no approved medical therapy; the morbidity of the operation with current strategies is minimal, and the benefits for the patient are tremendous. A recent large series reported that the cure rate at 6 months in nonimaged patients was greater than 98% and not significantly different from patients who had positive imaging results [10]. Imaging studies can facilitate minimally invasive surgery, such as allowing the operation to be performed under conscious sedation, but should never determine who is referred for surgery, because the results are equivalent in experienced hands.

References

[1] Okerlund MD, Sheldon K, Corpuz S, et al. New method with high sensitivity and specificity for localization of abnormal parathyroid glands. Ann Surg 1984;200(3):381–8.
[2] Mohebati A, Shaha AR. Imaging techniques in parathyroid surgery primary hyperparathyroidism. Am J Otolaryngol 2012;33(4):457–68.
[3] Udelsman R, Åkerström G, Biagini C, et al. The surgical management of asymptomatic primary hyperparathyroidism: proceedings of the Fourth International Workshop. J Clin Endocrinol Metab 2014;99:3595–606.
[4] Bilezikian JP, Brandi ML, Eastell R, et al. Guidelines for the management of asymptomatic primary hyperparathyroidism: summary statement from the Fourth International Workshop. J Clin Endocrinol Metab 2014;99:3561–9.

[5] Fraker DL, Harsono H, Lewis R. Minimally invasive parathyroidectomy: benefits and requirements of localization, diagnosis, and intraoperative PTH monitoring. Long-term results. World J Surg 2009;33:2256–65.
[6] Udelsman R, Lin Z, Donovan P. The superiority of minimally invasive parathyroidectomy based on 1650 consecutive patients with primary hyperparathyroidism. Ann Surg 2011;253(3):585–91.
[7] Hodin R, Angelos P, Carty S, et al. No need to abandon unilateral parathyroid surgery. J Am Coll Surg 2012;215(2):297.
[8] Norman J, Lopez J, Politz D. Abandoning unilateral parathyroidectomy: why we reversed our position after 15,000 parathyroid operations. J Am Coll Surg 2012;214:260–9.
[9] Doppman JL, Miller DL. Localization of parathyroid tumors in patients with asymptomatic hyperparathyroidism and no previous surgery. J Bone Miner Res 1991;6(suppl2):S153–8.
[10] Wachtel H, Bartlett EK, Kelz RR, et al. Primary hyperparathyroidism with negative imaging: a significant clinical problem. Ann Surg 2014;260:474–82.
[11] Wharry LI, Yip L, Armstrong MJ, et al. The final intraoperative parathyroid hormone level: how low should it go? World J Surg 2014;38(3):558–63.
[12] Ryan S, Courtney D, Timon C. Co-existent thyroid disease in patients treated for primary hyperparathyroidism: implications for clinical management. Eur Arch Otorhinolaryngol 2015;272(2):419–23.
[13] Kwon JH, Kim E, Lee HS, et al. Neck ultrasonography as preoperative localization of primary hyperparathyroidism with an additional role of detecting thyroid malignancy. Eur J Radiol 2013;82:e17–21.
[14] Sloan DA, Davenport DL, Eldridge RJ, et al. Surgeon-driven thyroid interrogation of patients presenting with primary hyperparathyroidism. J Am Coll Surg 2014;218(4):674–83.
[15] Van Husen R, Kim LT. Accuracy of surgeon-performed ultrasound in parathyroid localization. World J Surg 2004;28:1122–6.
[16] Solbiati L, Osti V, Cova L, et al. Ultrasound of the thyroid, parathyroid glands, and neck lymph nodes. Eur Radiol 2001;11:2411–24.
[17] Attie JN, Rumancik WM, Moskowitz GW, et al. Preoperative localization of parathyroid tumors. Am J Surg 1988;156:323–6.
[18] Whelan PJ, Rotstein LE, Rosen IB, et al. Do we really need another localizing technique for parathyroid glands? Am J Surg 1989;158:382–4.
[19] Kohri K, Ishikawa Y, Kodma M, et al. Comparison of imaging methods for localization of parathyroid tumors. Am J Surg 1992;164:140–5.
[20] Gilat H, Cohen M, Feinmesser R, et al. Minimally invasive procedure for resection of a parathyroid adenoma: the role of preoperative high resolution ultrasonography. J Clin Ultrasound 2005;33(6):283–7.
[21] Rodgers SE, Hunter GJ, Hamberg LM, et al. Improved preoperative planning for directed parathyroidectomy with 4-dimensional computed tomography. Surgery 2006;140: 932–41.
[22] Starker LF, Mahajan A, Björklund P, et al. 4D parathyroid CT as the initial localization study for patients with de novo primary hyperparathyroidism. Ann Surg Oncol 2011;18:1723–8.
[23] Agha A, Hornung M, Rennert J, et al. Contrast-enhanced ultrasonography for localization of pathologic glands in patients with primary hyperparathyroidism. Surgery 2012;151: 580–6.
[24] Rodriguez JM, Tezelman S, Siperstein AE, et al. Localization procedures in patients with persistent or recurrent hyperparathyroidism. Arch Surg 1994;129:870–5.
[25] Powell AC, Alexander HR, Chang R, et al. Reoperation for parathyroid adenoma: a contemporary experience. Surgery 2009;146:1144–55.
[26] Kettle AG, O'Doherty MJ. Parathyroid imaging: how good is it and how should it be done? Semin Nucl Med 2006;36:206–11.
[27] Witteveen JE, Kievit J, Stokkel MP, et al. Limitations of Tc99m-MIBI-SPECT imaging scans in persistent primary hyperparathyroidism. World J Surg 2011;35:128–39.

[28] Ciappuccini R, Morera J, Pascal P, et al. Dual-phase 99mTc sestamibi scintigraphy with neck and thorax SPECT/CT in primary hyperparathyroidism: a single-institution experience. Clin Nucl Med 2012;37(3):223–8.
[29] Untch BR, Adam MA, Scheri RP, et al. Surgeon-performed ultrasound is superior to 99Tc-sestamibi scanning to localize parathyroid adenomas in patients with primary hyperparathyroidism: results in 516 patients over 10 years. J Am Coll Surg 2011;212:522–9.
[30] Caldarella C, Treglia G, Pontecorvi A, et al. Diagnostic performance of planar scintigraphy using 99m Tc-MIBI in patients with secondary hyperparathyroidism: a meta-analysis. Ann Nucl Med 2012;26:794–803.
[31] Hunter GJ, Schellingerhout D, Vu TH, et al. Accuracy of 4-dimensional CT for the localization of abnormal parathyroid glands in patients with primary hyperparathyroidism. Radiology 2012;264(3):789–95.
[32] Kelly HR, Hamberg LM, Hunter GJ. 4D-CT for preoperative localization of abnormal parathyroid glands in patients with hyperparathyroidism: accuracy and ability to stratify patients by unilateral versus bilateral disease in surgery-naïve and re-exploration patients. AJNR Am J Neuroradiol 2014;35:176–81.
[33] Alvarado R, Meyer-Rochow G, Sywak M, et al. Bilateral internal jugular venous sampling for parathyroid hormone determination in patients with nonlocalizing hyperparathyroidism. World J Surg 2010;34:1299–303.
[34] Carneiro-Pla D. Effectiveness of "office"-based, ultrasound-guided differential jugular venous sampling (DJVS) of parathormone in patients with primary hyperparathyroidism. Surgery 2009;146:1014–20.

Advances in Surgery 49 (2015) 263–280

ADVANCES IN SURGERY

Abscess After Appendectomy

Predisposing Factors

Daniel E. Levin, MD[a], Walter Pegoli Jr, MD[b,*]

[a]Department of General Surgery, University of Rochester Medical Center, 601 Elmwood Avenue, Rochester, NY 14642, USA; [b]Department of General Surgery, Golisano Children's Hospital, University of Rochester Medical Center, 601 Elmwood Avenue, Rochester, NY 14642, USA

Keywords

• Acute appendicitis • Perforated appendicitis • Intra-abdominal abscess
• Organ space infection • Predisposing factors

Key points

- Perforated appendicitis is the single greatest predisposing factor for the development of postappendectomy intra-abdominal abscess (IAA).
- Preoperative elevations in C-reactive protein (CRP) and leukocyte count are associated with increased risk of postoperative complications, including formation of IAA.
- Several recent meta-analyses suggest a slight increase in IAA formation after laparoscopic appendectomy (LA) compared with open appendectomy.
- Postoperative antibiotics are not necessary for nonperforated appendicitis; 3 to 5 days of postoperative antibiotics are sufficient for perforated appendicitis to reduce risk of postoperative IAA.
- Techniques for appendiceal stump closure, routine peritoneal saline lavage, and routine peritoneal drain placement do not decrease risk of IAA formation in nonperforated or perforated appendicitis.

INTRODUCTION

According to the Centers for Disease Control and Prevention, approximately 325,000 appendectomies are performed in the United States each year [1]. In a majority of these cases, patients wake up in the recovery room noting immediate relief of their index symptoms. They spend an average of 1 day in the hospital [2] and, after a single follow-up visit with the surgeon's office, resume

The authors have nothing to disclose.

*Corresponding author. *E-mail address*: Walter_Pegoli@URMC.rochester.edu

0065-3411/15/$ – see front matter
http://dx.doi.org/10.1016/j.yasu.2015.03.010

their lives with little negative effect on their subsequent quality of life [3,4]. In some patients, unpleasant and potentially life-threatening complications of their disease have an impact.

Overall, complications after appendectomy occur in approximately 5% to 20% of patients and include a broad range of conditions, from ileus and wound infection to pneumonia and death [5]. Research on appendicitis is extensive. A search of the pubmed.gov database using the search term, "appendicitis", reveals 5239 articles during the 10-year period from 2004 through 2013. This is an average of 1.4 appendicitis articles per day for the past 10 years. The aim of this article is to evaluate and identify predisposing or predictive factors for the development of intra-abdominal infections after appendectomy. Approximately 1% to 10% of all patients develop an IAA after surgery for appendicitis [6] and a significant amount of research has been conducted in an attempt to identify those patients at greatest risk. Specifically, the following topics are examined:

NONPERFORATED VERSUS PERFORATED APPENDICITIS

In the modern era, rates of perforated appendicitis have been reported to be 15% to 20% for the general population. In a recent analysis of more than 32,000 appendectomy patients in the National Surgical Quality Improvement Program (NSQIP) database, the total rate of perforated appendicitis was 16.5% [2]. Similarly, in a review of 9048 adults from the Washington State Surgical Care and Outcomes Assessment Program who underwent appendectomy, 15.8% were perforated [7]. In children, rates of perforation often equal that of adults during adolescence; however, rates of perforation increase significantly under age 5 years (60%) and have been reported to be as high as 86% to 100% under age 3 years [8,9].

Among all perioperative factors, perforation status is the single greatest risk factor for the development of postoperative abscess. Based on data in Table 1,

Table 1
Rates of postoperative intra-abdominal abscess formation: nonperforated versus perforated appendicitis

Author (year)	Nonperforated appendicitis (%)	Perforated appendicitis (%)
van Rossem et al [16], 2014	1.8	7.9
Masoomi et al [5], 2014	0.3–1.2	1.6–3.6
Kelly et al [18], 2014	0.9	8.4
Romano et al [15], 2014	0.6	5.6
Markar et al [11], 2012	0.5	2.9
Asarias et al [10], 2011	0.9	5.4
Ingraham et al [2], 2010	Not available	5.7
Cueto et al [13], 2006	0.1	2.8
Kouwenhoven et al [14], 2005	2.5	7.2
Katkhouda et al [12], 2000	0.7	8.9

it is reasonable to give patients a 1.0% risk of postoperative abscess formation in cases of nonperforated appendicitis [5,10–15]. In comparison, perforated appendicitis carries an IAA rate of 5.0% to 10% [2,5,7,11–16]. Considering how many operations are done each year for appendicitis, this translates into a substantial number of patients annually who require treatment of IAA. Understandably, this generates interest in potential predisposing factors that may be identified and acted on to reduce the risk of postoperative abscess formation.

Clinical factors: adults

Determining which clinical factors may predispose or predict the development of an organ space infection (OSI) after appendectomy is challenging and has generated significant contradictory results in the literature. Fleming and colleagues [17] reviewed data obtained from the NSQIP database on 39,950 patients with appendicitis, revealing several clinical variables associated with the development of postoperative abscess. These results are demonstrated in Table 2 and suggest that male gender, history of smoking, systemic inflammatory response syndrome, mean preoperative WBC count, emergent procedure, higher wound classification and operative time greater than 60 minutes are all associated with higher incidence of OSI. Conversely, mean age, body mass index, history of diabetes mellitus, history of bleeding disorder and ASA class were not associated with any difference in rates of OSI on multivariate analysis [17].

Clinical factors: children

A similar study of 5097 children (ages 2–18 years) with appendicitis demonstrated that increased rates of OSI were associated with complicated appendicitis (peritonitis, perforation, or preoperative abscess), higher wound classification, sepsis, and operative time greater than 60 minutes. Unlike adults,

Table 2
Clinical variables predisposing to postoperative intra-abdominal abscess formation

Variable	Odds ratio (adults)	Odds ratio (children)
Intraoperative fecalith	Not available	8.8
Higher wound class	7.9	4.2
Diarrhea at presentation	Not available	3.6
Preoperative sepsis	1.5	2.2
Operative time >1 h	1.5	1.1
Male gender	1.3	1.1
Smoking	1.2	Not available
Emergent operation	1.3	0.8

Data from Refs [17,18,25].

there did not seem to be an increased rate of OSI between genders or with emergent operations [18].

Predisposing factors for complications after appendectomy

There are data to suggest that the patient population undergoing appendectomy is changing. The number of patients with obesity, multiple comorbidities, and age greater than 65 years is increasing. A retrospective review of more than 1.5 million appendectomy patients in the US National (Nationwide) Inpatient Sample from 2003 to 2011 demonstrated increased incidence of complications among men, people older than 52 years, nonteaching hospitals, rural locations, Medicare patients, and African American race [19]. Although this article could not comment on specific complications, such as IAA formation, others have investigated some of these patient populations.

Racial disparities

A 2012 review of 39,000 patients in the NSQIP database revealed that African American patients had statistically significant higher rates of postoperative abscess compared with white patients (2.7% vs 1.8%). The investigators conclude that more research is needed to identify the underlying cause [20]. Whatever the cause, it is important to recognize that this discrepancy exists so that all providers are educated and aware of this problem and more work can be done to eliminate the disparity.

Obesity

Because perforation is the greatest predisposing factor to postappendectomy IAA formation, it might be predicted that any circumstance that may result in a higher risk of perforation would, therefore, result in a higher rate of postoperative abscess formation. Obesity has been associated with a predisposition for perforated appendicitis, but this has not always translated to an increased risk of postoperative IAA [21,22]. Controversy exists, however, because other investigators have demonstrated an increased risk of postoperative IAA formation in obese children, as high as 35% [23], underscoring the need for additional research in this unique patient population.

Young age

As previously discussed, children under age 5 years are known to have increased rates of perforated appendicitis [8,24]. This higher rate of perforated appendicitis does not translate to increased IAA rates. Bansal and colleagues [8] found the postoperative OSI rate to be 3.2% in children under 5, and, despite that the rates of perforation for children ages less than 1 year, 1 to 2 years, and 2 to 3 years were 86%, 74%, and 60%, respectively (n = 6, 29, and 34, respectively), none of these infants or toddlers developed postoperative abscesses.

This study also corroborated the results of Henry and colleagues [25], who describe the presence of diarrhea at presentation as a predisposing factor for postoperative IAA development [8]. In addition to diarrhea on presentation, this multicenter case-control study also found the presence of intraoperative fecalith a predisposing factor for postappendectomy IAA formation, with an odds ratio (OR) of 8.77. They also concluded that duration of pain, type, and timing of antibiotics; the presence of an abscess at the time of surgery; and surgical technique were not predisposing factors for subsequent development of an abscess [25].

Old age

At the other end of the spectrum, patients older than 65 are at greater risk for perforation [26], but this has yet to be satisfactorily demonstrated as an independent risk factor for IAA formation.

Laboratory data predictive of intra-abdominal abscess formation

Articles have been published identifying various laboratory markers, such as WBC count, CRP, and bilirubin associated with perforated appendicitis [27]. There are, however, few data investigating the use of these values as predictors of postoperative IAA. Thereaux and colleagues [28] reviewed 141 appendectomies performed for diffuse appendicular peritonitis (defined by the presence of purulent intra-abdominal fluid) and found that preoperative leukocyte count of greater than 17,000 mm^{-3} and CRP concentration greater than 200 mg/dL were associated with increased rates of postoperative abscess formation. Gender, age, symptom duration, fever greater than 38°C, cecectomy, saline peritoneal irrigation, and presence or absence of a drain were not significantly associated with IAA formation. Other investigators have found the data regarding predictive value of WBC less convincing [17,18,29]. These data are summarized in Table 3.

Time to the operating room

As discussed previously, it is thought that any scenario resulting in a higher risk of perforation would likely result in a higher rate of postoperative abscess formation. One hypothesis, supported by historical research, suggests that delaying the

Table 3
Preoperative laboratory data predictive of postoperative intra-abdominal abscess formation

Author (year)	Comment
Preoperative CRP	
Thereaux et al [28], 2014	>200 mg/L is predictive of IAA (OR 16.4, $P = .02$)
Shelton et al [29], 2014	>150 mg/L is predictive of postoperative complication[a]
Preoperative WBC	
Thereaux et al [28], 2014	>17,000 mm^{-3} is predictive of IAA (OR 25.0, $P = .007$)
Shelton et al [29], 2014	Not predictive of postoperative complication[a]
Kelly et al [18], 2014	Not predictive of postoperative OSI[b]
Fleming et al [17], 2010	Not predictive of postoperative OSI[c]

[a] IAA was grouped into postoperative complication but not isolated for subgroup analysis.
[b] Univariate analysis revealed a difference in the mean WBC in the group with an OSI versus no OSI (17.0 vs 14.8 $P<.001$); however, on multivariate, this was not significantly associated with OSI.
[c] Univariate analysis revealed a difference in the mean WBC in the group with an OSI vs no OSI (15.2 vs 12.3 $P<.0001$); however, on multivariate, this translated to an OR of just 1.03 per 1000 mm^{-3} increase in WBC.

time to surgery increases rates of perforation and, therefore, the rates of postoperative abscess. A recent review confirmed that delaying operative intervention for greater than 12 hours increases the rates of perforation and postoperative IAA [30]. A review of more than 60,000 patients demonstrated the OR for development of perforated appendicitis increased with each hospital day [31].

Other studies, however, have suggested the contrary. Once antibiotics have been initiated, a delay in operation does not result in greater rates of perforation [7,32]. A meta-analysis published in 2014 concluded that delays of 12 to 24 hours had no impact on rates of complicated appendicitis or development of postoperative IAA. Delays beyond 48 hours did not increase rates of perforation but increased the likelihood of developing a surgical site infection or a 30-day adverse event. IAA was not isolated for subgroup analysis but was included as 1 of the 30-day adverse events [33].

Operative technique

Many investigators have sought to determine if the technique for removal of the appendix has any impact on the development of postoperative abscess, once patients are in an operating room. After McBurney described his method for appendectomy in 1894 [34], it became the technique of choice for approximately a century. In 1981, Semm performed the first LA [35]. For the past 30 years, surgeons have been debating the pros and cons of open versus minimally invasive techniques. With respect to the development of postoperative abscess, a significant body of work has been devoted to answering the question as to whether one technique is superior to the other.

Three-incision laparoscopy versus open surgery

The benefits of minimally invasive surgery (MIS) have made it the preferred method for appendectomy. With regard to postoperative abscess formation, however, current literature suggests that MIS is associated with greater rates of IAA in comparison with open surgery. One of the first meta-analyses to compare LA with open surgery was published in 1998. This study identified a trend suggesting higher rates of IAA after laparoscopic surgery (2.0%) versus open surgery (0.9%). This, however, failed to reach statistical significance [36]. Approximately a decade later, another meta-analysis examined all randomized controlled trials published from 1995 through 2006. The investigators identified a statistically significant OR of 2.26, demonstrating an increased risk of IAA after laparoscopic surgery (3.0%) versus open surgery (1.6%) [37].

Similar findings were highlighted in both a 2004 Cochrane review and a subsequent 2010 update, which identified an increased risk of postoperative abscess formation after laparoscopic surgery with ORs of 2.4 and 1.86, respectively [38,39]. Additionally, a 2010 review of the NSQIP database compared approximately 30,000 laparoscopic appendectomies with 9000 open appendectomies and also found an increased risk of OSI with an OR of 1.44 on multivariate analysis [17].

Nevertheless, there are data to refute this difference. Romy and colleagues [40] found no significant difference in OSI rates on multivariate analysis of 2468 patients. Similarly, a review of 1017 patients found rates of postoperative abscess formation in cases of complicated appendicitis to be lower in the laparoscopic group than historical data reported in the literature for open appendectomy [13].

Studies within the pediatric population suggest no difference in IAA formation between the 2 operative techniques. A recent meta-analysis reviewing only children found no difference in the rates of IAA after laparoscopic (2.9%) versus open appendectomy (2.7%). A recent meta-analysis published by Aziz and colleagues [41] found no difference in the rates of IAA formation when comparing laparoscopy with open surgery. Likewise, studies comparing the effects of appendectomy in older age found no statistical difference in IAA formation among patients older than 60 undergoing laparoscopic versus open appendectomy [42,43]. A summary of these meta-analyses and others is in Table 4.

Single-incision laparoscopic appendectomy

A 2014 meta-analysis comparing single-incision LA (SILA) with 3-incision LA in adult patients failed to demonstrate a difference in the rates of postoperative abscess. Although there was a trend toward higher incidence of abscess formation using SILA technique (2.7% vs 1.3%), this did not reach significance [44]. A meta-analysis published in 2013 included many of the same studies, including those conducted in the pediatric population and found no statistical difference in the rates of IAA among SILA patients (1.8%) and conventional laparoscopy (1.3%) [45]. Table 5 highlights these and other meta-analyses comparing SILA with LA.

Natural orifice translumenal endoscopic surgery

A relative paucity of data exists to support or refute the use of natural orifice translumenal endoscopic surgery (NOTES) for appendectomy. Recently, a prospective cohort study compared transvaginal appendectomy with traditional laparoscopic surgery. Each group had approximately 20 patients. One patient in the transvaginal group developed a postoperative abscess versus none in the laparoscopic group. Statistical comparison was not possible [46]. Additional research is required to determine the effect, if any, vaginal flora may contribute to the development of postoperative abscess formation. Additional NOTES or hybrid cases have been described, including transgastric appendectomy. Other than feasibility studies, no real data exist comparing the outcome of NOTES with traditional laparoscopy with regard to postoperative abscess formation [47].

Technique for appendiceal stump closure

Several studies have been performed in children comparing techniques for the closure of the appendiceal stump. In the era of laparoscopy, 2 of the most common techniques involve the use of either the endostapler or the endoloop. Several studies designed to compare these techniques have been performed. Two of these studies identified no difference between them [48,49], whereas another study found IAA more common in the stapled group versus the endoloop group [50].

Table 4
Summary of meta-analyses comparing postoperative intra-abdominal abscess formation: laparoscopic versus open appendectomy

Meta-analysis author (year)	No. and type of studies included	No. of patients	Patient population	Intra-abdominal abscess (%) laparoscopic appendectomy	Intra-abdominal abscess (%) open	Conclusion regarding postoperative intra-abdominal abscess formation
Markar et al [11], 2012	10 (RCT; PS; RR)	107,624	Pediatric	2.6	1.1	LA is associated with higher rates of IAA formation compared with open[a]
Woodham et al [69], 2012	2 (RCT; RR)	442	Obese adult	4.1	4.8	LA is equivalent to OA in rates of IAA formation
Li et al [70], 2010	17 (RCT)	3445	Adult and pediatric	Not Reported	Not Reported	OR 1.56, suggesting higher rates of IAA after LA vs OA
Sauerland et al [39], 2010	45 (RCT)	5577	Adult and pediatric	1.8	0.9	OR 1.87, LA is associated with higher rates of IAA formation compared with open
Markides et al [71], 2010	11 (RR)	2127	Adult and pediatric	5.9	4.6	OR 1.24, no statistical significant difference between LA and OA regarding rates of IAA formation
Bennett et al [37], 2007	25 (RCT)	4003	Adult and pediatric	3.0	1.6	OR 2.29, LA is associated with higher rates of IAA formation compared with open
Aziz et al [41], 2006	16 (PS, RR)	4385	Pediatric	3.8	3.4	OR 1.1, no statistical significant difference between LA and OA regarding rates of IAA formation[b]
Golub et al [36], 1998	14 (PS)	1585	Adult	2.0	0.9	Tendency toward increased IAA rates with LR but did not reach significance

Abbreviations: OA, open appendectomy; PS, prospective study; RCT, randomized controlled trial; RR, retrospective review.

[a] Results reveal this is attributed to difference observed with the treatment of perforated appendicitis. Nonperforated appendicitis demonstrated no significant difference when comparing LA with OA.

[b] Results of subgroup analysis comparing only RCTs reveals statistically significant difference. IAA incidence of 7.4% with LA vs 4.2% with OA (OR1.0).

Table 5
Summary of meta-analyses comparing postoperative intra-abdominal abscess formation: laparoscopic versus single-incision laparoscopic appendectomy

Meta-analysis author (year)	No. and type of studies included	No. of patients	Patient population	Intra-abdominal abscess (%) laparoscopic appendectomy	Intra-abdominal abscess (%) single-incision laparoscopic appendectomy	Conclusion regarding postoperative intra-abdominal abscess formation
Antoniou et al [44], 2014	5 (RCT)	746	Adult	3.0	2.7	SILA is equivalent to LA in rates of IAA formation
Markar et al [45], 2013	7 (RCT)	1108	Adult and pediatric	1.8	1.3	SILA is equivalent to LA in rates of IAA formation
Ding et al [72], 2013	6 (RCT; RR)	1004	Adult and pediatric	1.9	2.1	SILA is equivalent to LA in rates of IAA formation
Pisanu et al [73], 2013	13 (RCT; PS; RR)	893	Adult	1.0	1.7	Morbidity is greater in SILA, partly due to IAA rate Prospective RCTs are needed to better assess Outcomes
Gill et al [74], 2012	9 (RCT; PS; RR)	623	Adult	1.4	1.8	SILA is equivalent to LA in rates of IAA formation

Abbreviations: PS, prospective study; RCT, randomized controlled trial; RR, retrospective review.

Additional techniques for appendiceal stump closure include suture ligation, metal clips, and locking polymer clips. There seems to be no difference between the use of polyglactin suture ligation and metal clip application [51]. A 2014 review comparing 1100 patients with metal clips closure to 317 patients with locking polymer clip closure found no difference in the IAA formation (1.2% and 1.6%, respectively) [52]. Although the investigators did not compare these rates with more traditional closure techniques, the abscess rates seem comparable, suggesting that technique for stump closure is not a predisposing factor for IAA.

Routine drain placement versus no drain

Since the 1970s, most surgeons have abandoned placing drains in the peritoneal cavity for uncomplicated appendicitis [53,54]. Considerable present-day debate exits, however, regarding the merits of peritoneal drainage for complicated appendicitis. The most recent meta-analysis of randomized controlled trials comparing the use of drain versus no drain was published in 2004. Of the 5 studies identified, 4 were completed in the 1970s prior to the introduction of laparoscopic surgery and new-generation antibiotics. The fifth study was published in 1992. The investigators of the meta-analysis concluded that routine drainage for gangrenous or perforated appendicitis should not be performed and does not decrease the rates of postoperative IAA [55].

These data were corroborated in a more recent retrospective review comparing the outcomes of 209 patients operated on for complicated appendicitis. The investigators defined complicated appendicitis as the intraoperative finding of gangrenous or perforated appendicitis. Of these patients, 88 received a drain and 121 did not. There was no significant difference in the rates of postoperative abscess among the drained (8.0%) and undrained (10.7%) [56]. Therefore, the preponderance of the published data suggests that drainage of the peritoneal cavity for appendicitis is not necessary, irrespective of disease severity. It must be recognized, however, that level 1 data to support this claim in the modern era are not available.

Peritoneal irrigation versus no irrigation

Currently, few surgeons perform routine irrigation in cases of nonperforated appendicitis. To irrigate or not was the topic in a recent article of this journal, concluding that irrigation and suction demonstrate no benefit compared with suction alone [57]. A recent study investigating this question randomized 220 pediatric patients (age <18) with perforated appendicitis to either irrigation or suction without irrigation. The investigators found no significant difference in the rates of postoperative abscess formation in the irrigation group (18.3%) versus the suction-only group (19.1%) [58]. Retained fecolith has been identified as a cause of postoperative abscess formation [59,60].

Antibiotic duration-nonperforated appendicitis

A 2004 Cochrane review evaluating 45 studies and in more than 9000 adult and pediatric patients found that the use of antibiotics reduced the incidence of postoperative abscess formation [61]. More recent research has been aimed at determining the optimum antibiotic regimen and duration for the prevention of IAA. In cases of nonperforated appendicitis, a review of more than 700 patients determined that continuing antibiotics in the postoperative period may actually be harmful, increasing rates of *Clostridium difficile*, urinary tract infection, and length of stay [62].

The Surgical Infection Society (SIS) guidelines on antimicrobial therapy in children recommend preoperative antibiotics without postoperative antibiotics for nonperforated appendicitis. The choice of antibiotics must provide adequate gram-negative and anaerobic coverage. Common therapies include second-generation cephalosporins or extended-spectrum penicillins [63]. SIS guidelines in adults with nonperforated appendicitis suggest no postoperative antibiotics. Patients with gangrenous appendicitis without intraperitoneal contamination, however, may receive 24 hours of postoperative antibiotics [64]. A review of the adult literature published in 2013 also concluded that nonperforated appendicitis only requires a single dose of preoperative broad-spectrum antibiotics [65].

Antibiotic duration-perforated appendicitis

In cases of perforated appendicitis, the duration of antibiotics is controversial. The SIS guidelines in children with perforated appendicitis recommend broad-spectrum antibiotics until clinical evidence of recovery, namely 24 hours without fever, normal WBC and differential, and resolution of symptoms. Again, as long as antibiotics cover gram-negative and anaerobic bacteria, there is no preferential treatment [63]. The SIS guidelines in adults suggest that antibiotics be administered for no more than 7 days, unless source control has not been achieved. Examples of acceptable monotherapy include cefoxitin, ertapenem, and piperacillin-tazobactam [64].

Subsequent attempts to determine the duration of antibiotics have been explored. A 2014 review concluded that at least 3 to 5 days of intravenous antibiotics are recommended until there is clinical improvement. Markers of clinical improvement included a reduction in fever, CRP, and leukocytosis [65]. Moreover, a 2014 observational cohort study was designed to determine if there was a difference in 3 days versus 5 days of postoperative antibiotics with respect to IAA formation. It found no difference between the 2 groups. All patients were treated preoperatively and postoperatively with a second-generation cephalosporin and metronidazole [16]. Reducing the duration even further, Kimbrell and colleagues [66] demonstrated that there is no benefit in prescribing greater than 24 hours of postoperative antibiotics for patients with perforated appendicitis. This review, however, was limited by small sample size, and the investigators acknowledge the need for validation in larger randomized controlled studies.

Diagnosis and treatment

The diagnosis of IAA after appendectomy is less controversial. Fig. 1 demonstrates a common approach to diagnosis and treatment. In most instances, a patient develops recurrence of fevers, abdominal pain, and rising leukocytosis.

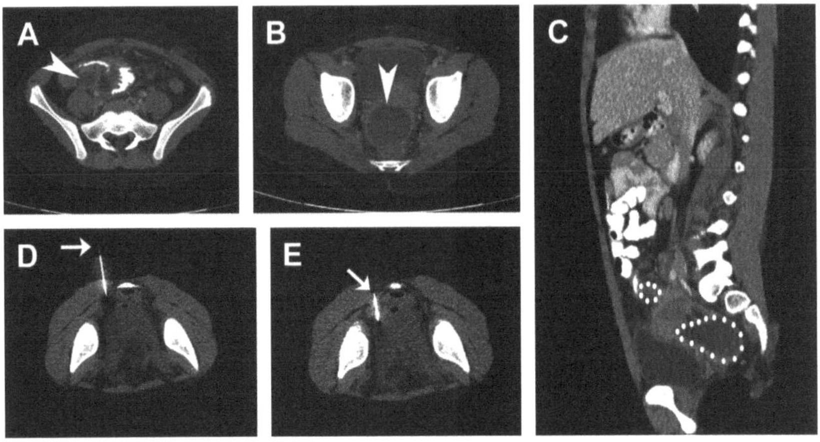

Fig. 1. CT scan demonstrating multiple postappendectomy abscesses and subsequent image guided percutaneous drainage. A female patient 10 days status post-LA presented with fevers, abdominal pain, and leukocytosis. CT scan revealed a well circumscribed, rim-enhancing IAA in the right lower quadrant (*A; arrowhead*) and a second abscess in the pelvis (*B; arrowhead*). The sagittal section (*C*) revealed the relationship of these abscesses to one another (*dotted lines*). With the patient in prone position and with CT guidance, interventional radiologists passed a needle through the skin (*D; arrow*) and into the larger abscess cavity (*E; arrow*) allowing placement of a drainage catheter via modified Seldinger technique.

When clinical suspicion is raised, CT is the preferred diagnostic imaging modality. If an abscess is identified, broad-spectrum antibiotics are continued or resumed and percutaneous drainage of the collection should be entertained. If this is not possible, then either surgical washout or continued antibiotic therapy may be indicated [67,68].

SUMMARY/DISCUSSION

Formation of IAA after appendectomy is an unpleasant complication of appendicitis. It occurs in approximately 1% of operations performed for acute, nonperforated appendicitis [4,10–15] and in 5% to 10% of operations performed for perforated appendicitis [2,5,7,12–16]. Box 1 attempts to stratify these predisposing factors but is limited by the lack of randomized controlled data for many of these variables. Perforation clearly predisposes to development of IAA, but it is beneficial to know if there are other predisposing factors. Higher wound class is associated with increased rates of IAA formation in both children (OR 4.2) and adults (OR 7.9,) which is likely a marker for perforation. Similarly, preoperative sepsis seems to increase this risk [17,18].

Knowing that perforation status is correlated with risk of IAA formation, it seems logical that factors that increase the risk of perforation would also predispose to development of postappendectomy OSI. This is supported by evidence that failure to treat appendicitis for greater than 48 hours is associated with increased postoperative complications [33]. Several other factors that are

Box 1: Summary of predisposing or predictive factors for development of postappendectomy intra-abdominal abscess

High risk
- Perforated appendicitis
- CRP greater than 200 mg/L
- Leukocyte greater than 17,000 mm^{-3}
- Intraoperative fecalith (children)

Moderate risk
- Preoperative sepsis
- Operative time greater than 1 hour
- Delay in operation greater than 48 hours from presentation[a]
- African American race
- Diarrhea at presentation (children)

Mild risk
- Adult male
- Smoking
- Obesity

[a] In patients not considered a candidate for nonoperative treatment.

associated with increased rates of perforation have been identified, such as obesity, black race, male gender, age less than 4 years, age greater than 65 years, lack of private insurance, and rural location [19]. Some of these have been demonstrated to result in increased rates of postoperative IAA as well.

Concerning data reveal that African American individuals have a higher incidence of postoperative IAA compared with white individuals (2.7% vs 1.8%) [20]. Similarly, there is some literature to suggest that obese individuals may also be at increased risk for IAA formation [23], although there are conflicting data in this regard [21,22]. Additional research is needed to better understand how these disparities arise and to better understand what role a person's age, gender, and insurance status may have on rates of postoperative IAA formation.

In addition to these variables, researchers have sought to identify laboratory variables that may identify at-risk patients. CRP levels greater than 200 mg/L and leukocyte count greater than 17,000 mm^{-3} have been implicated as predictors of postoperative IAA formation [28]. Once at-risk patients have been identified, it would be beneficial to identify strategies to decrease the rates of IAA formation. Box 2 summarizes some of these interventions based on whether or not they have any demonstrable benefit. For example, nonperforated appendicitis requires only preoperative antibiotics without the need for postoperative antibiotics. Patients with perforated appendicitis seem to benefit from 3 to 5 days of gram-negative and anaerobic antimicrobial coverage although randomized controlled trials are needed to determine the optimum duration. In

Box 2: Summary of interventions demonstrated to alter risk of postappendectomy intra-abdominal abscess formation

Decrease risk

- Preoperative antibiotics for both nonperforated and perforated appendicitis
- Antibiotics for 3–5 days in perforated appendicitis

Increase risk

- Minimally invasive appendectomy has a slight increase in risk compared with open appendectomy

No benefit

- Postoperative antibiotics for nonperforated appendicitis
- Technique for appendiceal stump closure
- Intraperitoneal drain placement
- Peritoneal irrigation with saline

all cases, patient clinical status should be monitored for improvements in symptoms, reduction in fever, and normalization of WBC and CRP [65].

Intense research has been directed at answering the question as to whether or not MIS results in greater IAA rates than open appendectomy. Although the literature is mixed, a majority of meta-analyses conducted to date demonstrate an increase in the IAA rates after MIS. Despite this, the many benefits of LA compared with open appendectomy make it the preferred method for most surgeons. The technique for appendiceal stump closure does not alter the risk of IAA formation [48,49] and should be chosen based on surgeon preference, availability, and cost-effectiveness. There is no apparent change in IAA rates based on intraperitoneal saline irrigation or drain placement [55,58].

During the postappendectomy recovery period, recurrence of or worsening abdominal pain, fever, and increasing or persistent elevations in WBC or CRP may be suggestive of IAA formation. Confirmation with CT scan is the most common diagnostic modality and provides the needed information for therapeutic guidance. This often includes continuation of antibiotics and possible image-guided drain placement versus operative drainage [67,68]. Overall, appendicitis and its complications continue to be a common scourge of people all over the world. It is an interesting entity that generates much debate and intellectual curiosity and, for now, remains in the purview of surgeons to treat.

References

[1] Hall MJ, DeFrances CJ, Williams SN, et al. National hospital discharge survey: 2007 summary. Natl Health Stat Report 2010;1–20, 24.

[2] Ingraham AM, Cohen ME, Bilimoria KY, et al. Comparison of outcomes after laparoscopic versus open appendectomy for acute appendicitis at 222 ACS NSQIP hospitals. Surgery 2010;148(4):625–35 [discussion: 635–7].

[3] Kapischke M, Friedrich F, Hedderich J, et al. Laparoscopic versus open appendectomy–quality of life 7 years after surgery. Langenbecks Arch Surg 2011;396(1):69–75.

[4] Koumarelas K, Theodoropoulos GE, Spyropoulos BG, et al. A prospective longitudinal evaluation and affecting factors of health related quality of life after appendectomy. Int J Surg 2014;12(8):848–57.
[5] Masoomi H, Nguyen NT, Dolich MO, et al. Laparoscopic appendectomy trends and outcomes in the United States: data from the nationwide inpatient sample (NIS), 2004–2011. Am Surg 2014;80(10):1074–7.
[6] Wilson DG, Bond AK, Ladwa N, et al. Intra-abdominal collections following laparoscopic versus open appendicectomy: an experience of 516 consecutive cases at a district general hospital. Surg Endosc 2013;27(7):2351–6.
[7] Drake FT, Mottey NE, Farrokhi ET, et al. Time to appendectomy and risk of perforation in acute appendicitis. JAMA Surg 2014;149(8):837–44.
[8] Bansal S, Banever GT, Karrer FM, et al. Appendicitis in children less than 5 years old: influence of age on presentation and outcome. Am J Surg 2012;204(6):1031–5 [discussion: 1035].
[9] Alloo J, Gerstle T, Shilyansky J, et al. Appendicitis in children less than 3 years of age: a 28-year review. Pediatr Surg Int 2004;19(12):777–9.
[10] Asarias JR, Schlussel AT, Cafasso DE, et al. Incidence of postoperative intraabdominal abscesses in open versus laparoscopic appendectomies. Surg Endosc 2011;25(8):2678–83.
[11] Markar SR, Blackburn S, Cobb R, et al. Laparoscopic versus open appendectomy for complicated and uncomplicated appendicitis in children. J Gastrointest Surg 2012;16(10): 1993–2004.
[12] Katkhouda N, Friedlander MH, Grant SW, et al. Intraabdominal abscess rate after laparoscopic appendectomy. Am J Surg 2000;180(6):456–9 [discussion: 460–1].
[13] Cueto J, D'Allemagne B, Vázquez-Frias JA, et al. Morbidity of laparoscopic surgery for complicated appendicitis: an international study. Surg Endosc 2006;20(5):717–20.
[14] Kouwenhoven EA, Repelaer van Driel OJ, van Erp WF. Fear for the intraabdominal abscess after laparoscopic appendectomy: not realistic. Surg Endosc 2005;19(7):923–6.
[15] Romano A, Parikh P, Byers P, et al. Simple acute appendicitis versus non-perforated gangrenous appendicitis: is there a difference in the rate of post-operative infectious complications? Surg Infect (Larchmt) 2014;15(5):517–20.
[16] van Rossem CC, Schreinemacher MH, Treskes K, et al. Duration of antibiotic treatment after appendicectomy for acute complicated appendicitis. Br J Surg 2014;101(6):715–9.
[17] Fleming FJ, Kim MJ, Messing S, et al. Balancing the risk of postoperative surgical infections: a multivariate analysis of factors associated with laparoscopic appendectomy from the NSQIP database. Ann Surg 2010;252(6):895–900.
[18] Kelly KN, Fleming FJ, Aquina CT, et al. Disease severity, not operative approach, drives organ space infection after pediatric appendectomy. Ann Surg 2014;260(3):466–71 [discussion: 472–3].
[19] Bliss LA, Yang CJ, Kent TS, et al. Appendicitis in the modern era: universal problem and variable treatment. Surg Endosc 2014. [Epub ahead of print].
[20] Scarborough JE, Bennett KM, Pappas TN. Racial disparities in outcomes after appendectomy for acute appendicitis. Am J Surg 2012;204(1):11–7.
[21] Blanco FC, Sandler AD, Nadler EP. Increased incidence of perforated appendicitis in children with obesity. Clin Pediatr (Phila) 2012;51(10):928–32.
[22] Deugarte DA, Stark R, Kaji AH, et al. Obesity does not impact outcomes for appendicitis. Am Surg 2012;78(2):254–7.
[23] Garey CL, Laituri CA, Little DC, et al. Outcomes of perforated appendicitis in obese and nonobese children. J Pediatr Surg 2011;46(12):2346–8.
[24] Bratton SL, Haberkern CM, Waldhausen JH. Acute appendicitis risks of complications: age and Medicaid insurance. Pediatrics 2000;106(1 Pt 1):75–8.
[25] Henry MC, Walker A, Silverman BL, et al. Risk factors for the development of abdominal abscess following operation for perforated appendicitis in children: a multicenter case-control study. Arch Surg 2007;142(3):236–41 [discussion: 241].

[26] Walker A, Hatch Q, Drake T, et al. Predictors of appendiceal perforation in an equal access system. J Surg Res 2014;190(1):87–92.
[27] Panagiotopoulou IG, Parashar D, Lin R, et al. The diagnostic value of white cell count, C-reactive protein and bilirubin in acute appendicitis and its complications. Ann R Coll Surg Engl 2013;95(3):215–21.
[28] Thereaux J, Veyrie N, Corigliano N, et al. Is laparoscopy a safe approach for diffuse appendicular peritonitis? Feasibility and determination of risk factors for post-operative intra-abdominal abscess. Surg Endosc 2014;28(6):1908–13.
[29] Shelton JA, Brown JJ, Young JA. Preoperative C-reactive protein predicts the severity and likelihood of complications following appendicectomy. Ann R Coll Surg Engl 2014;96(5):369–72.
[30] Busch M, Gutzwiller FS, Aellig S, et al. In-hospital delay increases the risk of perforation in adults with appendicitis. World J Surg 2011;35(7):1626–33.
[31] Papandria D, Goldstein SD, Rhee D, et al. Risk of perforation increases with delay in recognition and surgery for acute appendicitis. J Surg Res 2013;184(2):723–9.
[32] Teixeira PG, Sivrikoz E, Inaba K, et al. Appendectomy timing: waiting until the next morning increases the risk of surgical site infections. Ann Surg 2012;256(3):538–43.
[33] Bhangu A, United Kingdom National Surgical Research Collaborative. Safety of short, in-hospital delays before surgery for acute appendicitis: multicentre cohort study, systematic review, and meta-analysis. Ann Surg 2014;259(5):894–903.
[34] McBurney C IV. The incision made in the abdominal wall in cases of appendicitis, with a description of a new method of operating. Ann Surg 1894;20(1):38–43.
[35] Semm K. Endoscopic appendectomy. Endoscopy 1983;15(2):59–64.
[36] Golub R, Siddiqui F, Pohl D. Laparoscopic versus open appendectomy: a metaanalysis. J Am Coll Surg 1998;186(5):545–53.
[37] Bennett J, Boddy A, Rhodes M. Choice of approach for appendicectomy: a meta-analysis of open versus laparoscopic appendicectomy. Surg Laparosc Endosc Percutan Tech 2007;17(4):245–55.
[38] Sauerland S, Lefering R, Neugebauer EA. Laparoscopic versus open surgery for suspected appendicitis. Cochrane Database Syst Rev 2004;(4):CD001546.
[39] Sauerland S, Jaschinski T, Neugebauer EA. Laparoscopic versus open surgery for suspected appendicitis. Cochrane Database Syst Rev 2010;(10):CD001546.
[40] Romy S, Eisenring MC, Bettschart V, et al. Laparoscope use and surgical site infections in digestive surgery. Ann Surg 2008;247(4):627–32.
[41] Aziz O, Athanasiou T, Tekkis PP, et al. Laparoscopic versus open appendectomy in children: a meta-analysis. Ann Surg 2006;243(1):17–27.
[42] Southgate E, Vousden N, Karthikesalingam A, et al. Laparoscopic vs open appendectomy in older patients. Arch Surg 2012;147(6):557–62.
[43] Nataraja RM, Loukogeorgakis SP, Sherwood WJ, et al. The incidence of intraabdominal abscess formation following laparoscopic appendicectomy in children: a systematic review and meta-analysis. J Laparoendosc Adv Surg Tech A 2013;23(9):795–802.
[44] Antoniou SA, Koch OO, Antoniou GA, et al. Meta-analysis of randomized trials on single-incision laparoscopic versus conventional laparoscopic appendectomy. Am J Surg 2014;207(4):613–22.
[45] Markar SR, Karthikesalingam A, Di Franco F, et al. Systematic review and meta-analysis of single-incision versus conventional multiport appendicectomy. Br J Surg 2013;100(13):1709–18.
[46] Roberts KE, Solomon D, Mirensky T, et al. Pure transvaginal appendectomy versus traditional laparoscopic appendectomy for acute appendicitis: a prospective cohort study. Ann Surg 2012;255(2):266–9.
[47] Kaehler G, Schoenberg MB, Kienle P, et al. Transgastric appendicectomy. Br J Surg 2013;100(7):911–5.

[48] Naiditch J, Lautz T, Chin A, et al. Endoloop as the first line tool for appendiceal stump closure in children with appendicitis. Eur J Pediatr Surg 2013;25(2):155–9.
[49] Miyano G, Urao M, Lane G, et al. Appendiceal stump closure in children with complicated appendicitis: a prospective analysis of endoloops versus endostaples. Asian J Endosc Surg 2011;4(3):116–9.
[50] Safavi A, Langer M, Skarsgard ED. Endoloop versus endostapler closure of the appendiceal stump in pediatric laparoscopic appendectomy. Can J Surg 2012;55(1):37–40.
[51] Ates M, Dirican A, Ince V, et al. Comparison of intracorporeal knot-tying suture (polyglactin) and titanium endoclips in laparoscopic appendiceal stump closure: a prospective randomized study. Surg Laparosc Endosc Percutan Tech 2012;22(3):226–31.
[52] Bozkurt MA, Ünsal MG, Kapan S, et al. Two different methods for appendiceal stump closure: metal clip and Hem-o-lok clip. J Laparoendosc Adv Surg Tech A 2014;24(8):571–3.
[53] Magarey CJ, Chant AD, Rickford CR, et al. Clinical trial of the effects of drainage and antibiotics after appendicectomy. Br J Surg 1971;58(11):855–6.
[54] Stone HH, Hooper CA, Millikan WJ. Abdominal drainage following appendectomy and cholecystectomy. Ann Surg 1978;187(6):606–12.
[55] Petrowsky H, Demartines N, Rousson V, et al. Evidence-based value of prophylactic drainage in gastrointestinal surgery: a systematic review and meta-analyses. Ann Surg 2004;240(6):1074–84 [discussion: 1084–5].
[56] Rather SA, Bari SU, Malik AA, et al. Drainage vs no drainage in secondary peritonitis with sepsis following complicated appendicitis in adults in the modern era of antibiotics. World J Gastrointest Surg 2013;5(11):300–5.
[57] St Peter SD, Holcomb GW. Should peritoneal lavage be used with suction during laparoscopic appendectomy for perforated appendicitis? Adv Surg 2013;47:111–8.
[58] St Peter SD, Adibe OO, Iqbal CW, et al. Irrigation versus suction alone during laparoscopic appendectomy for perforated appendicitis: a prospective randomized trial. Ann Surg 2012;256(4):581–5.
[59] Strathern DW, Jones BT. Retained fecalith after laparoscopic appendectomy. Surg Endosc 1999;13(3):287–9.
[60] Rahili A, Habre J, Delotte J, et al. Retained fecalith after laparoscopic appendicectomy. Ann Chir 2003;128(5):326–8 [in French].
[61] Andersen BR, Kallehave FL, Andersen HK. Antibiotics versus placebo for prevention of postoperative infection after appendicectomy. Cochrane Database Syst Rev 2005;(3):CD001439.
[62] Coakley BA, Sussman ES, Wolfson TS, et al. Postoperative antibiotics correlate with worse outcomes after appendectomy for nonperforated appendicitis. J Am Coll Surg 2011;213(6):778–83.
[63] Nadler EP, Gaines BA, Therapeutic Agents Committee of the Surgical Infection Society. The Surgical Infection Society guidelines on antimicrobial therapy for children with appendicitis. Surg Infect (Larchmt) 2008;9(1):75–83.
[64] Solomkin JS. Evaluating evidence and grading recommendations: the SIS/IDSA guidelines for the treatment of complicated intra-abdominal infections. Surg Infect (Larchmt) 2010;11(3):269–74.
[65] Daskalakis K, Juhlin C, Påhlman L. The use of pre- or postoperative antibiotics in surgery for appendicitis: a systematic review. Scand J Surg 2014;103(1):14–20.
[66] Kimbrell AR, Novosel TJ, Collins JN, et al. Do postoperative antibiotics prevent abscess formation in complicated appendicitis? Am Surg 2014;80(9):878–83.
[67] Clark JJ, Johnson SM. Laparoscopic drainage of intraabdominal abscess after appendectomy: an alternative to laparotomy in cases not amenable to percutaneous drainage. J Pediatr Surg 2011;46(7):1385–9.
[68] Gupta R, Sample C, Bamehriz F, et al. Infectious complications following laparoscopic appendectomy. Can J Surg 2006;49(6):397–400.

[69] Woodham BL, Cox MR, Eslick GD. Evidence to support the use of laparoscopic over open appendicectomy for obese individuals: a meta-analysis. Surg Endosc 2012;26(9): 2566–70.
[70] Li X, Zhang J, Sang L, et al. Laparoscopic versus conventional appendectomy–a meta-analysis of randomized controlled trials. BMC Gastroenterol 2010;10:129.
[71] Markides G, Subar D, Riyad K. Laparoscopic versus open appendectomy in adults with complicated appendicitis: systematic review and meta-analysis. World J Surg 2010;34(9):2026–40.
[72] Ding J, Xia Y, Zhang ZM, et al. Single-incision versus conventional three-incision laparoscopic appendicectomy for appendicitis: a systematic review and meta-analysis. J Pediatr Surg 2013;48(5):1088–98.
[73] Pisanu A, Porceddu G, Reccia I, et al. Meta-analysis of studies comparing single-incision laparoscopic appendectomy and conventional multiport laparoscopic appendectomy. J Surg Res 2013;183(2):e49–59.
[74] Gill RS, Shi X, Al-Adra DP, et al. Single-incision appendectomy is comparable to conventional laparoscopic appendectomy: a systematic review and pooled analysis. Surg Laparosc Endosc Percutan Tech 2012;22(4):319–27.

Kolibri 360 GmbH
Ferdinand-Jühlke-Straße 7
99095 Erfurt, Deutschland
produktsicherheit@kolibri360.de